Temporary Skeletal Anchorage Devices

Ki Beom Kim
Editor

Temporary Skeletal Anchorage Devices

A Guide to Design and Evidence-Based Solution

Springer

Editor
Ki Beom Kim, DDS, MSD, PhD
Department of Orthodontics
Center for Advanced Dental Education
Saint Louis University
Saint Louis, MO
USA

ISBN 978-3-642-55051-5 ISBN 978-3-642-55052-2 (eBook)
DOI 10.1007/978-3-642-55052-2
Springer Heidelberg New York Dordrecht London

Library of Congress Control Number: 2014941940

Printed on acid-free paper

Springer is part of Springer Science+Business Media (www.springer.com)

Foreword

When a new textbook is written there should be a reason to do so, and those who read the book should derive benefit by considering the material within. Before you is a new book about the use of temporary skeletal anchorage devices (TSADs) in orthodontics and before one reads the work, you should know its intended purpose and potential significance.

It has been suggested that "temporary anchorage devices have revolutionized our ability to move teeth" (Kokich, 2012). While we have seen significant "advancements" and "improvements" over time in our knowledge, strategies, treatments, tools, and appliances (e.g., roentgenographic cephalometrics, direct bonded brackets, pre-torqued pre-angulated brackets, etc.) the pronouncement that TSADs represent a revolutionary change sounds significant indeed. Thus, it is perhaps appropriate to consider what "revolution" has occurred. In doing so, I will draw upon the thoughts of Thomas Kuhn who wrote a textbook in 1962 titled *The Structure of Scientific Revolutions*, but I will do so as his thoughts apply in the context of orthodontics.

In his publication, Kuhn describes the nature of a "paradigm" and a "paradigm shift." A paradigm refers to a model of reality that consists of distinct concepts, thought patterns, traditions, and practices that define a scientific discipline at a particular point in time. Through time, a new model of reality might emerge that replaces the original paradigm (i.e., paradigm shift). This change is often sudden, dramatic, and difficult and because of this Kuhn referred to this transition process as a "revolution."

As a frame of reference one could define an orthodontic paradigm called "traditional orthodontics" as the reality that exists during a period of time that includes distinct concepts, thought patterns, traditions, and practices that define the clinical and scientific activities of the discipline. When such conditions exist there is widespread consensus on terminology, methods, and practices. This consensus in thought, word, and deed also directs a focus on certain subjects and kinds of research that are considered likely to contribute additional knowledge to "traditional orthodontics." As a result, popular experiments are likely to be copied and, in some form, repeated. Such scientific experiments are also subject to bias in the form of preconceptions made prior to the conduct of the research and following the collection of data. Progress in science is generally viewed as the straightforward accumulation of acceptable facts and the reconfiguration of existing theories. The problems encountered in clinical practice and the issues of scientific endeavor thus are to be "solved" within the context of "traditional orthodontics." Inquiry outside this reality is seldom encouraged, and may be outwardly discouraged.

On the other hand, invention and scientific endeavor do allow opportunities for the production of new technology and information that could contradict and challenge the accepted model of reality. While a new development might be viewed with some initial curiosity and interest, acceptance might not be forthcoming depending on the degree of deviation from the current model of reality. Also a challenge is a conflict with the strongly held beliefs of "traditional orthodontics." For many members of the discipline, the need to function within the boundaries of "traditional orthodontics" is so strong that it normally renders even the possibility of exploring alternatives unconvincing, counter-intuitive, or even dangerous.

Revolution

Occasionally, invention or scientific discovery appears to produce an improvement, and if significant enough, an advancement that might even be considered revolutionary. We could call this potential new orthodontic reality "New Orthodontics" and expect that would define a new area of scientific inquiry and clinical practice. We would also expect this new reality will resolve some outstanding and significant problem that can be addressed in no other way. At the same time, to be accepted it must promise to preserve a relatively large part of the problem solving ability that has been previously developed.

Subsequently, it would be expected that many changes would occur. Some scientists in the field would change how they view and respond to "New Orthodontics." They would consider the new science in terms of what should be observed and scrutinized, what questions are regarded as vital and how they should be structured, how new theories are to be considered, what investigative methods and technology are needed, how research should be conducted, and what rules are to be used to interpret findings. In essence these scientists would "map" the direction of new research endeavors.

Clinically new intellectual options and practical applications become available. Importantly new opportunities for problem solving emerge, but there also may be the need to develop new procedures, new equipment and supplies, and new strategies for implementation within the context of "New Orthodontics." In both clinical and scientific settings new terminology often is developed, is argued, and then neologisms emerge. Notably, once a revolutionary shift has occurred new textbooks also need to be written.

TSADs

So, does the use of TSADs represent a revolutionary event in orthodontics? The answer is clear…yes, but in what way? It is obviously true that use of TSADs offers an advantage over some traditional mechanics in terms of patient compliance. It is also obviously true that TSADs offer new opportunities with regard to the point of force; although limited in some ways by anatomy, the point of force can be placed in many new locations. If that were all that TSADs offered, TSADs would represent an improvement or advancement in orthodontics but would not be considered revolutionary in nature.

Improvements in compliance and new locations for point of force applications…these are advancements to be sure. But the real revolution is that TSADs can be used to control anchorage so that pure dental, pure orthopedic, or some controlled combination of dentofacial movements can occur, at least potentially. They are a new means to an end, not defined previously. Thus, the promise of temporary skeletal anchorage devices is that they can serve as controllable and efficient anchors for any tooth movements the orthodontist would care to make. They are a completely new method of solving an old problem. Before TSADs, practitioners described the need for anchorage control using the terms of low, medium, and maximum. After the adoption of TSADs in orthodontics, the term "absolute anchorage" emerged. This then is the revolutionary characteristic that justifies greater attention in the literature.

Who are the leaders of this revolution? Of course there are those that served to "invent" and introduce TSADs to orthodontics, and those that followed who demonstrated the initial applications of TSADs initially in simple ways. These are the pioneers who had the mental flexibility, intellectual capacity, interest, and vision to accept the invention and understand the potential of TSADs.

Beyond the initial surge of interest, enthusiasm, and use of TSADs there are individuals that have assessed the invention, applied it to new situations, reported on their findings and are now pursuing the significance of TSADs. As this new textbook contains chapters written by some of the experienced users of TSADs they are the appropriate people to describe and demonstrate the positive qualities and potential of this new technology.

This new revolution applicable to clinical practice also changes and expands the science that needs to be considered in terms of the development of knowledge about TSADs. Those that were enlisted are scientists who possessed an exceptional ability to recognize the invention's potential; these were individuals whose preference and time shifted in favor of exploring the new design. Thus, a few scientists have recognized that the science needed for TSADs is new and incomplete. No system is perfect, so with each new invention its shortcomings must also be acknowledged and solutions sought. The challenge is that new scientific areas and ideas will need to be considered, new experimental protocols will need to be developed, and new methods of interpretation will need to be applied. Their contributions are also included in this book. In many of the chapters basic scientific knowledge will be presented as a foundation for clinical use. Consideration of the TSADs failures, screw materials and engineering, implant locations, and insertion techniques will be found in many places.

In terms of clinical applications, this textbook provides many applications including the distalization and protraction of teeth and en masse movement of the dental arches, orthopedic movements in the traverse and sagittal planes via fixed and fixed functional appliances, multidisciplinary treatment, and more using TSADs and miniplates. Questions of indications, contraindications, alternate treatments, and treatment timing will appear in many of the chapters included in this book.

In the end, the promise of TSADs is that practitioners can now place teeth where they want them to be placed. The following question will be "where do they want the teeth to be placed?" Perhaps the authors will provide guidance on this issue also.

References

Kokich VG. It's only a screw. Am J Orthod Dentofacial Orthop. 2012;142(1):1.
Kuhn TS. The structure of scientific revolution. 1st ed. University of Chicago Press; 1962.

Rolf G. Behrents
Department of Orthodontics
Center for Advanced Dental Education
Saint Louis University St Louis
MO, USA

Preface

Since Edward Angle, the father of modern orthodontics, introduced the edgewise appliance, there have been a few innovative developments in the field of orthodontics. Cephalometrics and the prescription bracket system are just two of the examples of such advancements. Many different appliances have been developed and used for efficient treatment over the years. Even with newer devices, orthodontists cannot be completely free from Newton's third law: for every action has an equal and opposite reaction. Anchorage control, which is controlling the unwanted opposite reaction, is one of the crucial factors that determine the success of the treatment. Although there have been many attempts to control anchorage, it remains a challenge for orthodontists. In recent years, temporary skeletal anchorage devices (TSADs) have made anchorage control both easier and have made some tooth movements not previously possible with traditional mechanics. For these reasons, TSADs can be considered as an example of innovative development in orthodontics. There have been an overwhelming number of case reports and TSADs related researches in the last ten years. Although numerous kinds of TSADs have been used, more information is needed to understand the scientific basis of TSADs.

Because of the lack of consensus based on evidence, it has been quite difficult for clinicians to choose TSADs and establish efficient treatment strategies. Some manufacturers have made claims based on less than a scientific basis for their TSADs. This makes the decision process more difficult for the clinician. With this in mind, the authors of this book have set out to make the job less difficult.

In addition, this book is designed to bring the most up-to-date evidence-based information possible to the reader by describing new concepts, treatment mechanics and techniques for many challenging cases.

Finally, I would like to express my gratitude towards my family, friends, and teachers for supporting this project.

Saint Louis, MO, USA — Ki Beom Kim

Contents

Considerations for Optimizing the Use of Miniscrew Implants in Orthodontic Practice

1

Peter H. Buschang and Ki Beom Kim

Abstract

Miniscrew implants (MSIs) have redefined how orthodontics is practiced. Not only do they provide absolute anchorage, but they also greatly enhance the possibilities of dentofacial orthopedics. It has been reported that approximately 13.5–16.4 % of the miniscrews placed fail. Such rates are excessive and deter many orthodontists, preventing them from, preventing them from taking advantage of these devices. To ameliorate failure rates, MSIs could be optimized by changing their characteristics and individualized depending on the sites where they are to be placed and how they are loaded. For example, increases in MSI length and width, decreases in pitch, and the addition of flutes provide ways to enhance both primary and secondary stability. Increasing the surface area of the screws also increases secondary stability. Excessive cortical bone thickness and density, which enhance primary stability, could be detrimental to secondary stability. Pilot holes can also be problematic and should only be used with thicker and denser bone. Orthodontists must also be meticulous about their placement techniques. They must carefully plan where the MSIs will be placed, they must take care to maintain the screw's position and orientation throughout the insertion phase, they must evaluate MSI stability after insertion and take corrective action when necessary, and they must ensure proper post-op hygiene. Placement techniques may well turn out to be as important, or even more important, for stability than the screw's physical characteristics or the characteristics of the placement sites.

P.H. Buschang, PhD (✉)
Department of Orthodontics,
Texas A & M University, Baylor College of Dentistry,
660677, Dallas, TX 75266-0677, USA
e-mail: phbuschang@bcd.tamhsc.edu

K.B. Kim, DDS, MSD, PhD
Department of Orthodontics, Center for Advanced
Dental Education, Saint Louis University,
3320 Rutger Street, Saint Louis, MO 63104, USA
e-mail: kkim8@slu.edu

K.B. Kim (ed.), *Temporary Skeletal Anchorage Devices*,
DOI 10.1007/978-3-642-55052-2_1, © Springer-Verlag Berlin Heidelberg 2014

1.1 Introduction

Miniscrew implants (MSIs) have become very popular among orthodontists. When appropriately used, they improve the quality of treatment [1] and open up new treatment alternatives. They make it possible to maintain anchorage, more precisely control the forces applied to the teeth, and produce orthopedic effects without reciprocal tooth movements. Their use goes well beyond the maintenance of anchorage. For example, MSIs make it possible to produce substantial orthopedic effects (e.g., advance the chin, decrease the mandibular plane angle, improve facial convexity, limit growth of lower anterior facial height) in growing, hyperdivergent retrognathic patients by selectively intruding the posterior teeth [2]. MSIs are the smallest skeletal anchorage devices available, which makes them extremely versatile. They can be easily placed by orthodontists in multiple locations; their removal is fast and typically uneventful; they are affordable, and they do not require a healing period prior to force activation. While patients initially believe that MSIs will be more painful and uncomfortable than other appliances, they actually turn out to not be painful, and they are less uncomfortable than other appliances [1].

MSIs were first used almost 70 years ago to experimentally retract canines [3]. This work showed, for the first time, that tooth movements with basal bone anchorage were possible. It was not until 1983 that MSIs were used again orthodontically, when a vitallium bone screw was placed below the anterior nasal spine and used for anchorage in a patient with severe deep bite malocclusion [4]. This led to the use of endosseous implants for orthodontic tooth movements. However, these implants never gained widespread acceptance due to their size, the costs of surgical placement and removal, and the delayed loading times involved. The problems associated with endosseous implants led Kanomi and coworkers [5] to use smaller – 1.2-mm wide and 6-mm long – implants, originally designed to stabilize surgical bone plates.

While they have been used extensively over the past 15 years, there is no consensus concerning the terminology that should be used for these devices. The terms *bone screws* and *miniature implants* are not sufficiently descriptive; the first set of terms provides no indication of size or osseointegration; the second set of terms does not specify the shape of the device. The prefix *micro*, as in *micro-implant* and *micro-screw implant*, is also inappropriate because micro denotes a factor of one millionth, which is far too small for MSIs. Temporary anchorage devices (*TADs*) do not provide an indication of size or shape. More importantly, the acronym is not specific enough because MSIs, headgears, lip bumpers, lingual arches, and numerous other orthodontic appliances also qualify as *TADs*. *Miniscrew implant* indicates size, shape, and osseointegration.

While variation is substantial, the majority of practicing orthodontists (approximately 67 %) report that MSIs fail less than 25 % of the time [1]. A recent systematic review of 19 studies reported success rates greater than 80 % when mobile and displaced MSIs are included [6]. A meta-analysis of 27 studies performed around the same time reported a failure rate of 16.4 % for MSIs, which was almost two times greater than the failure rates of palatal implants (10.5 %) and miniplates (7.3 %) [7]. Most recently, Papageorgiou et al. systematically evaluated 19 studies pertaining to 4,987 MSIs placed in 2,281 patients and reported an overall failure rate of 13.5 % [8]. While these reviews provide excellent summaries of the available literature, the individual studies were subject to various sources of uncontrolled variation and are not well suited for determining the causes of MSI instability. Well-controlled clinical and experimental studies provide the best means for determining the causal factors necessary to optimize the use of MSIs in orthodontics.

As originally defined by Brånemark et al. [9], MSIs osseointegrate. In other words, direct contact between the living bone and implant is evident under light microscopy (Fig. 1.1). However, the amount of integration that occurs around MSIs is highly variable, both between regions within a screw and between screws. One of the first studies to evaluate osseointegration of MSIs showed that bone-to-implant contact (BIC) ranged from approximately 10 to 58 %, depending on the duration of time after insertion [10].

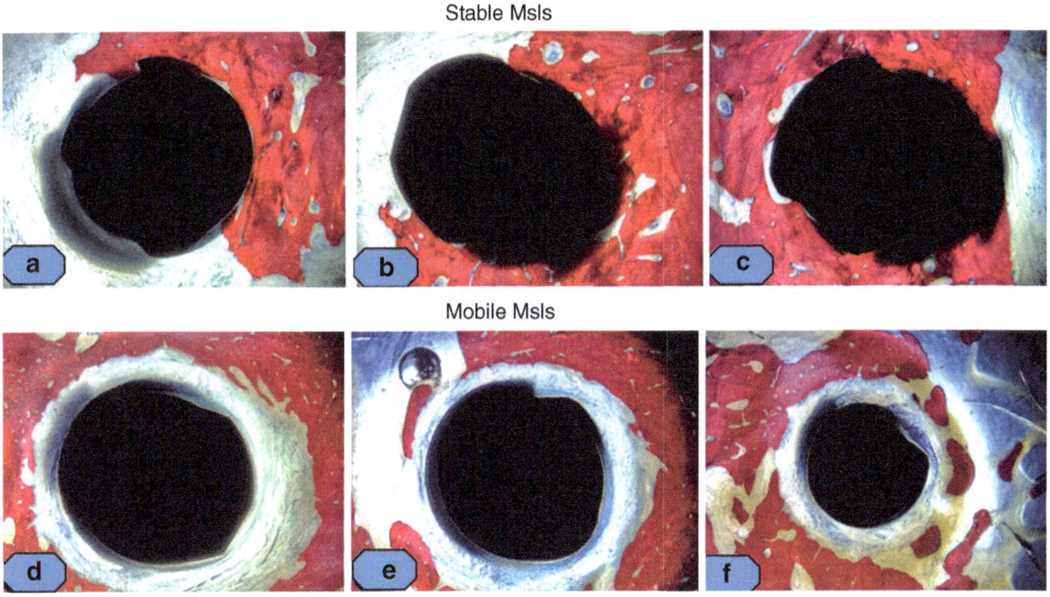

Fig 1.1 Photomicrographs showing osseointegration around stable MSIs (**a–c**) and fibrous tissues around mobile MSIs (**d–f**) MSIs (Adapted from Woods et al. [12])

As expected, osseointegration increases over time. In experimental animals, osseointegration increased from approximately 50 % after 22 days to 83 % after 70 days [11]. Woods and coworkers showed that BIC of stable MSIs ranged from 2.2 to 100 % after 110 days [12]. Importantly, they showed that stable MSIs always show some degree of osseointegration, albeit small. The high degrees of variability in BIC observed could be partially due to either their smooth machined surfaces or the limited ability of histology to quantify BIC (i.e. histology only captures a small portion of the MSI's surface area). Excessive variability in BIC could prove to be problematic for certain applications (e.g., young children with thin, less dense, cortices).

1.2 Primary and Secondary Stability

Long-term MSI stability depends on both primary and secondary stability, two closely related phenomena. Immediately after the MSI has been inserted, its retention is entirely mechanical, due primarily to the characteristics and amount of the bone contacting the MSI, particularly the cortical bone [13, 14]. This mechanical type of MSI retention is called primary stability. For orthodontists, primary stability is important because it allows MSIs to be immediately loaded. More importantly, primary stability is critical for the development of secondary stability. The endosseous literature has shown that primary stability is essential for the long-term success of implants [15]. MSI placement generates stresses and strains along the length of the screw that damage the surrounding bone. Too much damage can lead to micromotion of the implant and early loss due to lack of osseointegration. If MSIs are mobile after 5–6 weeks, they are probably surrounded by fibrous tissues and exhibit no bone-to-implant contact (Fig. 1.1) [12].

Both insertion torque and pullout force need to be measured when evaluating primary stability because their effects should not be expected to be equal. Increasing the shear forces along the screw increases the strain and microfractures, which might be expected to affect the healing process and lead to degeneration or necrosis at the interface. Bone damaged during MSI insertion requires repair, too much of which can result in

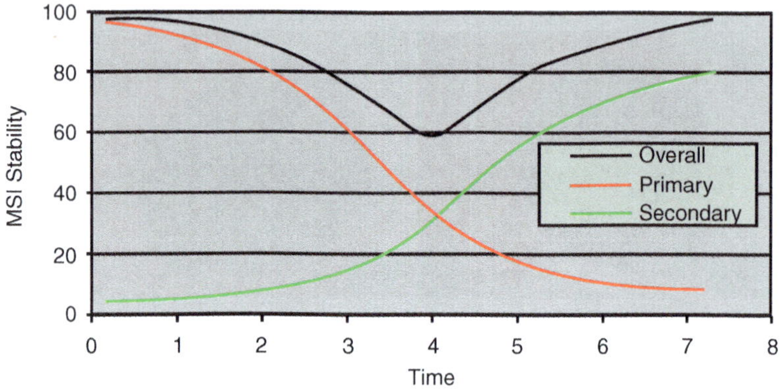

Fig. 1.2 Overall, primary and secondary stability curves of miniscrew implants (*MSIs*), showing the stability dip 4 weeks after insertion

screw loosening. Theoretically, primary stability can be optimized by minimizing insertion torque and maximizing pullout forces.

During the first few weeks after implant placement, primary stability decreases as osteoclasts remove older, damaged bone, and osteoblasts form new bone. As new bone is formed around the MSI, its stability increases. This second phase of increasing stability is referred to as secondary stability. Secondary stability is due to the osseointegration that occurs around MSIs. As healing and greater amounts of osseointegration occur, secondary stability increases.

Primary and secondary stability each exhibit characteristic curves (Fig. 1.2). The stability that the orthodontist observes clinically is the net or overall stability, composed of both primary and secondary stability. Initially, overall stability is due entirely to primary stability (i.e., there is no secondary stability). Overall stability decreases rapidly at first and then slows down as secondary stability takes over. The point at which the primary and secondary stability curves cross is when MSIs are least stable; it can be identified by the dip in the overall stability curve. At that time, primary stability is increasing rapidly. The rate at which secondary stability increases begins to slow down after 4–5 weeks of healing. After healing has occurred and the bone has remodeled, overall MSI stability is primarily due to secondary stability.

Theoretically, the overall stability of MSIs could be enhanced by either (1) delaying the decrease of primary stability that occurs after insertion or (2) accelerating the increases in secondary stability that occur with healing (Fig. 1.3). Unfortunately, increasing primary stability often damages the surrounding bone. Finite element analyses indicate that the insertion of MSIs produces bone strains well above physiologic limits [16], which damages the bone, increases remodeling requirements, and could have negative impacts on both primary and secondary stability. Ideally, MSIs should produce the least bone strain, heat, and damage (i.e., minimum insertion torque) while providing the greatest possible primary stability (maximum pullout force) immediately after insertion. Such conditions would establish a local environment that limits the damage of the bone around the MSIs and enhances the healing process.

Ure et al. described weekly changes in MSI stability [17]. Uniquely, their study measured MSI stability in vivo over time using the Osstell Mentor (Osstell AB, Göteborg, Sweden), a device that produces an electromagnetic signal that causes the MSI to vibrate via an attached magnetic peg. The results showed significantly greater decreases in the primary stability during the first 3 weeks for MSIs that failed than for those that remained stable (Fig. 1.3a). MSIs placed in nonkeratinized tissue – most of which eventually failed – exhibited significantly greater decreases in MSI stability during the first 3 weeks than MSIs placed in keratinized tissue (Fig. 1.3b). The stability of the MSIs placed in keratinized tissue also decreased during the first 3 weeks and increased significantly thereafter, indicated healing, and increased secondary stability (Fig. 1.4). This study was important because it showed that (1) MSI

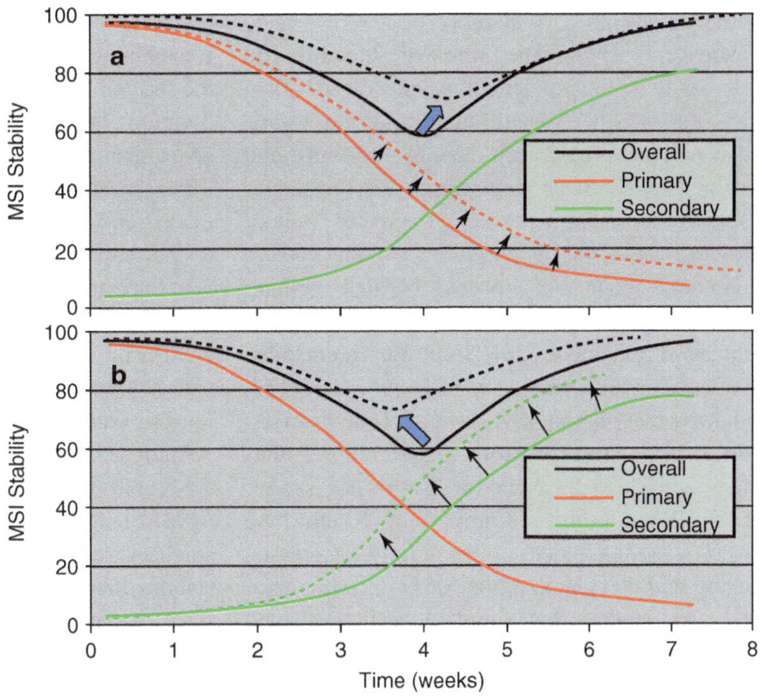

Fig 1.3 Increases in overall MSI stability associated with (**a**) decelerating the primary stability (old bone) curve and (**b**) accelerating the secondary stability (new bone) curve (Adapted from Ure et al. [17])

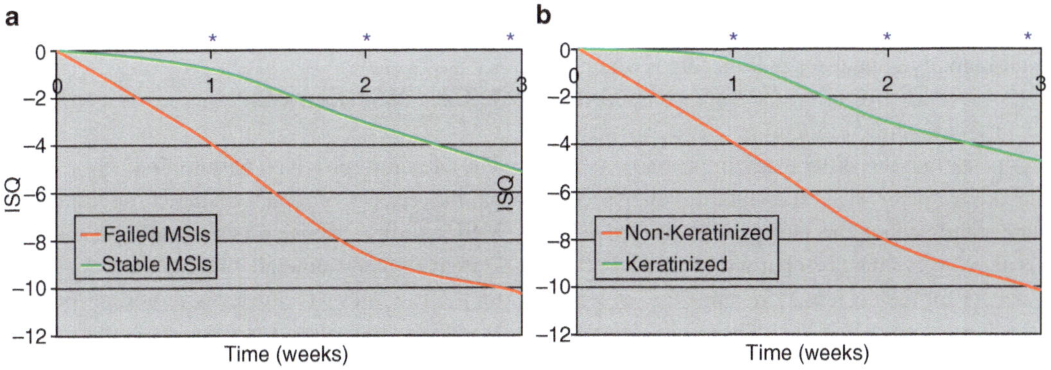

Fig 1.4 Differences (*$p<0.05$) in implant stability quotient (*ISQ*) of (**a**) MSIs that failed vs. those that did not fail and (**b**) MSIs placed in nonkeratinized vs. keratinized tissues (Adapted from Ure et al. [17])

failures can be predicted and (2) the primary and secondary stability curves of MSIs are similar to the curves previously described for endosseous implants [18].

1.3 MSI Characteristics

Ideally, MSIs should be designed to enhance their holding power (maximize pullout forces) and limit bone damage during insertion (minimize insertion torque), which together might be expected to maximize secondary stability and accelerate bone healing.

1.3.1 Effects of MSI Length

All other things being equal, the greater the surface area of the bone in contact with the MSI, the greater its primary stability. One of the easiest ways to increase the surface area, and therefore increase the primary stability of a screw, is to increase its length. The orthopedic literature has shown that implant length is one of the most important factors determining insertion torque and pullout force. When 12-mm-, 14-mm-, and 16-mm-long screws were compared, the longer screws consistently exhibited greater pullout forces [19]. The increases in holding power observed might be expected because holding power of a screw is proportional to the amount of thread engagement [20]. Insertion torque also increases with increased MSI length. Lim et al. showed that maximum insertion torque of cylindrical MSIs increased from 19.5 Ncm for 7-mm-long screws to 23 Ncm for 9-mm-long screws [21]. When 6-mm-, 8-mm-, and 10-mm-long MSIs were compared, insertion torque increased along with the length of the MSIs [22]. In one of the few studies that simultaneously evaluated insertion torque and pullout force, Shah and coworkers recently showed that the maximum insertion torque of 6-mm-long MSIs was 1.3–1.5 times greater than the insertion torque of identical 3-mm-long MSIs [23]. The effects of length were substantially greater for pullout force, which was 3.2–3.6 times greater for the 6-mm-long MSIs.

The literature evaluating long-term stability suggests that the differences in primary stability favoring longer MSIs translate in better secondary stability, but the evidence is limited. Chen et al., who evaluated 29 patients, reported 90.2 % success for their 8 mm MSIs and 72.2 % success for their 6 mm MSIs [24]. Other clinical studies have also reported greater success with longer screws, but the differences they reported were not statistically significant [25, 26].

Mortensen et al. experimentally compared 6-mm-long MSIs to identical, specially manufactured, 3-mm-long MSIs [27]. Success rates 6 weeks after immediately loading were significantly higher for the 6 mm (100 %) than the 3 mm (67 %) MSIs. However, the differences were partially due to the fact that the tips of some 3 mm MSIs sheared off during insertion, which might be expected to ream out the bone around the screw during insertion and decrease stability. Also, one of the dogs, which was described as unusually active and prone to chewing on the run bars and food bowls, accounted for 60 % of the 3 mm failures. Excluding all of the MSIs from that dog, as well as the sheared MSIs, increased the success rate of the 3 mm MSI to 90.6 %, which was still significantly lower than the success rate of the 6 mm screws. Three recent experiments using a total of 162 loaded and unloaded 3 mm MSIs confirmed an overall success rate of approximately 91 % [28–30]. Importantly, the length of the MSI shaft does not necessary equal the depth of its placement. Neither the 3 mm nor the 6 mm MSIs were completely inserted into the bone; postmortem evaluations showed that the 6 mm MSIs had been inserted 3.9 mm and the 3 mm MSIs had been inserted only 1.6 mm [31]. These findings indicate that the effect of MSI length on long-term stability is relatively small and probably related to the enhanced primary stability that longer screws provide. It also emphasizes the importance of the techniques used to insert shorter screws. While design changes are required to further enhance their stability, shorter MSI holds future potential for providing orthodontists greater versatility in terms of placement sites.

1.3.2 MSI Diameter

The literature provides only limited information on the effects of outer diameter on long-term MSI stability. Miniscrews currently on the market have outer diameters ranging from 1.2 to 2.0 mm [21, 32–43]. Diameter is important because MSIs are often placed into interradicular spaces. In order to avoid unwanted root damage by MSIs and increase the success rate, diameter is one of the factors that need to be considered in the selection of the correct dimension of MSIs.

Park et al. evaluated 227 miniscrews and showed no differences in success associated with outer diameter [44]. In contrast, Miyawaki et al., who compared MSIs with outer diameters of 1.0 mm, 1.5 mm, and 2.3 mm, reported that all of the 1.0-mm-wide MSIs failed, whereas the wider MSIs were 84–85 % successful [33]. Wiechmann et al. reported that 1.6 mm wide MSIs showed a higher success rate than the 1.1 mm MSIs [45]. Chen et al. suggested that MSIs with a diameter of less than 1.3 mm are unsuitable for insertion into a higher density bone [36]. According to Wu et al. [46], an MSI diameter equal to or less than 1.4 mm is recommended for the maxilla and an MSI diameter larger than 1.4 mm is recommended for the mandible. Poggio et al. reported that the ideal diameter for the interradicular space is 1.2–1.5 mm [43]. Based on a systematic review of the literature [35], it has been suggested that MSIs with less than 1.2 mm in diameter should be avoided.

The differences in diameter affect both the insertion torque and removal torque [14, 21, 36, 42, 45]. Using a synthetic bone model, DeCoster et al. showed that mean pullout forces increase in a linear fashion as the major diameter is increased [47]. When major diameter was doubled, pullout force almost tripled. Wider MSIs also produce higher insertion torque. Wilmes et al., who compared five different MSIs, showed that those with the largest diameters produced the greatest insertion torques [48].

Importantly, even small differences in outer diameter can have substantial effects of primary stability. Comparing 3-mm-long/1.75-mm outer diameter MSIs and 3-mm-long/2.0-mm outer diameter MSIs, Shah and coworkers showed that the extra one fourth of a mm increased insertion torque between 5.2 and 17.2 %, with greater increases in low-density than high-density bone [23]. They also showed that pullout forces increased between 15 and 27 %.

Minor diameter (i.e., inner or core diameter) of MSIs, which range between 1.2 and 1.6 mm, is also related to the holding strength of the MSI. Decoster et al. showed that when the minor diameter was increased while outer diameter was maintained, pullout forces decreased [47]. Pullout forces decreased because the major to minor diameter ratio decreased from 1.5 to 1.2. Increasing the major/minor ratio, while holding all other parameters constant, leads to small but measurable increases in pullout force. Importantly, Carano and coworkers indicated that a reduction in minor diameter of as little as 0.2 mm can reduce the screw's resistance to breakage by 50 % [49].

MSIs with smaller diameters tend to exhibit more loosening when subjected to orthodontic force, perhaps because they may have decreased removal torque [33, 50, 51] As the diameter increases, the microdamage in the cortical bone increases, which may cause failure of the MSIs [39, 52–56].

A few studies have suggested that the maximum insertion torque level should not be beyond between 5 and 10 Ncm [27, 57, 58], but there is some disagreement regarding the optimum torque level [59–61]. In a recent systemic review [62], no evidence was provided linking specific maximum insertion torque levels with higher success rate. Even though there is no consensus concerning the ideal maximum insertion torque value, a certain level of insertion torque needs to be achieved for initial stability. Since most of the MSIs are immediately loaded, the degree of mobility that would be considered acceptable to withstand initial force remains uncertain.

When it has been determined that the best strategic location for an MSI is between roots, the available space should be carefully measured. There are differing ideas on how much alveolar bone should be left around MSIs [43, 63–65]. Root proximity is considered a major factor for MSI failure, and increasing the distance from the MSI is recommended to improve the success rate [66, 67].

However, if a MSI with a smaller diameter is selected in order to prevent root contact, it may increase the fracture risk. In an animal study, Buchter et al. [68] reported that eight of 200 MSIs were fractured at the time of insertion and two failed at the time of removal. In a human study, Park et al. reported that eight of 227 MSIs were fractured in 87 consecutive patients [44]. The fracture risk increases as the diameter of MSIs decreased [36, 40, 57, 69, 70]. The core diameter seems to be a more important factor for fracture torque than the outer diameter [70, 71].

The larger the difference between the maximum insertion torque and/or maximum removal torque and maximum fracture torque, the smaller the fracture risk. If a MSI with a smaller diameter has to be used because of a limited amount of space, a pilot hole may be necessary in order to reduce the fracture risk. According to the recent study [72], the diameter does not have a significant effect on the amount of linear microdamage with pilot drilling.

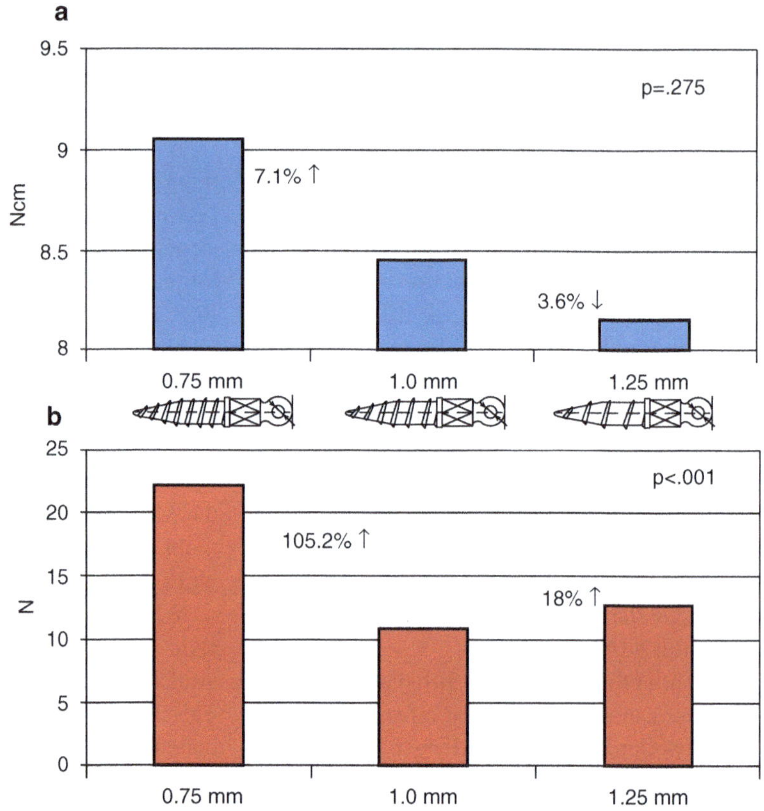

Fig 1.5 The effects of MSI pitch on (**a**) insertion torque and (**b**) pullout strength testing using synthetic bone, with percent changes based on the 1.0 mm pitch MSI (Adapted from Brinley et al. [75])

Duaibis et al. [38] evaluated the various types of stress in the cortical bone around MSIs using a three-dimensional finite element study. They concluded that the most critical MSI design factors affecting the stability are the diameter and extra-bony head length, with larger diameters and shorter heads developing less stress in the cortical bone surrounding the MSI. Another study [73] evaluating risk factors showed that diameter was not related to primary stability. Park et al. [44] and Wu et al. [46] reported that diameter did not make any difference with respect to success rates.

1.3.3 Effects of Pitch

Another way to increase the surface area and primary stability of MSIs is to decrease their pitch (i.e., the distance between the threads). It is well established that pitch increases the purchase strength of screws in porous materials. Decreasing pitch increases the pullout forces of bone screws [47, 74]. Migliorati and coworkers reported that pitch had a significant effect on maximum insertion torque (i.e., the smaller the pitch, the greater the torque), but not on pullout forces [14]. However, their results were potentially confounded because they compared four screws that differed in terms of their major diameter, length, as well as the depth of thread.

Brinley and coworkers compared MSIs that differed only in terms of pitch [75]. All of the MSIs were made of surgical grade titanium, they were 6-mm long, and they were self-drilling and self-tapping. The MSIs had major and minor diameters of 1.8 mm and 1.6 mm, respectively, the threads had a 90° asymmetric buttress design, and the apical 3 mm of the MSIs were tapered. MSIs with 1.0-mm, 0.75-mm, and 1.25-mm pitch were compared. When the MSIs were placed in synthetic bone, insertion torque increased with decreases in pitch. However, the differences were small and not statistically significant ($p=0.275$). Compared to the 1.0-mm pitch screws, the insertion torque of the 0.75- and 1.25-mm pitch MSIs were only 7.2 % greater and 3.6 % less, respectively (Fig. 1.5). In contrast, pullout forces were over 105 % greater with the 0.75-mm than 1.0-mm pitch MSIs; the pullout forces of 1.25-mm pitch MSIs were approximately 18 % greater than the 1.0-mm MSI. The effects of pitch on pullout were clearly associated with bone density. When the MSIs were inserted in denser human cadaver bone, the differences were still significant, but insertion torque and pullout forces were only 11.8 % and 7.1 % greater, respectively, for the 0.75-mm than for the 1.0-mm pitch MSIs. Together, these results suggest that changes in pitch might be an effective approach for increasing stability in patients with immature or thin cortical bone.

1.3.4 Thread Design

The thread design of an MSI can vary in pitch, depth, and shape. Modification of thread designs can substantially affect the mechanical properties. Wilmes et al. [71] reported that the thread shape affects the MSI's primary stability. The thread design influenced the resistance to pullout of the MSIs [76, 77]. There are reports of MSIs with asymmetric thread designs showing better mechanical properties [49, 78]. The buttress reverse thread shape has been shown to produce higher pullout strength values than the other designs [76]. Duaibis et al. [38] reported that the thread depth affected the stress in the cortical bone, but the thread shape and pitch did not influence the stress in the cortical bone.

MSIs with greater thread depth exhibit higher primary stability [47, 74, 79]. The ratio between thread depth and pitch has been described as a thread-shape factors [80], with smaller pitch and greater depth showing greater pullout strength [14, 74, 81]. If the thread depth is increased while the external diameter is maintained, the pullout strength is increased up to a certain point. However, this may increase the fracture risk depending on the reduction in core diameter. Chang et al. [77] suggested that MSIs perform better with a core/external diameter ratio of 0.68.

Dual or double thread-shape MSIs have two different pitches. A smaller pitch is on the upper part of the MSI to increase the contact between the upper part of the MSI and the cortical bone (Fig. 1.6). The dual thread shape showed a lower insertion torque and a higher removal torque than either the cylindrical or conical shapes [82]. The dual thread shape exhibited a more gradual increase of insertion torque and a more gradual decrease of removal torque. It also had higher removal torque than the single thread shape. This suggests that the dual thread MSIs might be less harmful to the surrounding bone tissue and improve the stability. However, the dual thread shape needs a longer insertion time which might create excessive heat and lead to tissue damage. Pilot drilling and slower rotational maneuvering during MSI insertion may be helpful for preventing possible negative effects on the tissues.

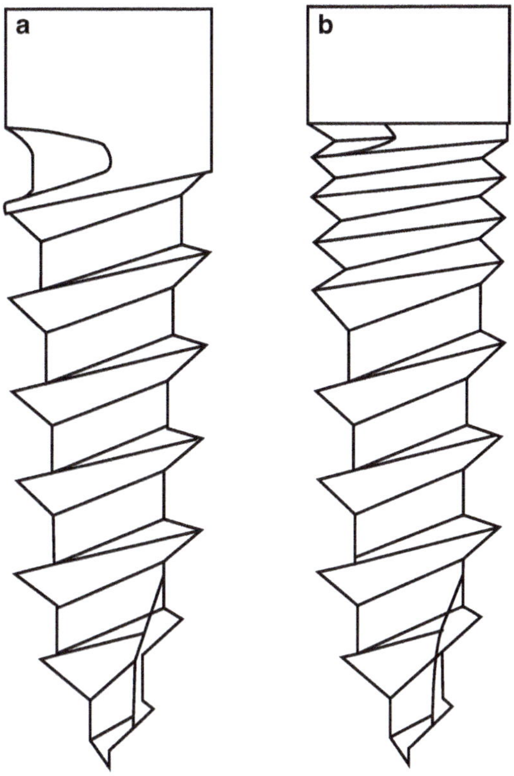

Fig 1.6 (**a**) Single thread shape MSI, (**b**) dual thread shape MSI

1.3.5 Fluting

Flutes might be expected to either decrease insertion torque if they increase the clearance of bone

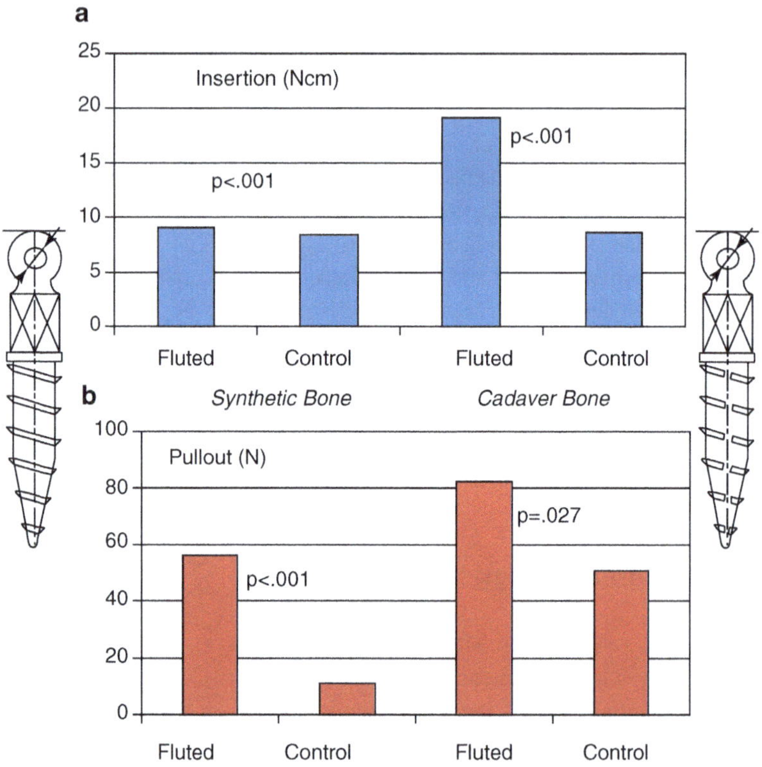

Fig 1.7 The effects of MSI longitudinal fluting on (**a**) insertion torque and (**b**) pullout strength testing using synthetic and cadaver bone, with percent changes based on the 1.0 mm pitch MSI (Adapted from Brinley et al. [75])

debris accumulating around the threads or increase torque if the flute dimensions allow bone chips and debris to accumulate around the threads [79, 83]. This could explain why flutes have been reported to both decrease [84, 85] and increase [83, 86, 87] pullout forces of endosseous and surgical screws. Wu et al. showed that fluting (depending on the shape) played a significant role in reducing the insertion torque of endosseous implants [88]. Decreased insertion torque and cortical damage have been shown to occur with increases in the number and lengths of cutting flutes at the bottom of cortical bone screws [83]. In contrast, the number and length of the flutes increased pullout forces.

Brinley and coworkers evaluated the effects of three longitudinal flutes, extending the full length of the threaded portion of an MSI, on insertion torque and pullout forces [75]. The depth of the flutes, which were 0.25-mm wide, extended through the threads to the core; the surfaces of the flutes were cut to facilitate placement and removal. Results showed even more pronounced differences between synthetic and cadaver bone for fluting than for pitch. In the softer synthetic bone, insertion torque and pullout were 15 and 400 % larger, respectively, for the fluted MSIs (Fig. 1.7). In the denser cadaver bone, insertion torque increased 120 %, while pullout increased only 65 %. Once again, this suggests that fluting might be used to enhance the primary stability of screws placed in thinner, less dense bone.

1.3.6 SLA Surface Treatment

Surface modifications of endosseous implants have proven to be one of the best ways to increase surface area, accelerate secondary stability, and enhance osseointegration. Endosseous implants with surfaces that are sandblasted large grit and acid etched (SLA) exhibit significantly greater shear strength than machined surfaces [89]. SLA surfaces also increase the rate of osseointegration

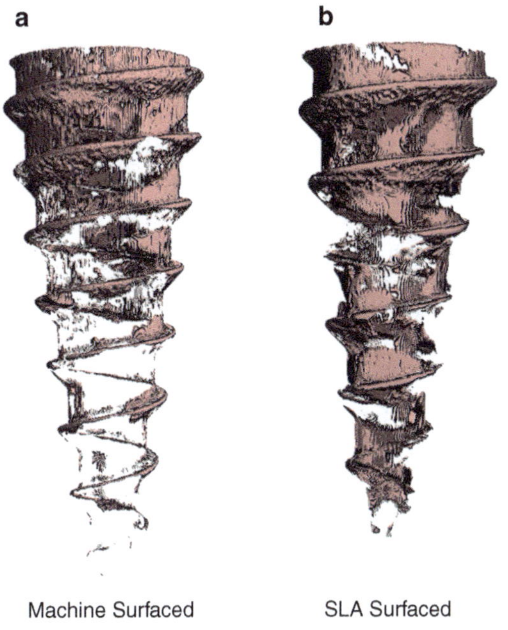

Fig 1.8 Micro-CT of bone located 6–24 μm from the surface of (**a**) machine-surfaced and (**b**) sandblasted large-grit acid-etched (SLA) MSIs (Adapted from Ikeda et al. [94])

[90, 91]. The effects that SLA surfaces have on MSIs are controversial and studies remain limited. Kim and coworkers reported significantly lower insertion torque and significantly higher total removal energy (energy [J] required to remove MSI from maximum torque thru time of removal) for SLA than machined MSIs, but no differences in removal torque [92]. Based on 144 MSIs placed in rabbit tibias, Chang et al. reported considerably higher BIC after 12 weeks for those that had SLA surfaces than those with machined surfaces [91]. More recently, Mo and coworkers showed that SLA MSIs (9.5 × 1.8 mm) produced significantly greater removal torque than machined MSIs (8.2 vs. 5.8 Ncm, respectively) during the first 6 weeks after placement, but no differences after 10 weeks [93]. The actual effects of SLA modification on the bone in the vicinity of the MSI remain poorly understood.

Using a split-mouth design, 21 SLA MSIs were compared to 21 machine-surfaced MSIs [94]. The MSIs were placed in seven mature foxhounds and immediately loaded with a 200-g force, which was maintained for 9.2 weeks. Micro-CT (μCT) was used to determine the absolute and relative amounts of bone surrounding the MSI. Two very thin layers of bone surrounding the MSI were evaluated; one layer included the bone located 6–24 μm from the MSI surface; the other layer included the bone located 24–42 μm from the MSI. The results showed significantly ($p<0.05$) greater amount of the bone (5–21 %) around the SLA than machined MSIs (Fig. 1.8). SLA coating had the greatest effects in the most coronal aspects of both the cortical and non-cortical sections evaluated, which were the regions exhibiting the greatest bone volume to total volume.

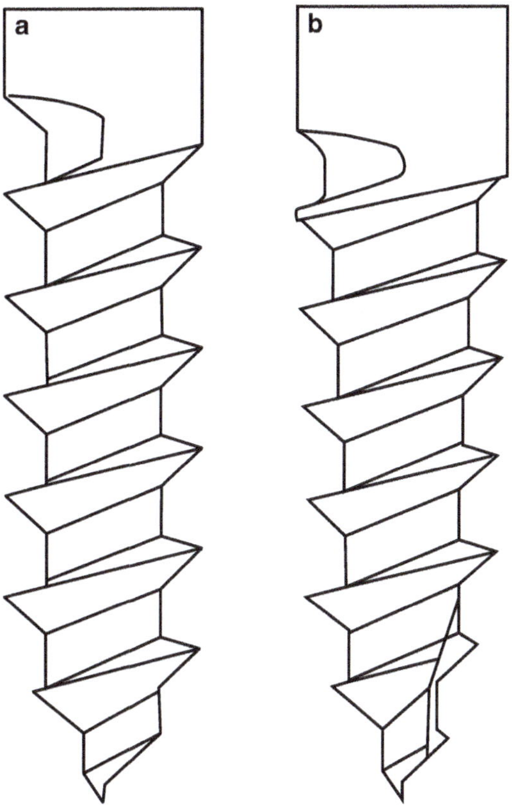

Fig 1.9 Shaft design. (**a**) Cylindrical shaft MSI, (**b**) Conical shaft MSI

1.3.7 Shaft Design

Conical and cylindrical shafts are the most common shapes of MSIs (Fig. 1.9). The conical MSIs showed a higher insertion torque and greater primary stability than the cylindrical

MSIs [39, 71, 95–100]. A conical shape provides tight contact between the tissue and the MSI because the upper part of the screw has a larger diameter than the lower part [101]. Drago and Del Castillo reported that the conical MSIs have less surface area than cylindrical shape MSIs [102], and small surface contact area with the bone may compromise MSI stability [100, 103]. However, Kim et al. [100] reported that there was no significant difference in bone-to-implant contact and bone area between conical and cylindrical MSIs.

The effects of shaft design remain controversial. One study reported that the cylindrical MSIs showed a greater pullout strength [95]. Conversely, another study showed that conical MSIs showed greater pullout resistance than cylindrical MSIs [104].

The conical-shaped MSIs produced higher stress in the cortical bone during insertion than the cylindrical shape [105]. This explains why conical MSIs caused greater microdamage to the cortical bone than cylindrical MSIs [39]. As previously indicated, tight contact can cause excessive insertion torque which may lead to microfracture, ischemia of the surrounding bone, delayed bone healing, and eventually the failure of the MSIs [53, 54, 99, 106].

While conical MSIs require greater maximum removal torque, torque values decrease more rapidly during the removal procedure than with cylindrical MSIs [82]. Perhaps this is why it has been suggested that the conical shape has less risk of fracture during the removal procedure [107].

Considering all the results from the various studies, the conical MSI has an advantage regarding primary stability. However, the cylindrical MSI is better in terms of secondary stability. It causes less tissue damage because it produces lower maximum insertion torque [39, 105]. Sakoh et al. [99] reported that conical MSIs showed higher failure rates than cylindrical MSIs in an in vitro study. In one animal study, there was no difference in the failure rates [100]. Another animal study [97] showed that the conical MSIs had better primary stability compared to cylindrical MSIs, but no difference between the two screws in secondary stability [39]. A human study evaluating, 324 MSIs in 144 patients found no significant difference in the success rate between the cylindrical and conical shape [108].

Kim et al. [100] suggested that the conical shape may require modifications in the thread structure and the insertion technique in order to reduce the excessive insertion torque while maintaining a high resistance to removal. Chang et al. [77] reported that increasing the core diameter of the uppermost threads to create a conical core design could reduce the stress concentration effects at the neck while improving the pullout resistance.

It is still not clear which shaft design has an advantage for clinical success. Further research is needed to improve the primary stability without sacrificing the secondary stability.

1.4 Placement Site Characteristics

As previously indicated, the anchorage an implant provides depends on its interaction with the bone into which it has been inserted. Differences in the quality and quantity of bone into which MSIs are placed might therefore be expected to influence both their primary and secondary stability. It has been suggested that cortical bone quantity and quality are two of the most important determinants of primary stability [33, 50].

1.4.1 Bone Density/Quality

Bone density is positively related to both insertion torque and pullout strength [13, 109–114]. The higher the density of the bone, the greater the primary stability. This can again be explained by higher initial bone-to-implant contact.

In order to better understand how bone density affects the primary stability of MSIs, Hung et al. evaluated the insertion torque and pullout forces of MSIs placed in synthetic cortical bone

[115]. Cortical densities of 0.8 and 0.64 g/cc (the density of the human mandible has been reported to be 0.66 g/cc) were compared (Fig. 1.10). While the MSIs placed in more dense bone exhibited significantly greater insertion torque and pullout force than the MSIs placed in less dense bone, the effects were greater on insertion torque (156 % increase) than on pullout force (135 % increase).

In their recent meta-analysis of 17 studies, Papageorgiou et al. reported greater MSI failures in the mandible than maxilla (19.3 vs. 12.0 %) [8]. Greater numbers of failures might be expected for denser bone due to increases in microfractures. Moreover, greater MSI failures in the mandible than maxilla might be due to ischemia and necrosis associated with overheating when drilling into denser bone [116, 117]. Increased microfractures, ischemia, and necrosis might be expected because bone mineral density has consistently been shown to be greater in the human mandible than maxilla [118–120].

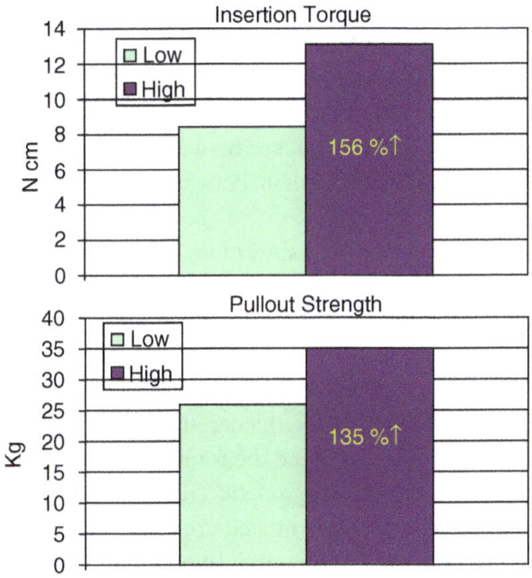

Fig 1.10 Effects of synthetic cortical bone density [high (0.8 g/cc) vs. low (0.64 g/cc)] on the insertion torque and pullout strength of 6-mm-long MSIs (Adapted from Hung et al. [115])

Experimental studies make it possible to better evaluate stability by controlling confounding variables. A total of 106 immediately loaded MSIs (6-mm long and 1.8-mm wide) were placed and followed for either 98 [121, 122] or 105 days [123]. Of the 53 MSIs that were placed in the maxillary, 52 (98.1 %) remained stable compared to 49 (92.5 %) of their counterparts placed in the mandible (Table 1.1). This suggests that failures may be higher in the mandible, but the differences between jaws were small and not statistically significant ($p=0.119$). Another experimental study (Fig. 1.11) comparing 3-mm MSI loaded with 600 g also showed significantly ($p<0.001$) greater stability over a 6-week observation period for MSI placed in the maxillas (80 % success) than for those placed in the mandibles (60 % success) of the same dogs [27].

1.4.2 Cortical Bone Thickness

Clinical failures of MSIs have been commonly attributed to thick cortical bone [33, 82, 109, 124]. On the other hand, thin cortical bone can also be problematic. For example, Papageorgiou et al. reported significantly more failures in cortical bone that was <1-mm thick than in thicker cortical bone (21.3 vs. 8.3 %) [8]. Thin cortical bone could explain the higher failure rates that have been attributed to younger patients [110, 124–126]. There are also differences in cortical

Table 1.1 Differences in the stability of immediately loaded MSIs (6-mm long × 1.8-mm wide) placed in the maxilla and mandible

Study	Maxilla	Stability (%)	Mandible	Stability (%)
1	Control	14/14 (100 %)	Control	13/14 (92.8 %)
1	25 g	7/7 (100 %)	25 g	5/7 (71.4 %)
2	50 g	16/16 (100 %)	50 g	16/16 (100 %)
2	100 g	15/16 (93.8 %)	100 g	15/16 (93.8 %)
Total		52/53 (98.1 %)		49/53 (92.5 %)

Adapted from Owens et al. [124] and Carrillo et al. [121, 122]

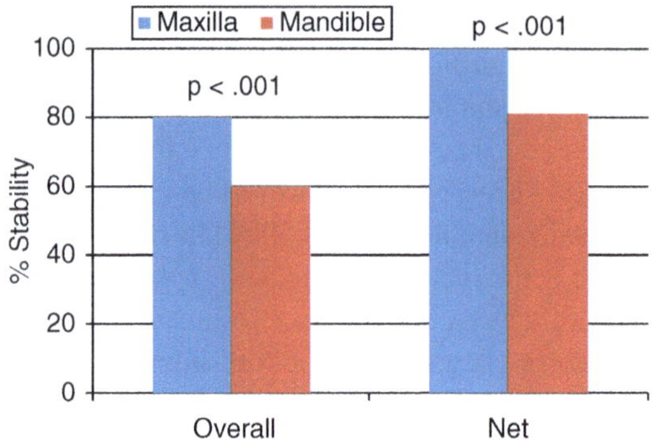

Fig 1.11 Overall and net stability of MSIs placed without pilot holes in the maxillas and mandibles of mature beagle dogs and immediately loaded with 600 g (Adapted from Mortensen et al. [27])

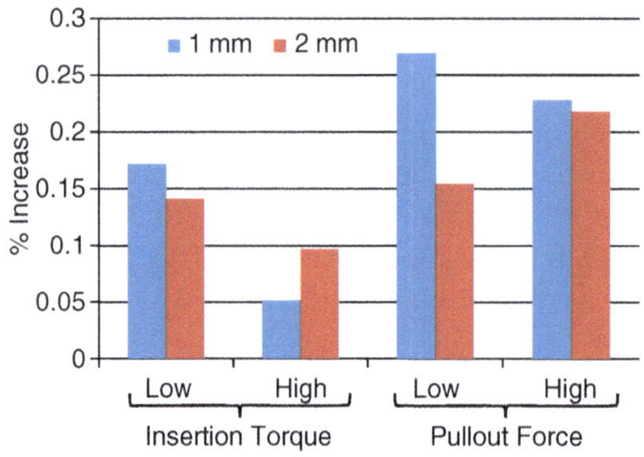

Fig. 1.12 Relative increases of insertion torque and pullout force by increasing the major diameter of 3-mm-long MSIs by ¼ mm (Adapted from Shah et al. [23])

thickness between jaws and within regions of each jaw that hold important clinical implications [127–131].

The thicker the cortical bone, the higher the insertion torque and pullout force [13, 111] indicating greater primary stability. For example, Pithon et al. showed that insertion torque was approximately 4 times greater in 6-mm than 1-mm-thick cortical bone [22]. Using synthetic bone to control extraneous sources of variation, Shah et al. showed that increasing cortical thickness from 1 to 2 mm increased both insertion torque and pullout force [23]. Importantly, the effects were greater on insertion torques than pullout force (Fig. 1.12).

Because there had been no comprehensive comparisons of cortical bone thickness at common placement sites of the maxilla and mandible, Farnsworth et al. quantified cortical bone thickness at 16 commonly used sites [132]. Cone beam computed tomography (CBCT) images of 26 adolescents (11–16 years of age) and 26 adults (20–45 years of age) showed that adult cortical bone was significantly thicker (0.12–0.56 mm) at all sites except the infrazygomatic crest, the most posterior palatal site, and the mandibular buccal site between the 6 and 7. Cortical bone at the buccal mandibular sites was significantly thicker in the posterior than anterior regions; the cortex was more than twice as thick between the first and second molar (2.4–2.5 mm) than between the lateral incisors and canines (0.9–1.2 mm) (Fig. 1.13). Cortical bone in the buccal aspect of the maxilla tended to be thinner than in the buccal aspect of the mandible. Also, differences between sites were much smaller in the maxilla; the cortex was only slightly thicker between 5–6 (1.0–1.5) and 4–5 (1.1–1.3) than between 2–3 (1.0–1.2) and 6–7 (0.9–1.2). Cortical bone thickness and differences between sites in the lingual region of the maxilla were similar to the buccal region of the maxilla. Paramedian palatal cortex was slightly thicker 3 mm (1.3–1.4 mm) than 6 mm (1.1–1.2 mm) behind the incisive foramen, which was in turn slightly thicker than bone located 9 mm (1.0–1.2) behind the foramen. The cortical bone in the infrazygomatic crest (1.4–1.6 mm) more closely approximated cortical thickness of the mandible than maxilla. Importantly, variability in cortical thickness among individuals was substantial; it would not be unusual for an adolescent patient to present with maxillary cortices less than 1.0-mm thick, which could be problematic for MSI retention. Conversely, it is not uncommon for mandibular cortices between the first and second molars to be more than 2.5-mm thick, which could also be problematic when the bone is dense.

It has also recently been shown that the cortical bone and the alveolar ridge are thicker in hypodivergent than in hyperdivergent subjects [133]. In the maxillary buccal region, differences were

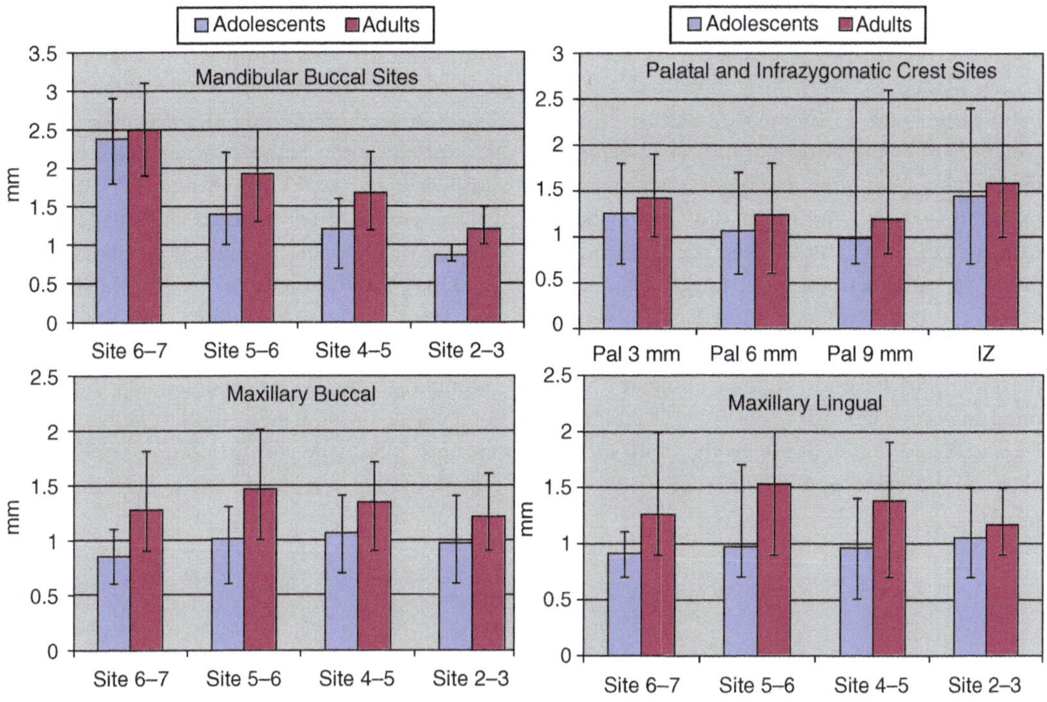

Fig. 1.13 Cortical bone thickness (means and ranges) for mandibular and maxillary interradicular MSI sites (Adapted from Farnsworth et al. [132])

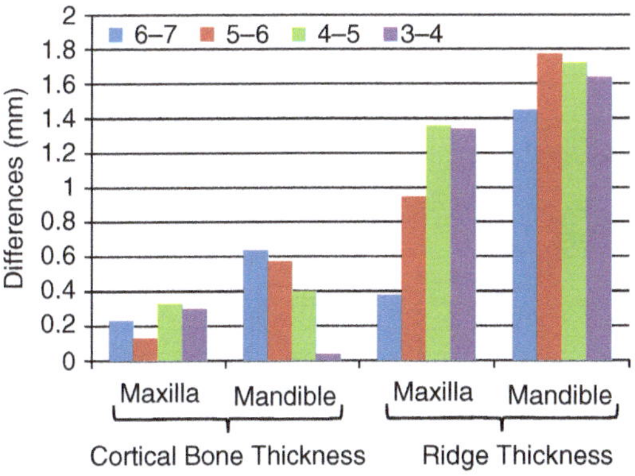

Fig. 1.14 Differences between hyper- and hypodivergent adults in buccal cortical bone and dentoalveoloar ridge thickness (Adapted from Horner et al. [115])

small, ranging from 0.13 to 0.33 mm (Fig. 1.14). Differences were larger in the maxilla, especially between the molars. The thickness of the dentoalveolar ridges measured 5 mm from the crests were up to 1.77-mm thicker in hypodivergent adults, and the differences were due primarily to differences in cortical rather than medullary bone thickness. They also showed that lingual cortical bone was consistently thicker in the mandible than maxilla; in the mandible, bone in the posterior region was thicker.

1.4.3 MSI Orientation

In one of the first studies evaluating MSI orientation, two different MSIs were inserted at seven different angles (30°, 40°, 50°, 60°, 70°, 80°, and 90°) into cadaver bone. The results demonstrated that the angle of MSI insertion had a significant impact on insertion torque [71]. MSIs angled between 60° and 70° produced the highest insertion torque values. Very oblique insertion angles (30°) resulted in reduced primary stability. Based on the differences observed, the authors hypothesized that an oblique insertion of MSIs might be advantageous in regions with reduced bone quality.

One of the earliest studies designed to evaluate the effects of MSI orientation on pullout forces placed MSIs (6-mm long and 1.8-mm outer diameter) in human mandibles [134]. Ninety MSIs were allocated into nine groups of ten each and placed in nine fresh human cadaver mandibles. A 1.1-mm pilot hole was drilled using a guide, and the MSIs were inserted at either 90° angles to the bone surface, angled at 45° to the bone surface and oriented along the maximum axis of stiffness or angled at 45° to the bone surface and oriented along the minimum axis of bone stiffness (Fig. 1.15). Pullout forces were oriented at 90° to the bone surface; shear forces were applied parallel to the bone surface along either the maximum and minimum axes of bone stiffness. The pullout tests showed that the implants aligned at 90° to the bone surface required significantly greater amounts of force before failing (34.2 kg) than those oriented at 45° (10.8 and 14.1 kg). The differences in force reflected differences in the amount of bone that remained in contact with the MSI after failure. For the 90° MSIs, bone that broke off after failure surrounded the implant more or less symmetrically and had an elliptical shape. MSIs oriented at 45° to the bone surface produced a smaller wedge of bone on only one side of the screw, oriented at approximately 135° to the MSI. The shear force

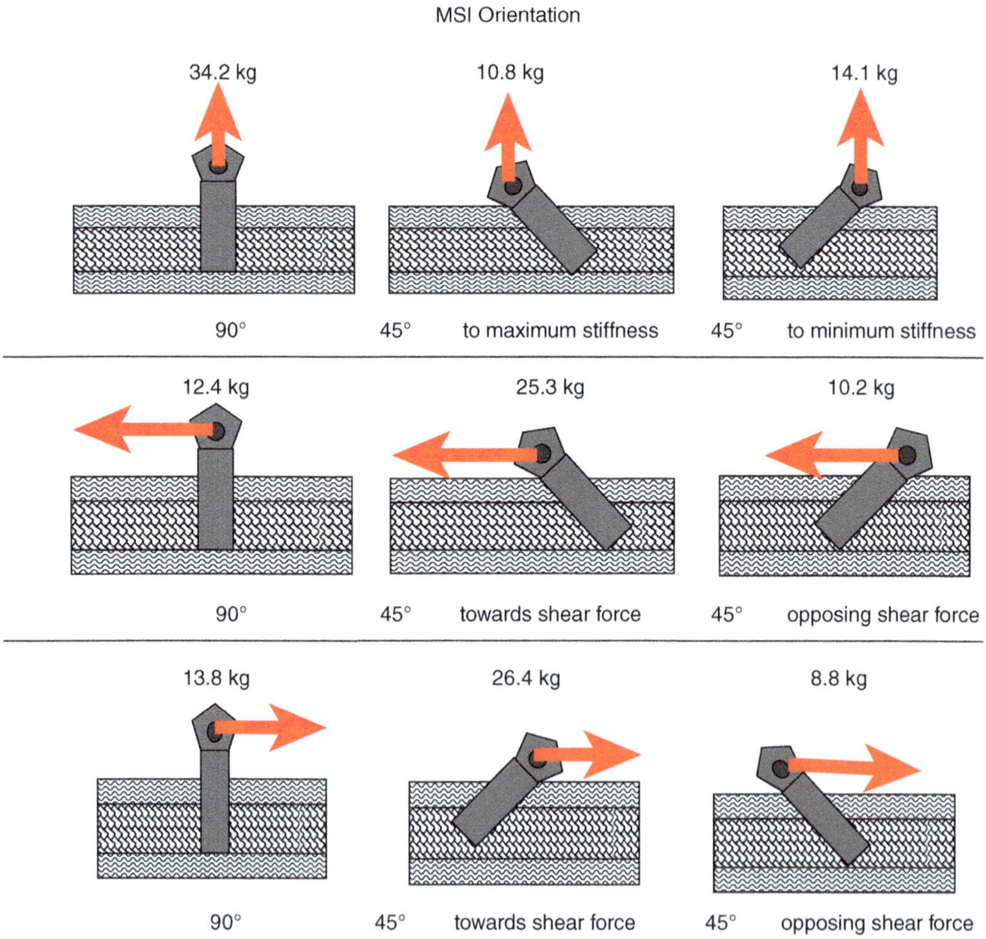

Fig. 1.15 Maximum pullout and shear forces at failure of 6 mm MSI placed perpendicular and at 45° toward shear force (Adapted from Pickard et al. [135])

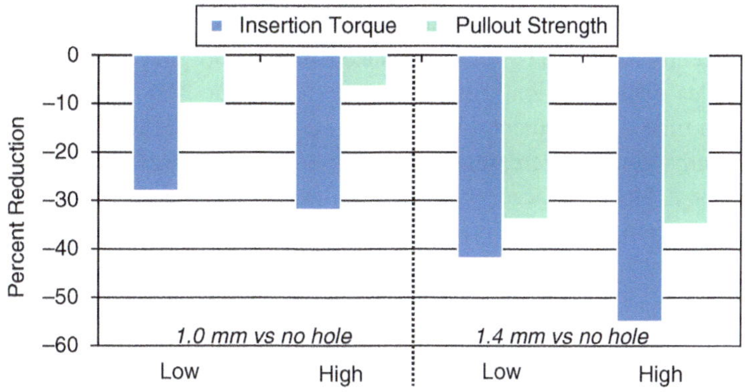

Fig. 1.16 Decreases in insertion torque and pullout strength of MSIs (6-mm long and 1.8-mm wide) associated with pilot hole size (1.0 and 1.4 mm) (Adapted from Hung et al. [115])

tests showed that the MSIs that were angled at 45° in the same direction as the line of force required significantly more force before failing (25.3 and 26.4 kg) than the MSIs oriented at 90° (12.4 and 13.8 kg); the MSIs oriented at 45° away from the line of force (tent peg) displayed the lowest forces at failure (8.8 and 10.2 kg). The tent-peg orientations produce stress concentrations near the cortical surface at 135° between the MSI and bone, which decreased their stability.

Recent finite element analyses confirmed that 90° provides the best anchorage resistance to pullout forces [135]. Using cadaver mandibular bone, the finite analysis showed that maximum anchorage resistance for MSIs placed at 90° to the bone surface was 5.5 and 1.4 times greater than for MSIs placed at 30° and 60° to the bone surface.

1.4.4 Pilot Hole Size

Decreases in insertion torque have been previously reported with increases in the size of pilot holes drilled for inserting bones screws [136, 137] and MSIs [109, 138]. Insertion torque decreases with pilot holes due to the decreased amounts of bone that needs to be displaced during insertion. Larger pilot holes require less bone to be displaced during MSI insertion, resulting in less compression of the adjacent bone. Pullout force has also been reported to decrease with increasing pilot hole size [137, 138]. The ideal pilot hole should provide the greatest decreases in insertion torque and the smallest decreases in pullout force.

Hung and coworkers recently evaluated the effects of pilot holes on insertion torque and pullout force [115]. The MSIs they tested were 6-mm long, with inner and outer diameters of 0.9 and 1.6 mm, respectively. As expected, insertion torque and pullout force were significantly smaller with, than without, pilot holes (Fig. 1.16). Importantly, the relative reductions in insertion torque associated with increasing pilot hole size were consistently greater than the relative reductions in pullout force observed, indicating that pilot holes reduce the initial trauma associated with MSI insertion without compromising stability proportionately. In comparison with no pilot hole, the 1-mm pilot holes produced substantially greater relative reductions in insertion torque than pullout force; the relative reductions were also greater for insertion torque with 1.4-mm pilot holes, but the differences between insertion torque and pullout force were much smaller. These findings strongly suggest that – depending on the MSI characteristics – there is an optimal pilot hole size, which substantially reduces the stresses caused during insertion but maintains the screws' holding power. Moreover, these effects are most pronounced in denser bone, which might be expected to benefit most from pilot holes.

Using a randomized split-mouth design, the effects that pilot holes have on (1) the longitudinal stability of MSIs measured with the Osstell

Mentor and (2) bone surrounding MSIs were recently studied [139]. MSIs placed with pilot holes exhibited significantly greater stability at the time of placement, but they showed significantly greater decreases in stability over time than MSIs placed without pilot holes. Microcomputed tomographic analyses showed that, after 7 weeks of healing, the most coronal aspects of the layer of cortical bone 6–24 μm from the MSIs placed with pilot holes, as well as all of three layers (6–24 μm, 24–42 μm, and 42–60 μm) of trabecular bone surrounding the MSIs placed without pilot holes, exhibited significantly more bone. These findings indicated greater primary stability for MSIs placed with pilot holes, but also greater losses of stability due primarily to less surrounding trabecular bone. These findings indicate that bone damage associated with the drilling process is detrimental to the long-term stability of MSIs.

Experimentally, Okazaki et al. placed 1.2-mm-wide (major diameter) MSIs in 1.0-mm- and 1.2-mm-wide pilot holes and measured removal torque 1, 3, 6, 9, and 12 weeks post-insertion [140]. For the MSIs placed in the 1.0-mm pilot holes, removal torque decreased over the first 6 weeks and then remained at the same level for the remainder of the experiment. For the MSIs placed in the 1.2-mm pilot holes, removal torque values were initially 11 times lower than those of the 1.0-mm pilot holes; they increased thereafter and were similar to the 1.0 pilot hole values at 6, 9, and 12 weeks post-insertion.

1.5 Loading Characteristics

While the influence of the heavy forces on the peri-implant tissue has been established for endosseous implant applications, [141, 142] the effects of orthodontic force on MSIs remains poorly understood. Orthodontic forces placed on MSI, which are considerably lower than the occlusal forces placed on dental implants, might be expected to produce much less strain and have lesser effects. While excessive loads could affect MSI stability, there appears to be no clear pattern of association between the amount of load (ranging from 100 to 500 cN) and bone-to-implant contact [12, 57]. Most of the available literature comparing loaded vs. unloaded control MSIs also shows little or no differences in osseointegration or in failure rates [143, 144]. Garfinkle et al. did report higher success rate for loaded than for unloaded MSIs [126].

1.5.1 The Effects of Force

Using split-mouth designs, the effects of force on the stability of 142, 6-mm long, MSIs placed in the maxillas and mandibles of 15 beagle dogs have been evaluated experimentally [121–123]. The overall stability of the MSIs was 97.2 % (Table 1.2); the MSI on the side of the mouth immediately loaded with lighter forces (100 % stable) were only slightly, but significantly, more stable than those subjected to heavier forces (94.4 % stable). In contrast (Fig. 1.17), significantly ($p<0.001$) higher (100 %) success has been reported for 3-mm-long MSIs loaded with 100 and 200 g, than for the same MSIs loaded with 50 g (77 %); success rates were also significantly lower for unloaded (75 %) MSIs than those loaded with 100 or 200 g [29]. Conflicting results such as these suggest interactions with other factors that could have been responsible for the different success rates observed (i.e., it is possible that the amount of force – within limits – does not matter).

Because they are loaded so differently, the literature showing the effects of force on endosseous implants is not applicable to MSIs. The earlier studies comparing the effects of different forces on MSIs suggest that osseointegration is independent of force magnitudes [10, 12]. Studies comparing applied forces to no forces have also shown no significant histological differences in the bone surrounding the MSIs [143, 145]. This could be due to the fact that histomorphometry only provides a limited two-dimension representation of the bone around implants. For example, a 10-μm slice represents less than 0.14 % of an 8-mm MSI. This necessarily increases the variation and makes it more difficult to identify the effects of force.

Table 1.2 Split-mouth comparisons of the stability of 6-mm-long MSIs loaded immediately with lighter or heavier immediate forces (chi square = 4.23; $p = 0.039$)

Study	Lighter	Stability (%)	Heavier	Stability (%)
1	Mandible 25 g	7/7 (100 %)	Mandible 50 g	5/7 (71.4 %)
2	Mandible 25 g	16/16 (100 %)	Mandible 50 g	16/16 (100 %)
2	Mandible 50 g	16/16 (100 %)	Mandible 100 g	15/16 (93.8 %)
2	Mandible 25 g	16/16 (100 %)	Mandible 100 g	16/16 (100 %)
2	Maxilla 50 g	16/16 (100 %)	Maxilla 100 g	15/16 (93.8 %)
2		71/71 (100 %)		67/71 (94.4 %)

Data from Owens et al. [124] and Carrillo et al. [121, 122]
Overall stability = 138/142 (97.2 %)

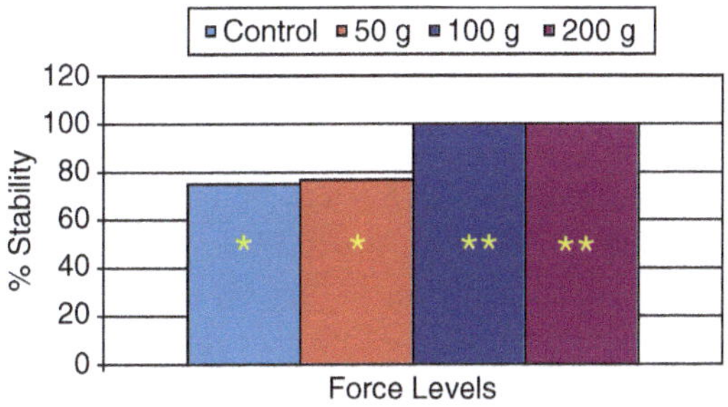

Fig. 1.17 Percent stability of 3 mm control and immediately loaded MSIs over a 42-day experimental period (different number of * indicates significant $p < 0.001$ differences) (Adapted from Liu et al. [30])

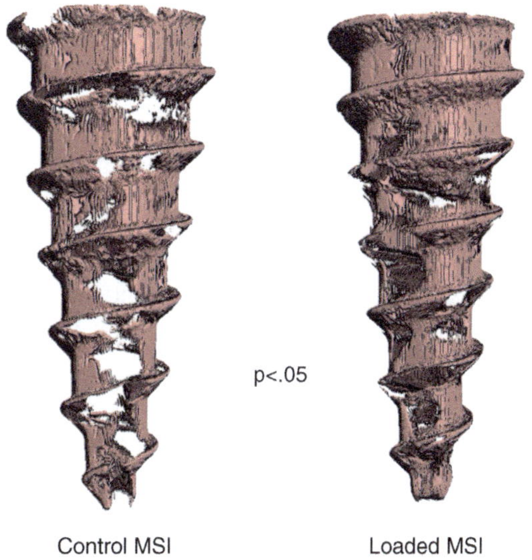

Fig. 1.18 Bone 6–24-μm thick surrounding the MSI of unloaded control and loaded SLA-surfaced MSIs (Adapted from Ikeda et al. [94])

Based on μ-CT evaluations, significantly greater peri-BIC was reported for loaded (200 g), 6-mm-long sandblasted and acid-etched surfaced MSIs, than for their unloaded counterparts [94]. The differences were greatest in the regions with the greatest bone-volume-to-total-volume (i.e., the more coronal aspects of the cortical and non-cortical regions), for which the loaded MSIs showed 3–13 % more peri-bone-to-implant contact than the unloaded MSIs (Fig. 1.18).

The application of force, amount of force, and the direction of force all affect the amount of bone produced around miniscrew implants [146]. The amount of cortical bone around the apical aspects of unloaded MSIs is greater than the amount of cortical bone around loaded MSIs. However, the amount of non-cortical bone is greater around loaded implants. MSIs loaded with 200 g showed greater amounts of non-cortical bone surrounding them than MSIs loaded with 600 g. The regions around the MSI under compression also exhibited more bone than the regions that were not under compression. Together, these findings suggest that there is an optimal range of force (i.e., you need force but not too much) for optimal secondary stability.

1.5.2 Potential Root Injuries

While there are various reasons why orthodontists do not place their own MSIs (Fig. 1.19), the most common reason is the risk of root damage [1]. The risk of root damage was deemed to be more important than time, training, pain, or the

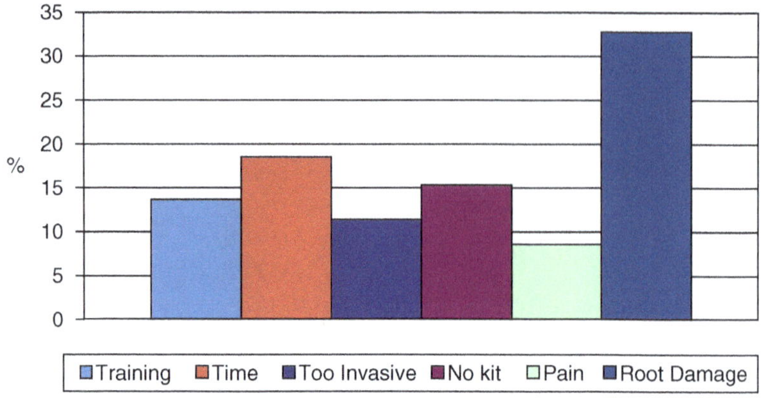

Fig. 1.19 Responses to a survey of 451 orthodontists to the question "Why don't you place your own MSIs?" (Adapted from Buschang et al. [1])

availability of a kit. Potential damage to the roots has been well documented with dental implants and fixation screws. Implant placements have resulted in loss of tooth vitality [147] and transection of root apices [148]. Fixation screws have also been shown to damage the roots in up to 43 % of the cases [141, 149]. Importantly, the periodontal literature shows that repair can occur following root and PDL damage [150]. Until very recently, our understanding of the healing effects on structures damaged with MSIs was very limited. Chen et al. reported increased failure rates when MSIs contact roots; they also showed that roots repair by cementum deposition and that bone regenerates if the MSIs are removed and the sites are allowed to heal [151].

In order to evaluate the immediate, short-term (6 weeks) and long-term (12 weeks) damage caused by MSIs that are left in situ, intentional damage was inflicted to the roots of the maxillary second, third, and fourth premolars of seven mature beagle dogs with self-tapping MSI (8 mm × 1.8 mm) [152]. The results showed that the placement of MSIs can produce immediate and extensive damage of the teeth, periodontium, and bone; the short- and long-term damage was similar to the immediate damage caused. Importantly, it was shown that the tactile resistance felt by the operator increases suddenly when the MSI contacts the tooth, with resistance approximately doubling when the MSI contacts the tooth. Changes in resistance felt during insertion may be a better indication of root contact than radiographs. Histology showed that approximately 75 % of the teeth had been damaged by the MSIs (Fig. 1.20). Damage varied from the displacement of bone and periodontal ligament (7.2 %) to invasion of the pulp chamber (14.2 %) – dentinal damage was the most common (26.2 %), followed by cementum damage (19 %). Immediate damage usually produced clean cuts through both the cementum and dentinal layers. There was evidence of both short- and long-term healing, even though the MSIs remained in place throughout the experiment. Placement of MSIs into the pulp produced detrimental and irreversible damage. Such damage usually requires either root canal therapy or tooth extractions [153]. Based on the extent of damage that is possible, orthodontists should have a thorough knowledge of the underlying structures before MSI placement, and they should obtain informed consent from their patients.

A companion study evaluated healing of the roots and surrounding structures after damage was caused by MSIs that were immediately removed after having been inserted into the teeth [154]. As previously indicated, insertion torque doubled when the MSIs contacted the roots. Approximately 67.9 % of the teeth showed damage of the dentin, 19.6 % showed damage of the cementum, and 12.5 % showed damage of the pulp. Most of the damaged teeth (64.3 %) displayed normal healing (Fig. 1.21). Healing was evident by 6 weeks and continued through

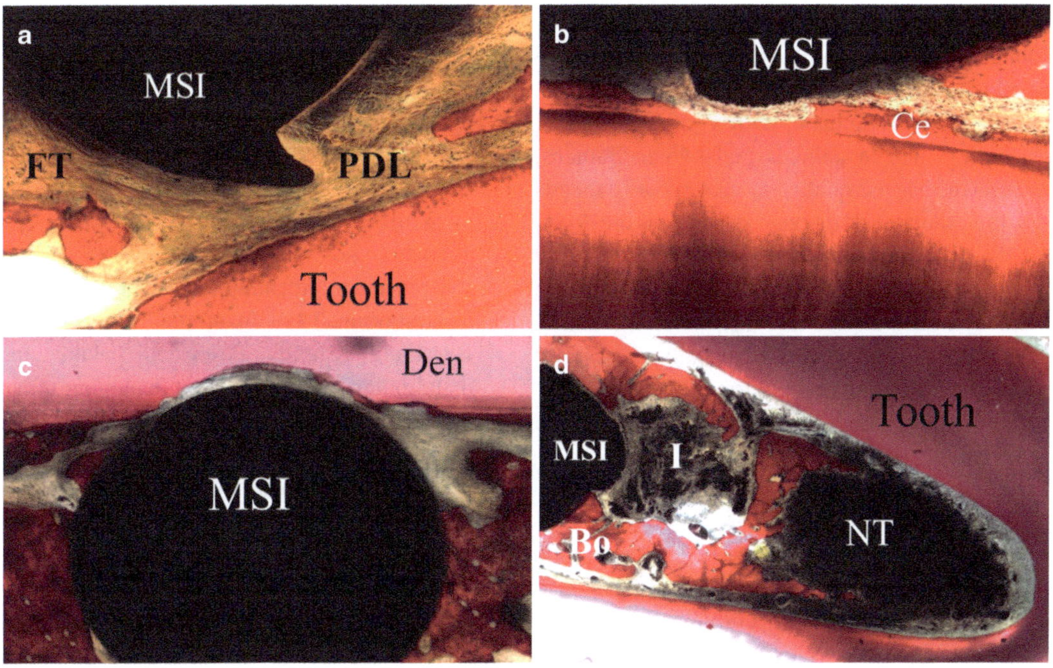

Fig. 1.20 Short- and long-term damage caused by MSI placement to the (**a**) PDL, (**b**) cementum (*Ce*), (**c**) dentin (*Den*), and (**d**) furcation, causing inflammation (*I*), necrotic tissue (*NT*), and loss of bone (*Bo*) (Adapted from Hembree et al. [153])

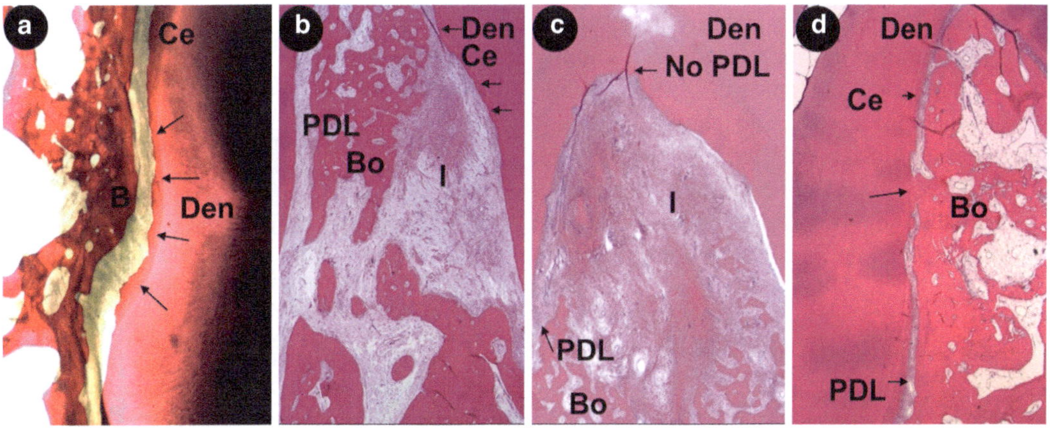

Fig. 1.21 (**a**) Normal healing after damage caused by MSI inserted into the dentin (*Den*) with a new cementum (*Ce*) layer, PDL restored to functional width, and bone (*Bo*) regeneration in the area of damage, (**b**) new cementum but no PDL or bone regeneration around the dentin defect (*arrows*); (**c**) degeneration in the furcation area; (**d**) lack of a layer of cementum and PDL with direct contact between the bone and dentin. Note the inflammatory infiltrate (*I*) in both (b) and (c) (Adapted from Briceno et al. [154])

12 weeks. New cementum approximately doubled between 6 and 12 weeks of healing. After 12 weeks of healing, the new bone, PDL, and cementum appeared similar to the adjacent, undamaged structures. Abnormal healing, including lack of PDL, lack of bone regeneration, bone degeneration in the furcation area, ankylosis, and the lack of healing due to inflammatory infiltrate or pulpal invasion, was evident in 35.7 % of the damaged teeth. The lack of healing

observed further emphasizes the importance of obtaining informed consent from patients prior to MSI placement.

A recent systematic review of 11 articles, including nine in animals and two in humans, indicated that the quality of root repair depends on the amounts of damage caused by the MSIs [155]. The best available studies consistently show that when the damage is limited to the cementum and dentin, and there is no inflammatory infiltrate, normal healing usually occurs. But it does not always occur. Normal healing is substantially less likely to occur when the MSIs are inserted into the pulp.

Conclusions

Based on the evidence presently available, MSIs used by orthodontists could be optimized in various ways (Table 1.3). The fact that pullout forces increase relatively more than insertion torque suggests that increases in MSI length and width, decreases in pitch, and the addition of flutes are all beneficial features that might be expected to increase primary and secondary stability. SLA surface treatment also enhances secondary stability by increasing the amount of BIC. While greater bone density and cortical thickness increase primary stability, excessively thick or dense cortical bone appears to be detrimental to long-term MSI stability. There is undoubtedly an ideal range of acceptable cortical thicknesses and bone densities associated with long-term stability. While pilot holes decrease insertion torque, they pose problems for long-term MSI stability and should therefore only be used with thicker and denser bone.

While the MSI and placement site characteristics are important for MSI stability, placement techniques are probably just as important. For example, Carrillo and Buschang recently described palatal and mandibular MSI placement techniques that produce success rates above 90 % [156]. Their techniques emphasize careful planning, maintenance of MSI position and orientation throughout the insertion phase, evaluation of stability after insertion, and post-op hygiene instructions and daily rinses with chlorhexidine for 5 days. MSI placement techniques must be taken seriously by the orthodontist. If they are not, the MSIs could fail, regardless of their characteristics or the characteristics of the placement sites.

Table 1.3 Increases (+) and decreases (–) in insertion torque, pullout force, and stability associated with various MSI and placement site characteristics

Characteristics	Insertion torque	Pullout force	Stability
↑Length	+	++	+
↑Width	+	++	NE
↓Pitch	+	++	NE
↑Thread depth	++	+	NE
Fluting	+	++	NE
SLA surface treatment	–	NE	+
↑Bone density	++	+	IRV
↑Cortical thickness	++	+	IRV
Pilot holes	–	–	–

NE not evaluated, *IRV* ideal range of values

References

1. Buschang PH, Carrillo R, Ozenbaugh B, Rossouw PE. 2008 survey of AAO members on miniscrew usage. J Clin Orthod. 2008;42(9):513–8.
2. Buschang PH, Carrillo R, Rossouw PE. Orthopedic correction of growing hyperdivergent, retrognathic patients with miniscrew implants. J Oral Maxillofac Surg. 2011;69(3):754–62.
3. Gainsforth B, Higley L. A study of orthodontic anchorage possibilities in basal bone. Am J Orthod Oral Surg. 1945;31:406–517.
4. Creekmore TD, Eklund MK. The possibility of skeletal anchorage. J Clin Orthod. 1983;17(4):266–9.
5. Kanomi R. Mini-implant for orthodontic anchorage. J Clin Orthod. 1997;31(11):763–7.
6. Reynders R, Ronchi L, Bipat S. Mini-implants in orthodontics: a systematic review of the literature. Am J Orthod Dentofac Orthop. 2009;135(5):564.e1–19.
7. Schätzle M, Männchen R, Zwahlen M, Lang NP. Survival and failure rates of orthodontic temporary anchorage devices: a systematic review. Clin Oral Implants Res. 2009;20(12):1351–9.
8. Papageorgiou SN, Zogakis IP, Papadopoulos MA. Failure rates and associated risk factors of orthodontic miniscrew implants: a meta-analysis. Am J Orthod Dentofacial Orthop. 2012;142(5):577–595.e7.

9. Brånemark PI, Adell R, Breine U, Hansson BO, Lindström J, Ohlsson A. Intra-osseous anchorage of dental prostheses. I. Experimental studies. Scand J Plast Reconstr Surg. 1969;3(2):81–100.
10. Melsen B, Costa A. Immediate loading of implants used for orthodontic anchorage. Clin Orthod Res. 2000;3(1):23–8.
11. Büchter A, Wiechmann D, Gaertner C, Hendrik M, Vogeler M, Wiesmann HP, et al. Load-related bone modelling at the interface of orthodontic micro-implants. Clin Oral Implants Res. 2006;17(6):714–22.
12. Woods PW, Buschang PH, Owens SE, Rossouw PE, Opperman LA. The effect of force, timing, and location on bone-to-implant contact of miniscrew implants. Eur J Orthod. 2009;31(3):232–40.
13. Huja SS, Litsky AS, Beck FM, Johnson KA, Larsen PE. Pull-out strength of monocortical screws placed in the maxillae and mandibles of dogs. Am J Orthod Dentofacial Orthop. 2005;127(3):307–13.
14. Migliorati M, Benedicenti S, Signori A, Drago S, Barberis F, Tournier H, et al. Miniscrew design and bone characteristics: an experimental study of primary stability. Am J Orthod Dentofac Orthop. 2012;142(2):228–34.
15. Ivanoff CJ, Sennerby L, Lekholm U. Influence of initial implant mobility on the integration of titanium implants. An experimental study in rabbits. Clin Oral Implants Res. 1996;7(2):120–7.
16. Nam O, Yu W, Kyung H. Cortical bone strain during the placement of orthodontic microimplant studies by 3D finite element analysis. Kor J Orthod. 2008;38:228–39.
17. Ure DS, Oliver DR, Kim KB, Melo AC, Buschang PH. Stability changes of miniscrew implants over time. Angle Orthod. 2011;81(6):994–1000.
18. Ersanli S, Karabuda C, Beck F, Leblebicioglu B. Resonance frequency analysis of one-stage dental implant stability during the osseointegration period. J Periodontol. 2005;76(7):1066–71.
19. Hitchon PW, Brenton MD, Coppes JK, From AM, Torner JC. Factors affecting the pullout strength of self-drilling and self-tapping anterior cervical screws. Spine. 2003;28(1):9–13.
20. Lyon WF, Cochran JR, Smith L. Actual holding power of various screws in bone. Ann Surg. 1941;114(3):376–84.
21. Lim S-A, Cha J-Y, Hwang C-J. Insertion torque of orthodontic miniscrews according to changes in shape, diameter and length. Angle Orthod. 2008;78(2):234–40.
22. Pithon MM, Figueiredo DSF, Oliveira DD. Mechanical evaluation of orthodontic mini-implants of different lengths. J Oral Maxillofac Surg. 2013;71(3):479–86.
23. Shah AH, Behrents RG, Kim KB, Kyung H-M, Buschang PH. Effects of screw and host factors on insertion torque and pullout strength. Angle Orthod. 2012;82(4):603–10.
24. Chen C-H, Chang C-S, Hsieh C-H, Tseng Y-C, Shen Y-S, Huang I-Y, et al. The use of microimplants in orthodontic anchorage. J Oral Maxillofac Surg. 2006;64(8):1209–13.
25. Park H-S, Lee S-K, Kwon O-W. Group distal movement of teeth using microscrew implant anchorage. Angle Orthod. 2005;75(4):602–9.
26. Kuroda S, Sugawara Y, Deguchi T, Kyung H-M, Takano-Yamamoto T. Clinical use of miniscrew implants as orthodontic anchorage: success rates and postoperative discomfort. Am J Orthod Dentofacial Orthop. 2007;131(1):9–15.
27. Mortensen MG, Buschang PH, Oliver DR, Kyung H-M, Behrents RG. Stability of immediately loaded 3- and 6-mm miniscrew implants in beagle dogs–a pilot study. Am J Orthod Dentofacial Orthop. 2009;136(2):251–9.
28. Liu SS-Y, Opperman LA, Buschang PH. Effects of recombinant human bone morphogenetic protein-2 on midsagittal sutural bone formation during expansion. Am J Orthod Dentofacial Orthop. 2009;136(6):768.e1–8; discussion 768–9.
29. Liu SS-Y, Opperman LA, Kyung H-M, Buschang PH. Is there an optimal force level for sutural expansion? Am J Orthod Dentofacial Orthop. 2011;139(4):446–55.
30. Liu SS-Y, Kyung H-M, Buschang PH. Continuous forces are more effective than intermittent forces in expanding sutures. Eur J Orthod. 2010;32(4):371–80.
31. Caraway D. Shear force at failure of immediately-loaded 3 mm and 6 mm miniscrew implants at six weeks post-insertion [Master's thesis]. Saint Louis: Center for Advanced Dental Education, Saint Louis University; 2007.
32. Liou EJW, Pai BCJ, Lin JCY. Do miniscrews remain stationary under orthodontic forces? Am J Orthod Dentofacial Orthop. 2004;126(1):42–7.
33. Miyawaki S, Koyama I, Inoue M, Mishima K, Sugahara T, Takano-Yamamoto T. Factors associated with the stability of titanium screws placed in the posterior region for orthodontic anchorage. Am J Orthod Dentofac Orthop. 2003;124(4):373–8.
34. Motoyoshi M, Uemura M, Ono A, Okazaki K, Shigeeda T, Shimizu N. Factors affecting the long-term stability of orthodontic mini-implants. Am J Orthod Dentofac Orthop. 2010;137(5):588.e1–5.
35. Crismani AG, Bertl MH, Celar AG, Bantleon H-P, Burstone CJ. Miniscrews in orthodontic treatment: review and analysis of published clinical trials. Am J Orthod Dentofacial Orthop. 2010;137(1):108–13.
36. Chen Y, Kyung HM, Gao L, Yu W-J, Bae E-J, Kim S-M. Mechanical properties of self-drilling orthodontic micro-implants with different diameters. Angle Orthod. 2010;80(5):821–7.
37. Liu T-C, Chang C-H, Wong T-Y, Liu J-K. Finite element analysis of miniscrew implants used for orthodontic anchorage. Am J Orthod Dentofac Orthop. 2012;141(4):468–76.
38. Duaibis R, Kusnoto B, Natarajan R, Zhao L, Evans C. Factors affecting stresses in cortical bone around miniscrew implants. Angle Orthod. 2012;82;875–80.

39. Lee N-K, Baek S-H. Effects of the diameter and shape of orthodontic mini-implants on microdamage to the cortical bone. Am J Orthod Dentofac Orthop. 2010;138(1):8.e1–8.
40. Barros SE, Janson G, Chiqueto K, Garib DG, Janson M. Effect of mini-implant diameter on fracture risk and self-drilling efficacy. Am J Orthod Dentofac Orthop. 2011;140(4):e181–92.
41. Florvaag B, Kneuertz P, Lazar F, Koebke J, Zöller JE, Braumann B, et al. Biomechanical properties of orthodontic miniscrews. An in-vitro study. J Orofac Orthop. 2010;71(1):53–67.
42. Holm L, Cunningham SJ, Petrie A, Cousley RRJ. An in vitro study of factors affecting the primary stability of orthodontic mini-implants. Angle Orthod. 2012;82(6):1022–8.
43. Poggio PM, Incorvati C, Velo S, Carano A. "Safe zones": a guide for miniscrew positioning in the maxillary and mandibular arch. Angle Orthod. 2006;76(2):191–7.
44. Park H-S, Jeong S-H, Kwon O-W. Factors affecting the clinical success of screw implants used as orthodontic anchorage. Am J Orthod Dentofac Orthop. 2006;130(1):18–25.
45. Wiechmann D, Meyer U, Büchter A. Success rate of mini- and micro-implants used for orthodontic anchorage: a prospective clinical study. Clin Oral Implants Res. 2007;18(2):263–7.
46. Wu T-Y, Kuang S-H, Wu C-H. Factors associated with the stability of mini-implants for orthodontic anchorage: a study of 414 samples in Taiwan. J Oral Maxillofac Surg. 2009;67(8):1595–9.
47. DeCoster TA, Heetderks DB, Downey DJ, Ferries JS, Jones W. Optimizing bone screw pullout force. J Orthop Trauma. 1990;4(2):169–74.
48. Wilmes B, Su Y-Y, Drescher D. Insertion angle impact on primary stability of orthodontic mini-implants. Angle Orthod. 2008;78(6):1065–70.
49. Carano A, Lonardo P, Velo S, Incorvati C. Mechanical properties of three different commercially available miniscrews for skeletal anchorage. Prog Orthod. 2005;6(1):82–97.
50. Costa A, Raffainl M, Melsen B. Miniscrews as orthodontic anchorage: a preliminary report. Int J Adult Orthod Orthognath Surg. 1998;13(3):201–9.
51. Kim J-W, Ahn S-J, Chang Y-I. Histomorphometric and mechanical analyses of the drill-free screw as orthodontic anchorage. Am J Orthod Dentofac Orthop. 2005;128(2):190–4.
52. Motoyoshi M, Hirabayashi M, Uemura M, Shimizu N. Recommended placement torque when tightening an orthodontic mini-implant. Clin Oral Implants Res. 2006;17(1):109–14.
53. Huja SS, Katona TR, Burr DB, Garetto LP, Roberts WE. Microdamage adjacent to endosseous implants. Bone. 1999;25(2):217–22.
54. Martin RB. Fatigue microdamage as an essential element of bone mechanics and biology. Calcif Tissue Int. 2003;73(2):101–7.
55. Wawrzinek C, Sommer T, Fischer-Brandies H. Microdamage in cortical bone due to the overtightening of orthodontic microscrews. J Orofac Orthop. 2008;69(2):121–34.
56. Meredith N. Assessment of implant stability as a prognostic determinant. Int J Prosthodont. 1998; 11(5):491–501.
57. Büchter A, Wiechmann D, Koerdt S, Wiesmann HP, Piffko J, Meyer U. Load-related implant reaction of mini-implants used for orthodontic anchorage. Clin Oral Implants Res. 2005;16(4):473–9.
58. Viwattanatipa N, Thanakitcharu S, Uttraravichien A, Pitiphat W. Survival analyses of surgical miniscrews as orthodontic anchorage. Am J Orthod Dentofacial Orthop. 2009;136(1):29–36.
59. Chaddad K, Ferreira AH, Geurs N, Reddy MS. Influence of surface characteristics on survival rates of mini-implants. Angle Orthod. 2008;78(1):107–13.
60. Asscherickx K, Vannet BV, Bottenberg P, Wehrbein H, Sabzevar MM. Clinical observations and success rates of palatal implants. Am J Orthod Dentofacial Orthop. 2010;137(1):114–22.
61. Hong C, Lee H, Webster R, Kwak J, Wu BM, Moon W. Stability comparison between commercially available mini-implants and a novel design: part 1. Angle Orthod. 2011;81(4):692–9.
62. Meursinge Reynders RA, Ronchi L, Ladu L, van Etten-Jamaludin F, Bipat S. Insertion torque and success of orthodontic mini-implants: a systematic review. Am J Orthod Dentofacial Orthop. 2012;142(5):596–614.e5.
63. Maino BG, Maino G, Mura P. Spider screw: skeletal anchorage system. Prog Orthod. 2005;6(1):70–81.
64. Schnelle MA, Beck FM, Jaynes RM, Huja SS. A radiographic evaluation of the availability of bone for placement of miniscrews. Angle Orthod. 2004; 74(6):832–7.
65. Huang L-H, Shotwell JL, Wang H-L. Dental implants for orthodontic anchorage. Am J Orthod Dentofacial Orthop. 2005;127(6):713–22.
66. Min K-I, Kim S-C, Kang K-H, Cho J-H, Lee E-H, Chang N-Y, et al. Root proximity and cortical bone thickness effects on the success rate of orthodontic micro-implants using cone beam computed tomography. Angle Orthod. 2012;82(6):1014–21.
67. Kuroda S, Yamada K, Deguchi T, Hashimoto T, Kyung H-M, Takano-Yamamoto T. Root proximity is a major factor for screw failure in orthodontic anchorage. Am J Orthod Dentofacial Orthop. 2007; 131(4 Suppl):S68–73.
68. Büchter A, Wiechmann D, Koerdt S, Wiesmann HP, Piffko J, Meyer U. Belastungsbedingte Reaktionen von Mini-Implantaten, welche für orthodontische Verankerungen verwendet werden. Clin Oral Implants Res. 2005;16(4):473–9.
69. Mah J, Bergstrand F. Temporary anchorage devices: a status report. J Clin Orthod. 2005;39(3):132–6.
70. Jolley TH, Chung CH. Peak torque values at fracture of orthodontic miniscrews. J Clin Orthod. 2007; 41(6):326–8.

71. Wilmes B, Ottenstreuer S, Su Y-Y, Drescher D. Impact of implant design on primary stability of orthodontic mini-implants. J Orofac Orthop/Fortschr Kieferorthop. 2008;69(1):42–50.
72. Liu SS-Y, Cruz-Marroquin E, Sun J, Stewart KT, Allen MR. Orthodontic mini-implant diameter does not affect in-situ linear microcrack generation in the mandible or the maxilla. Am J Orthod Dentofac Orthop. 2012;142(6):768–73.
73. Lim H-J, Eun C-S, Cho J-H, Lee K-H, Hwang H-S. Factors associated with initial stability of miniscrews for orthodontic treatment. Am J Orthod Dentofac Orthop. 2009;136(2):236–42.
74. Chapman JR, Harrington RM, Lee KM, Anderson PA, Tencer AF, Kowalski D. Factors affecting the pullout strength of cancellous bone screws. J Biomech Eng. 1996;118(3):391–8.
75. Brinley CL, Behrents R, Kim KB, Condoor S, Kyung H-M, Buschang PH. Pitch and longitudinal fluting effects on the primary stability of miniscrew implants. Angle Orthod. 2009;79(6):1156–61.
76. Gracco A, Giagnorio C, Incerti Parenti S, Alessandri Bonetti G, Siciliani G. Effects of thread shape on the pullout strength of miniscrews. Am J Orthod Dentofac Orthop. 2012;142(2):186–90.
77. Chang JZ-C, Chen Y-J, Tung Y-Y, Chiang Y-Y, Lai EH-H, Chen W-P, et al. Effects of thread depth, taper shape, and taper length on the mechanical properties of mini-implants. Am J Orthod Dentofac Orthop. 2012;141(3):279–88.
78. Hou S-M, Hsu C-C, Wang J-L, Chao C-K, Lin J. Mechanical tests and finite element models for bone holding power of tibial locking screws. Clin Biomech (Bristol Avon). 2004;19(7):738–45.
79. Johnson NL, Galuppo LD, Stover SM, Taylor KT. An in vitro biomechanical comparison of the insertion variables and pullout mechanical properties of 6.5-mm standard cancellous and 7.3-mm self-tapping, cannulated bone screws in foal femoral bone. Vet Surg. 2004;33(6):681–90.
80. Migliorati M, Signori A, Silvestrini-Biavati A. Temporary anchorage device stability: an evaluation of thread shape factor. Eur J Orthod. 2012;34(5): 582–6.
81. Migliorati M, Benedicenti S, Signori A, Drago S, Cirillo P, Barberis F, et al. Thread shape factor: evaluation of three different orthodontic miniscrews stability. Eur J Orthod. 2013;35(3):401–5.
82. Kim Y-K, Kim Y-J, Yun P-Y, Kim J-W. Effects of the taper shape, dual-thread, and length on the mechanical properties of mini-implants. Angle Orthod. 2009;79(5):908–14.
83. Yerby S, Scott CC, Evans NJ, Messing KL, Carter DR. Effect of cutting flute design on cortical bone screw insertion torque and pullout strength. J Orthop Trauma. 2001;15(3):216–21.
84. Bechtol C, Ferguson A, Lang P. Internal fixation with plates and screws. In: Bechtol CO, Ferguson AB, Laing PG, editors. Metals and engineering in bone and joint surgery. Williams & Wilkins Company, Baltimore; 1959. p. 162–4.
85. Koranyi E, Bowman CE, Knecht CD, Janssen M. Holding power of orthopedic screws in bone. Clin Orthop Relat Res. 1970;72:283–6.
86. Boyle 3rd JM, Frost DE, Foley WL, Grady JJ. Torque and pullout analysis of six currently available self-tapping and "emergency" screws. J Oral Maxillofac Surg. 1993;51(1):45–50.
87. Evans M, Spencer M, Wang Q, White SH, Cunningham JL. Design and testing of external fixator bone screws. J Biomed Eng. 1990;12(6):457–62.
88. Wu S-W, Lee C-C, Fu P-Y, Lin S-C. The effects of flute shape and thread profile on the insertion torque and primary stability of dental implants. Med Eng Phys. 2012;34(7):797–805.
89. Buser D, Nydegger T, Oxland T, Cochran DL, Schenk RK, Hirt HP, et al. Interface shear strength of titanium implants with a sandblasted and acid-etched surface: a biomechanical study in the maxilla of miniature pigs. J Biomed Mater Res. 1999;45(2):75–83.
90. Abrahamsson I, Berglundh T, Linder E, Lang NP, Lindhe J. Early bone formation adjacent to rough and turned endosseous implant surfaces. An experimental study in the dog. Clin Oral Implants Res. 2004;15(4):381–92.
91. Chang C-S, Lee T-M, Chang C-H, Liu J-K. The effect of microrough surface treatment on miniscrews used as orthodontic anchors. Clin Oral Implants Res. 2009;20(10):1178–84.
92. Kim S-H, Lee S-J, Cho I-S, Kim S-K, Kim T-W. Rotational resistance of surface-treated mini-implants. Angle Orthod. 2009;79(5):899–907.
93. Mo S-S, Kim S-H, Kook Y-A, Jeong D-M, Chung K-R, Nelson G. Resistance to immediate orthodontic loading of surface-treated mini-implants. Angle Orthod. 2010;80(1):123–9.
94. Ikeda H, Rossouw PE, Campbell PM, Kontogiorgos E, Kontogirogos E, Buschang PH. Three-dimensional analysis of peri-bone-implant contact of rough-surface miniscrew implants. Am J Orthod Dentofacial Orthop. 2011;139(2):e153–63.
95. Florvaag B, Kneuertz P, Lazar F, Koebke J, Zöller JE, Braumann B, et al. Biomechanical properties of orthodontic miniscrews. In Vitro Study J Orofac Orthop/. 2010;71(1):53–67.
96. Yano S, Motoyoshi M, Uemura M, Ono A, Shimizu N. Tapered orthodontic miniscrews induce bone-screw cohesion following immediate loading. Eur J Orthod. 2006;28(6):541–6.
97. Cha J-Y, Takano-Yamamoto T, Hwang C-J. The effect of miniscrew taper morphology on insertion and removal torque in dogs. Int J Oral Maxillofac Implants. 2010;25(4):777–83.
98. Mischkowski RA, Kneuertz P, Florvaag B, Lazar F, Koebke J, Zöller JE. Biomechanical comparison of four different miniscrew types for skeletal anchorage in the mandibulo-maxillary area. Int J Oral Maxillofac Surg. 2008;37(10):948–54.

99. Sakoh J, Wahlmann U, Stender E, Nat R, Al-Nawas B, Wagner W. Primary stability of a conical implant and a hybrid, cylindric screw-type implant in vitro. Int J Oral Maxillofac Implants. 2006;21(4):560–6.
100. Kim JW, Baek SH, Kim TW, Chang YI. Comparison of stability between cylindrical and conical type mini-implants. Angle Orthod. 2008;78(4):692–8.
101. Martinez H, Davarpanah M, Missika P, Celletti R, Lazzara R. Optimal implant stabilization in low density bone. Clin Oral Implants Res. 2001;12(5): 423–32.
102. Drago CJ, Del Castillo RA. A retrospective analysis of osseotite NT implants in clinical practice: 1-year follow-up. Int J Periodontics Restor Dent. 2006; 26(4):337–45.
103. Heidemann W, Terheyden H, Gerlach KL. Analysis of the osseous/metal interface of drill free screws and self-tapping screws. J Craniomaxillofac Surg. 2001;29(2):69–74.
104. Abshire BB, McLain RF, Valdevit A, Kambic HE. Characteristics of pullout failure in conical and cylindrical pedicle screws after full insertion and back-out. Spine J. 2001;1(6):408–14.
105. Siegele D, Soltesz U. Numerical investigations of the influence of implant shape on stress distribution in the jaw bone. Int J Oral Maxillofac Implants. 1989;4(4):333–40.
106. O'Sullivan D, Sennerby L, Meredith N. Influence of implant taper on the primary and secondary stability of osseointegrated titanium implants. Clin Oral Implants Res. 2004;15(4):474–80.
107. Melsen B. Mini-implants: where are we? J Clin Orthod. 2005;39(9):539–47, quiz 531–2.
108. Giuliano Maino B, Pagin P, Di Blasio A. Success of miniscrews used as anchorage for orthodontic treatment: analysis of different factors. Prog Orthod. 2012;13(3):202–9.
109. Wilmes B, Rademacher C, Olthoff G, Drescher D. Parameters affecting primary stability of orthodontic mini-implants. J Orofac Orthop. 2006;67(3):162–74.
110. Motoyoshi M, Yoshida T, Ono A, Shimizu N. Effect of cortical bone thickness and implant placement torque on stability of orthodontic mini-implants. Int J Oral Maxillofac Implants. 2007;22(5):779–84.
111. Cleek TM, Reynolds KJ, Hearn TC. Effect of screw torque level on cortical bone pullout strength. J Orthop Trauma. 2007;21(2):117–23.
112. Koistinen A, Santavirta SS, Kröger H, Lappalainen R. Effect of bone mineral density and amorphous diamond coatings on insertion torque of bone screws. Biomaterials. 2005;26(28):5687–94.
113. Friberg B, Sennerby L, Gröndahl K, Bergström C, Bäck T, Lekholm U. On cutting torque measurements during implant placement: a 3-year clinical prospective study. Clin Implant Dent Relat Res. 1999;1(2):75–83.
114. Hughes AN, Jordan BA. The mechanical properties of surgical bone screws and some aspects of insertion practice. Injury. 1972;4(1):25–38.
115. Hung E, Oliver D, Kim KB, Kyung H-M, Buschang PH. Effects of pilot hole size and bone density on miniscrew implants' stability. Clin Implant Dent Relat Res. 2012;14(3):454–60.
116. Tehemar SH. Factors affecting heat generation during implant site preparation: a review of biologic observations and future considerations. Int J Oral Maxillofac Implants. 1999;14(1):127–36.
117. Eriksson AR, Albrektsson T. Temperature threshold levels for heat-induced bone tissue injury: a vital-microscopic study in the rabbit. J Prosthet Dent. 1983;50(1):101–7.
118. Devlin H, Horner K, Ledgerton D. A comparison of maxillary and mandibular bone mineral densities. J Prosthet Dent. 1998;79(3):323–7.
119. Park H-S, Lee Y-J, Jeong S-H, Kwon T-G. Density of the alveolar and basal bones of the maxilla and the mandible. Am J Orthod Dentofacial Orthop. 2008;133(1):30–7.
120. Gulsahi A, Paksoy CS, Ozden S, Kucuk NO, Cebeci ARI, Genc Y. Assessment of bone mineral density in the jaws and its relationship to radiomorphometric indices. Dentomaxillofac Radiol. 2010;39(5): 284–9.
121. Carrillo R, Rossouw PE, Franco PF, Opperman LA, Buschang PH. Intrusion of multiradicular teeth and related root resorption with mini-screw implant anchorage: a radiographic evaluation. Am J Orthod Dentofacial Orthop. 2007;132(5):647–55.
122. Carrillo R, Buschang PH, Opperman LA, Franco PF, Rossouw PE. Segmental intrusion with mini-screw implant anchorage: a radiographic evaluation. Am J Orthod Dentofacial Orthop. 2007;132(5): 576.e1–6.
123. Owens SE, Buschang PH, Cope JB, Franco PF, Rossouw PE. Experimental evaluation of tooth movement in the beagle dog with the mini-screw implant for orthodontic anchorage. Am J Orthod Dentofacial Orthop. 2007;132(5):639–46.
124. Park H-S, Kwon T-G, Sung J-H. Nonextraction treatment with microscrew implants. Angle Orthod. 2004;74(4):539–49.
125. Chen Y-J, Chang H-H, Huang C-Y, Hung H-C, Lai EH-H, Yao C-CJ. A retrospective analysis of the failure rate of three different orthodontic skeletal anchorage systems. Clin Oral Implants Res. 2007;18(6):768–75.
126. Garfinkle JS, Cunningham Jr LL, Beeman CS, Kluemper GT, Hicks EP, Kim M-O. Evaluation of orthodontic mini-implant anchorage in premolar extraction therapy in adolescents. Am J Orthod Dentofacial Orthop. 2008;133(5):642–53.
127. Schwartz-Dabney CL, Dechow PC. Variations in cortical material properties throughout the human dentate mandible. Am J Phys Anthropol. 2003; 120(3):252–77.
128. Peterson J, Wang Q, Dechow PC. Material properties of the dentate maxilla. Anat Rec A Discov Mol Cell Evol Biol. 2006;288(9):962–72.

129. Deguchi T, Nasu M, Murakami K, Yabuuchi T, Kamioka H, Takano-Yamamoto T. Quantitative evaluation of cortical bone thickness with computed tomographic scanning for orthodontic implants. Am J Orthod Dentofacial Orthop. 2006;129(6):721.e7–12.
130. Katranji A, Misch K, Wang H-L. Cortical bone thickness in dentate and edentulous human cadavers. J Periodontol. 2007;78(5):874–8.
131. Ono A, Motoyoshi M, Shimizu N. Cortical bone thickness in the buccal posterior region for orthodontic mini-implants. Int J Oral Maxillofac Surg. 2008;37(4):334–40.
132. Farnsworth D, Rossouw PE, Ceen RF, Buschang PH. Cortical bone thickness at common miniscrew implant placement sites. Am J Orthod Dentofacial Orthop. 2011;139(4):495–503.
133. Horner KA, Behrents RG, Kim KB, Buschang PH. Cortical bone and ridge thickness of hyperdivergent and hypodivergent adults. Am J Orthod Dentofac Orthop. 2012;142(2):170–8.
134. Pickard MB, Dechow P, Rossouw PE, Buschang PH. Effects of miniscrew orientation on implant stability and resistance to failure. Am J Orthod Dentofac Orthop. 2010;137(1):91–9.
135. Woodall N, Tadepalli SC, Qian F, Grosland NM, Marshall SD, Southard TE. Effect of miniscrew angulation on anchorage resistance. Am J Orthod Dentofacial Orthop. 2011;139(2):e147–52.
136. Daftari TK, Horton WC, Hutton WC. Correlations between screw hole preparation, torque of insertion, and pullout strength for spinal screws. J Spinal Disord. 1994;7(2):139–45.
137. Heidemann W, Gerlach KL, Gröbel KH, Köllner HG. Influence of different pilot hole sizes on torque measurements and pullout analysis of osteosynthesis screws. J Craniomaxillofac Surg. 1998;26(1):50–5.
138. Gantous A, Phillips JH. The effects of varying pilot hole size on the holding power of miniscrews and microscrews. Plast Reconstr Surg. 1995;95(7):1165–9.
139. Carney L. The effect of pilot holes on longitudinal miniscrew stability and bony adaptation [Master's thesis]. Dallas: Texas A&M University Baylor College of Dentistry; 2013.
140. Okazaki J, Komasa Y, Sakai D, Kamada A, Ikeo T, Toda I, et al. A torque removal study on the primary stability of orthodontic titanium screw mini-implants in the cortical bone of dog femurs. Int J Oral Maxillofac Surg. 2008;37(7):647–50.
141. Duyck J, Rønold HJ, Van Oosterwyck H, Naert I, Vander Sloten J, Ellingsen JE. The influence of static and dynamic loading on marginal bone reactions around osseointegrated implants: an animal experimental study. Clin Oral Implants Res. 2001;12(3):207–18.
142. Berglundh T, Abrahamsson I, Lindhe J. Bone reactions to longstanding functional load at implants: an experimental study in dogs. J Clin Periodontol. 2005;32(9):925–32.
143. Freire JNO, Silva NRFA, Gil JN, Magini RS, Coelho PG. Histomorphologic and histomorphometric evaluation of immediately and early loaded mini-implants for orthodontic anchorage. Am J Orthod Dentofacial Orthop. 2007;131(6):704.e1–9.
144. Vande Vannet B, Sabzevar MM, Wehrbein H, Asscherickx K. Osseointegration of miniscrews: a histomorphometric evaluation. Eur J Orthod. 2007;29(5):437–42.
145. Ohmae M, Saito S, Morohashi T, Seki K, Qu H, Kanomi R, et al. A clinical and histological evaluation of titanium mini-implants as anchors for orthodontic intrusion in the beagle dog. Am J Orthod Dentofacial Orthop. 2001;119(5):489–97.
146. Massey CC, Kontogiorgos E, Taylor R, Opperman L, Dechow P, Buschang PH. Effect of force on alveolar bone surrounding miniscrew implants: a 3-dimensional microcomputed tomography study. Am J Orthod Dentofacial Orthop. 2012;142(1):32–44.
147. Margelos JT, Verdelis KG. Irreversible pulpal damage of teeth adjacent to recently placed osseointegrated implants. J Endod. 1995;21(9):479–82.
148. Rubenstein JE, Taylor TD. Apical nerve transection resulting from implant placement: a 10-year follow-up report. J Prosthet Dent. 1997;78(6):537–41.
149. Farr DR, Whear NM. Intermaxillary fixation screws and tooth damage. Br J Oral Maxillofac Surg. 2002;40(1):84–5.
150. Helldén L. Periodontal healing following experimental injury to root surfaces of human teeth. Scand J Dent Res. 1972;80(3):197–205.
151. Chen Y-H, Chang H-H, Chen Y-J, Lee D, Chiang H-H, Yao C-CJ. Root contact during insertion of miniscrews for orthodontic anchorage increases the failure rate: an animal study. Clin Oral Implants Res. 2008;19(1):99–106.
152. Hembree M, Buschang PH, Carrillo R, Spears R, Rossouw PE. Effects of intentional damage of the roots and surrounding structures with miniscrew implants. Am J Orthod Dentofacial Orthop. 2009;135(3):280.e1–9; discussion 280–1.
153. Kim SG. Implant-related damage to an adjacent tooth: a case report. Implant Dent. 2000;9(3):278–80.
154. Brisceno CE, Rossouw PE, Carrillo R, Spears R, Buschang PH. Healing of the roots and surrounding structures after intentional damage with miniscrew implants. Am J Orthod Dentofacial Orthop. 2009;135(3):292–301.
155. Alves Jr M, Baratieri C, Araújo MTS, Souza MMG, Maia LC. Root damage associated with intermaxillary screws: a systematic review. Int J Oral Maxillofac Surg. 2012;41(11):1445–50.
156. Carrillo R, Buschang P. Palatal and mandibular miniscrew implant placement techniques. J Clin Orthod. 97 (12):737–43..

Surface-Treated Two-Component C-Implant: Revisited

2

Kyu-Rhim Chung, Yong Kim, and Seong-Hun Kim

Abstract

C-implant is a two-component orthodontic mini-implant with 1.8 mm diameter and 8.5 mm length. It is surface treated with sandblasting and acid etching to reduce implant failure. The head portion of the C-implant is detachable and functions as a buccal tube of a fixed appliance to allow archwire to pass through the hole in the head portion. Osseointegration of C-implants widened the clinical treatment modality by allowing multidirectional orthodontic force applications for intended orthodontic tooth movement. Rotation resistance increased the efficiency and efficacy of force control during orthodontic treatment. C-implant is especially useful for Biocreative Orthodontics, defined as independent en masse retraction of the anterior teeth while avoiding orthodontic appliances on the posterior segments during the retraction period. This alternative approach is beneficial in maximum anchorage cases that present with a poor dental health status such as severe dental caries, advanced periodontal disease, or missing posterior teeth.

C-implant was first introduced in 2000 and the design of the mini-implant has not been modified since then. Design of C-implant is similar to orthodontic miniscrews, and also it is analogous to the miniature version of endosseous implant. The difference of C-implant from orthodontic miniscrews is that it has been surface treated by sandblasting and acid etching to increase the bone to implant osseointegration potential. The similarity of the C-implant to endosseous implant is that it is composed of two separate parts: the screw part in the bone and head part in the oral cavity (Fig. 2.1). The screw part is 1.8 mm in diameter and 8.5, 9.5, 10.5 mm in length. The entire surface, except for the upper 2 mm, is sandblasted and acid etched (SLA) for optimal osseointegration because partial osseointegration reduces the risk of implant failure [1–3]. The head portion of the C-implant is detachable from the screw

K.-R. Chung, DMD, MSD, PhD
Division of Orthodontics, School of Medicine, Ajou University, Wonchun-dong 5, Youngtong-Ku, Suwon 443-380, South Korea
e-mail: speedor@hotmail.com

Y. Kim, DDS • S.-H. Kim, DDS, MSD, PhD (✉)
Department of Orthodontics, School of Dentistry, Kyung Hee University, #1 Hoegi-dong, Dongdaemun-gu, Seoul 130-701, South Korea
e-mail: yong_korea@hotmail.com; bravortho@gmail.com, bravortho@khu.ac.kr

K.B. Kim (ed.), *Temporary Skeletal Anchorage Devices*,
DOI 10.1007/978-3-642-55052-2_2, © Springer-Verlag Berlin Heidelberg 2014

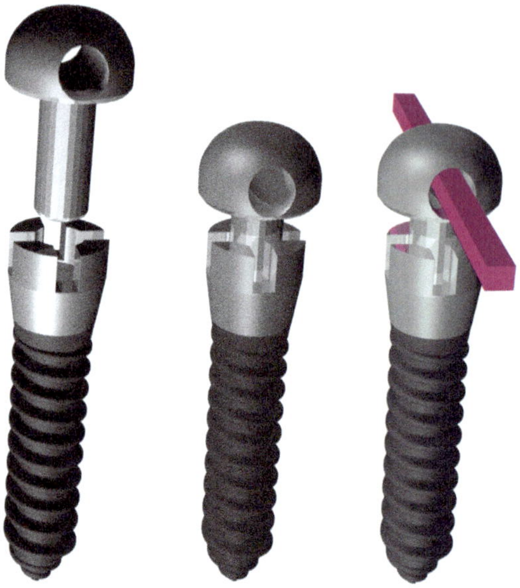

Fig. 2.1 The design of the C-implant

part. The head portion can function as a buccal tube of the fixed appliance that allows archwire to pass through the hole (0.08″ diameter) in the head portion (Fig. 2.2). The C-implant lacks self-drilling ability unlike orthodontic miniscrews, so manual drilling with driver is required before placing the C-implant. Before placing the screw part of the C-implant, pilot hole is drilled through the gingiva into the bone to guide direction of the C-implant. A 1.5-mm-diameter guide hand drill is connected to the screw handle. The pointed tip of the drill permits manual screwing. Lastly, the head portion is tapped into lock in the screw part.

The C-implant opened up new paradigm of skeletal anchorage in orthodontic treatment. The osseointegration potential has been studied clinically and histologically. Moreover, the survival rate and the clinical applications of C-implants were reported, and these generated changes in orthodontic treatment modalities. First, the SLA-treated C-implants were proved

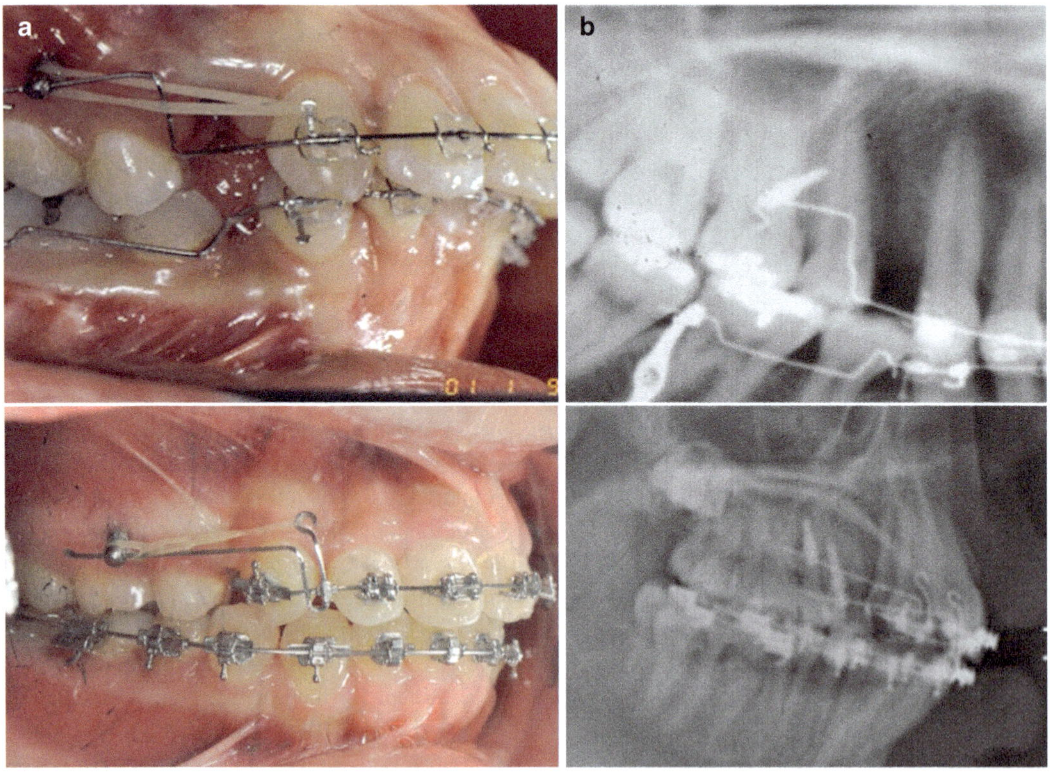

Fig. 2.2 Clinical (**a**) and radiographic (**b**) pictures demonstrating the wire insertion at the head part of the C-implant

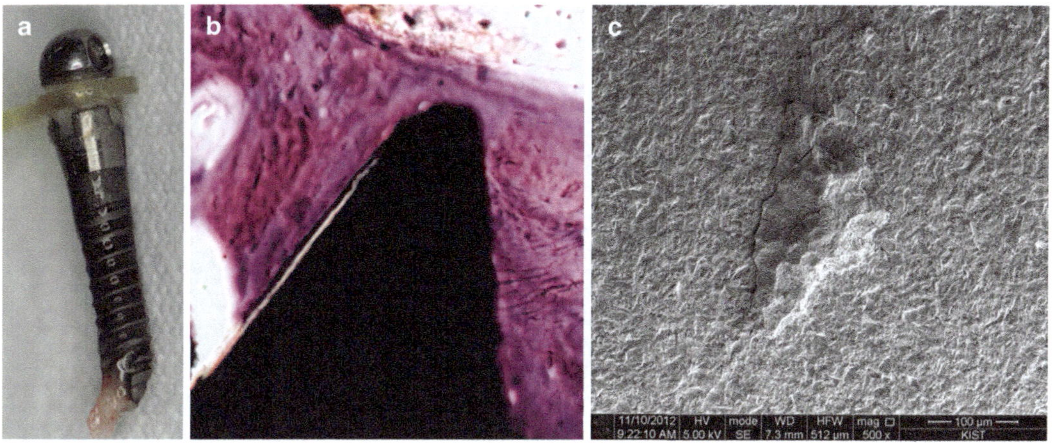

Fig. 2.3 (**a**) Showing the visible alveolar bone attachment upon C-implant removal. (**b**) SEM image demonstrating the intimate osseointegration between thread and bone. (**c**) TEM image

Fig. 2.4 Animal study comparing the machined miniscrews and SLA-treated miniscrews on rotational force and the removal toque value experiment. (**a**) Machined group, (**b**) SLA-treated group

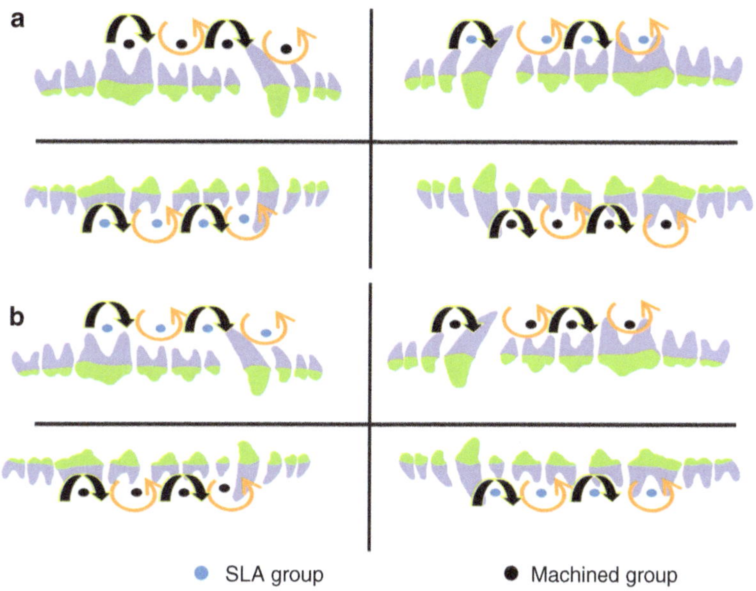

to have osseointegration with the bone (Fig. 2.3). As a measurement of osseointegration potential and related stability of miniscrews, the removal torque values (RTV) of C-implants were studied by Kim et al. to compare the difference in RTV between machined and SLA-treated (C-implant) miniscrews on clockwise and counterclockwise force application on experimental animal model (Figs. 2.4 and 2.5) [4]. Also, it was proved to have increased RTV with longer duration of C-implant placement [5]. There have been debates whether miniscrews remain absolute skeletal anchorage or not with applied orthodontic forces. The positional stability of C-implants was examined with superimposition of the CBCT images, and the result clarified that the C-implants remained absolutely stationary [6]. So, C-implants remain stationary through treatment and, as a result, resist multidirectional orthodontic forces. Since the osseointegrated endosseous prosthetic implant has known to have positional stability, the finding from the CBCT study implies the osseointegration of C-implants. In recent study of Lee et al. on survival rate of the C-implant, they found that

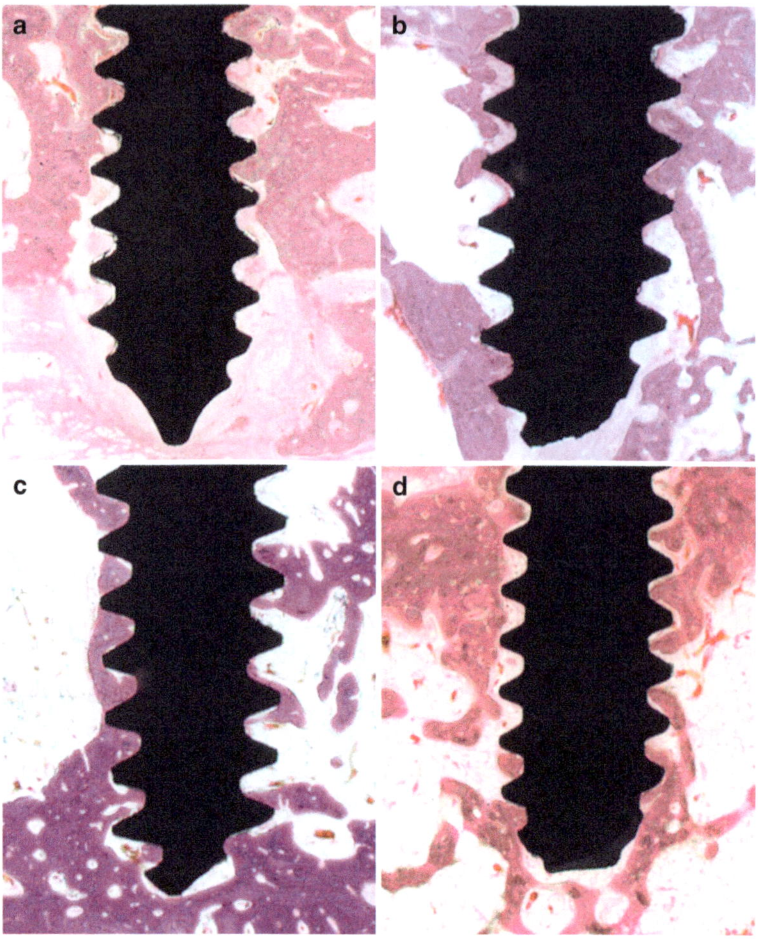

Fig. 2.5 (**a**) Machined clockwise rotational force. (**b**) Machined counterclockwise rotational force. (**c**) SLA-treated clockwise rotational force. (**d**) SLA-treated counterclockwise rotational force. Histological images showing osseointegration of both machined and SLA-treated miniscrews

the decrease in hazard function can successfully suggest the osseointegration of the orthodontic C-implants [7]. Lastly, in the backscatter SEM examination of the removed C-implants, the direct bone attachment to the implant surface was identified [8].

Osseointegration of C-implants widened clinical treatment modality by allowing multidirectional orthodontic force applications for intended orthodontic tooth movement. Rotation resistance increased the efficiency and efficacy of force control during orthodontic treatment. Biocreative Orthodontics Strategy (BO) is based on the ability of osseointegrated absolute skeletal anchorage control with C-implant. Ideal patient selections for Biocreative Orthodontics treatment are those who have stable posterior occlusion with anterior crowding with lip protrusion. Without altering the posterior occlusion, BO uses skeletal anchorage for en masse retraction without posterior dental anchorage support. The example of the Biocreative treatment is described below:

A 24-year-old woman presented with the chief complaints of lip protrusion and crowding (Fig. 2.6). Her prior medical and dental history revealed no significant systemic problems and absence of significant temporomandibular joint disorders. The initial clinical findings showed a convex facial profile associated with a retrognathic mandible and protrusive lips. The patient had a large overjet (6.0 mm) and significant amount of crowding in both arches (maxilla 20.0 mm; mandible 11.0 mm). The patient had class I molar relationship with the dental midline of lower arch deviated 4.0 mm to the right relative to the facial midline. Cephalometric analysis indicated a skeletal Class

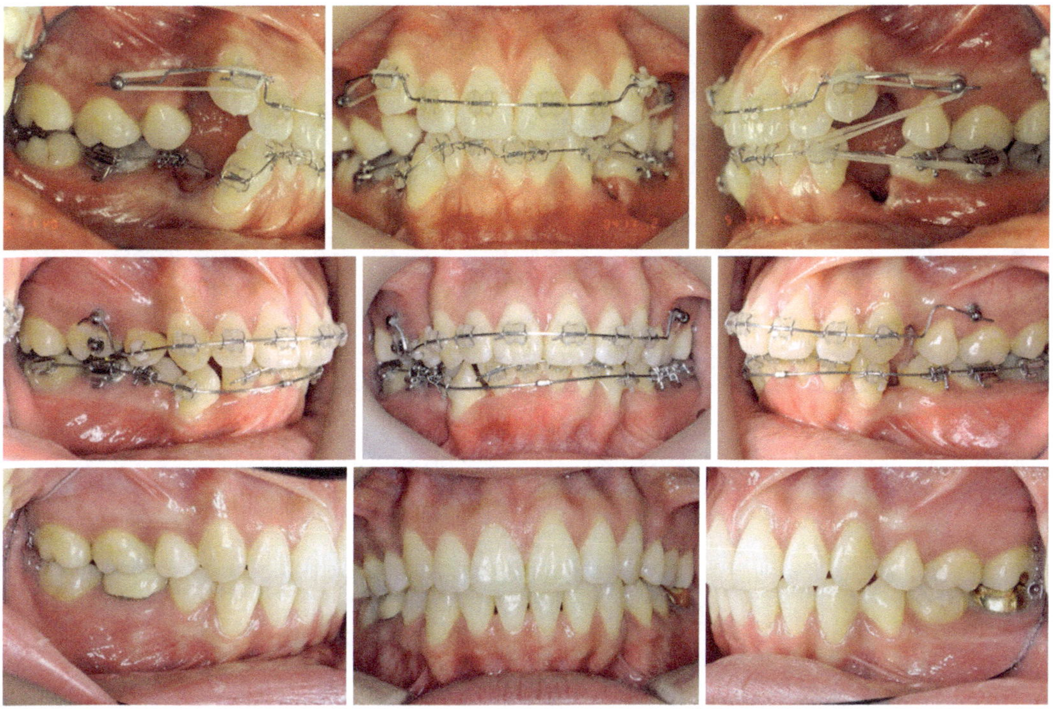

Fig. 2.6 Case treated with two C-implants in the maxillary arch with Biocreative Orthodontics Strategy

II, a hyperdivergent profile with steep mandibular plane angle, and upright maxillary and mandibular incisors. The patient was diagnosed with skeletal Class II protrusion with severe crowding.

Four first premolars were extracted. Two C-implants were placed between the second premolar and first molar in the maxilla. Brackets were bonded only on six anterior teeth in the maxilla during the initial stage of en masse retraction. Upper archwire was bent upward from distal of canines to pass through the head portion of the C-implant. Retraction of six anterior teeth and correction of the midline were performed by elastics. Class III elastic was placed between the maxillary C-implant and lower canine in the right side. When the extraction space was almost closed on the right side, the bracket was bonded on the upper second premolar and the button was bonded on the upper first molar. For detailing, brackets were bonded on all remaining teeth. At the completion of the treatment, soft tissue profile was dramatically improved. Panoramic x-ray revealed acceptable root parallelism without any other complications.

With C-implants, intrusive force can be created from resistance to rotation. The application of intrusive force is described using mousetrap appliance for molar intrusion (Figs. 2.7, 2.8, and 2.9).

In a patient who needed minor tooth movement for molar intrusion, two C-implants were placed between the second premolar and molar in the buccal and palatal areas. Mousetrap appliance made with TMA archwire is held in the occlusal surface of the molar for intrusion, and 150–300 g of intrusive force is immediately applied. Osseointegration of the C-implant resists the rotational force and is converted into the intrusive force, which then is applied to the molar to intrude the palatal cusp. Because C-implant was identified to be osseointegrated into the bone, the mousetrap appliance can be successfully used with the assurance of resistance to rotational force created by intrusion.

Furthermore, the C-implant can be used in general dentistry as a provisional implant due to the proof of osseointegration. The C-implant design is analogous to endosseous prosthetic implant with the screw part and head part and

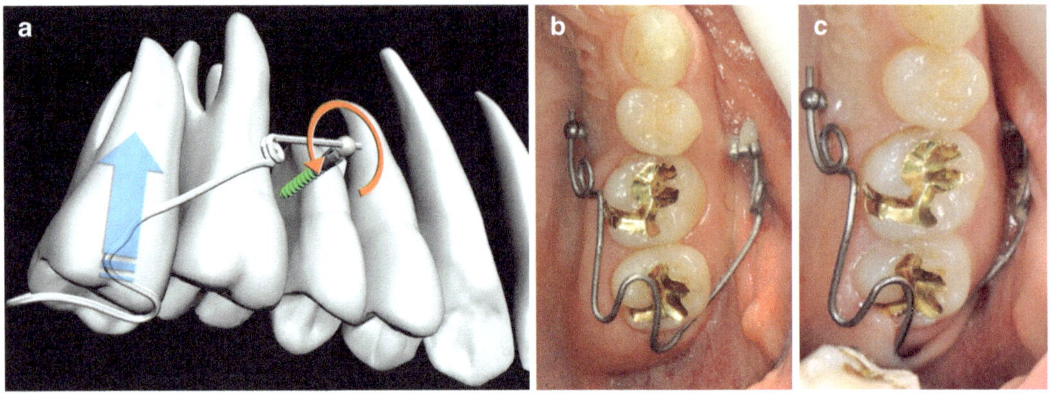

Fig. 2.7 (**a**) Mousetrap appliance diagram illustrating the conversion of rotational force to intrusive force. (**b**) Clinical picture of mousetrap appliance for intrusion of the maxillary second molar. (**c**) The intrusion of the maxillary second molar shown

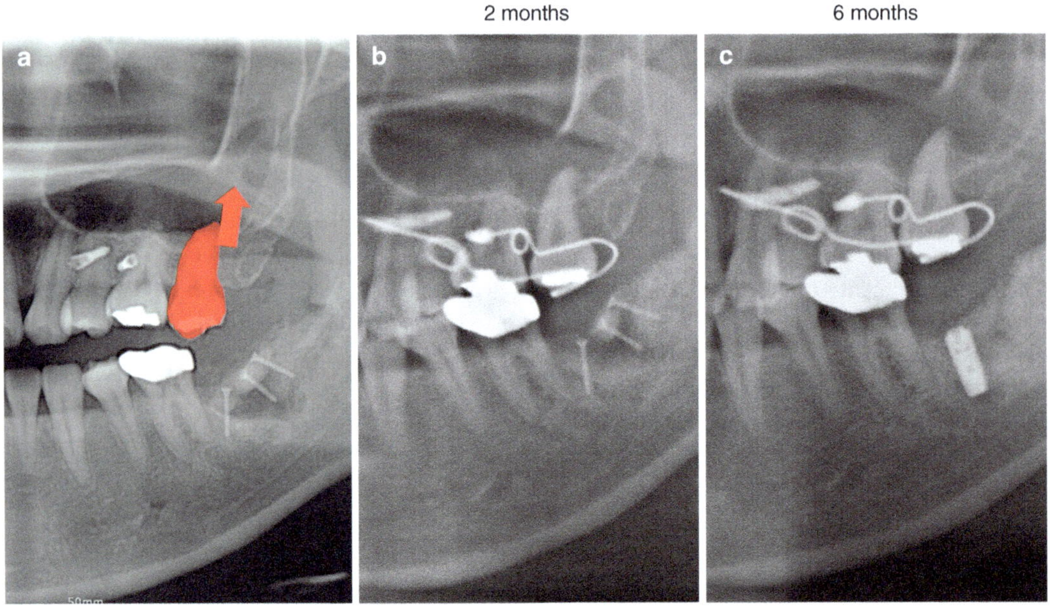

Fig. 2.8 (**a**) Illustrating the expected result of the mousetrap appliance. (**b**) Two months of application shows intruded second maxillary molar. (**c**) After 6 months of the mousetrap appliance, maxillary second molar intrusion is completed without any complication and the space for the opposing implant site is prepared

used for provisional implant system (Figs. 2.10 and 2.11). The head part can be replaced with implant custom-made abutment and tapped into the endosseous screw part. The provisional crown can be fabricated to evaluate the function and esthetic of the final implant crown. It is useful in growing child to maintain space, to function as a provisional crown, and to enhance esthetics until the termination of growth for the future recipient of endosseous implant. If in case of the limited edentulous space for the endosseous implant, the C-implant can act as replacement of choice.

Here are case presentations of the C-implants applied in orthodontic treatment.

Case 1 (Figs. 2.12, 2.13, 2.14, 2.15, 2.16, 2.17, 2.18, and 2.19)

A 12-year-old male presented at the orthodontic department of Kyung Hee University with the chief complaint of protrusive lips.

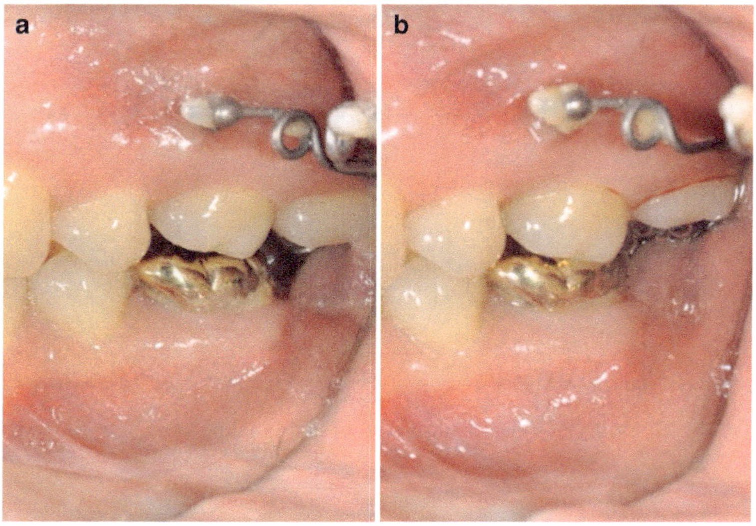

Fig. 2.9 Clinical pictures showing the initial (**a**) and final (**b**)

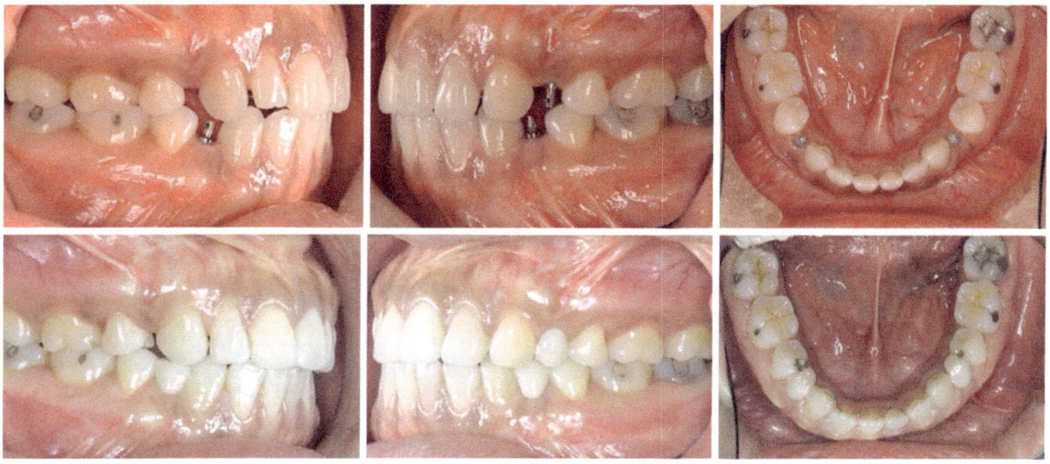

Fig. 2.10 C-implants working as a provisional implant fixture and custom-made abutment illustrated on the *upper row*. The finished provisional implant crown in place shows esthetic result in the *bottom row*

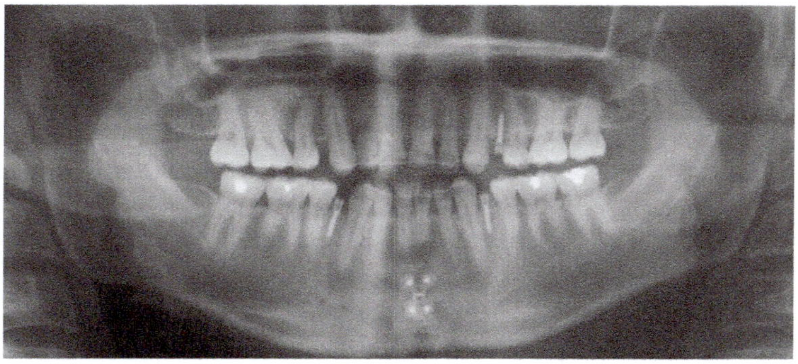

Fig. 2.11 The panoramic radiograph with three C-implants placement without custom abutment and crown portion

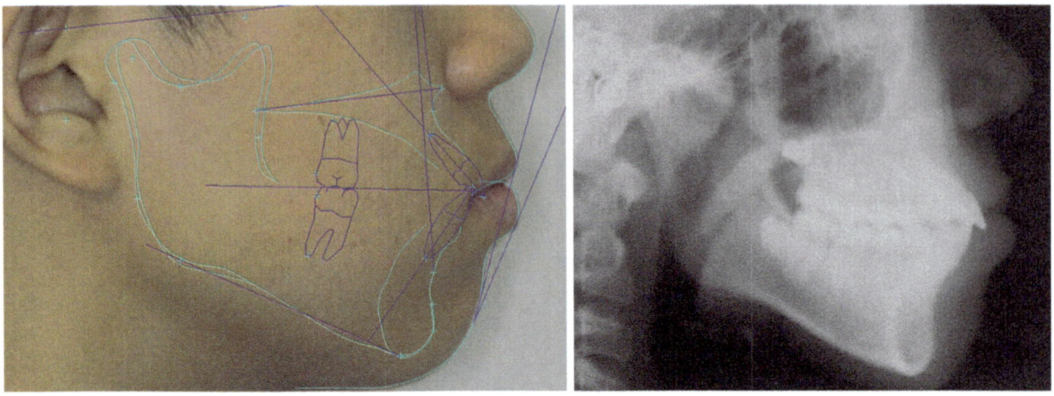

Fig. 2.12 Case 1 of Biocreative treatment. Lateral facial photograph with lateral cephalometric tracing and lateral cephalogram

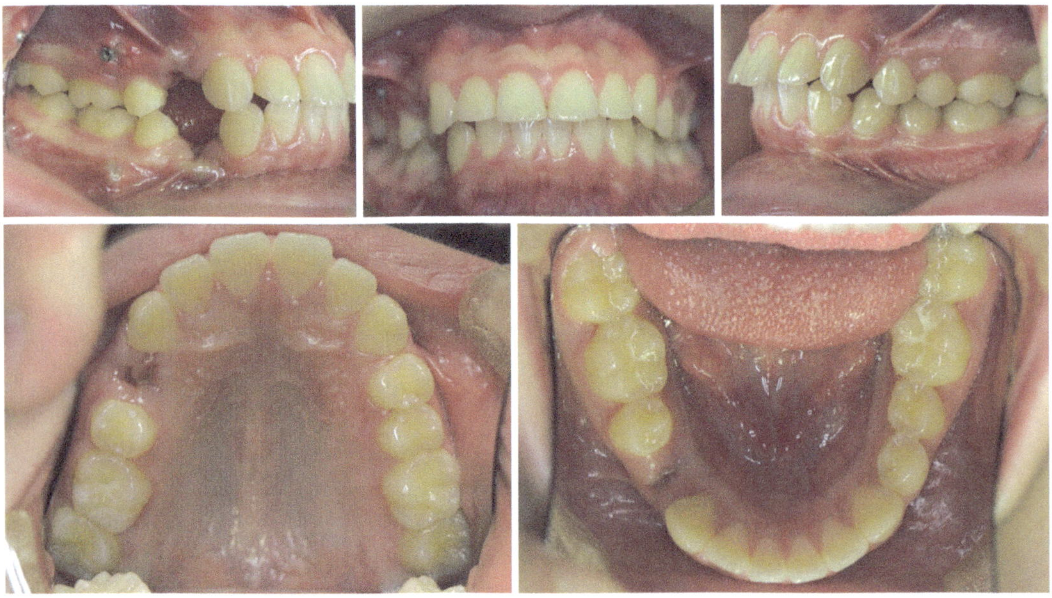

Fig. 2.13 Right maxillary C-implant placement between the second premolar and first molar with upper and lower right first premolar extraction. Notice Class I molar relationship in both right and left sides

Clinical examination showed a convex profile, incompetent lips with incisal exposure of 5 mm at rest, decreased nasolabial angle, deep labiomental sulcus, and normal lower facial height. Intraoral examination revealed Class I molar and Class II canine relationship, with an overjet of 6 mm and an overbite of 2 mm (Fig. 2.12). All third molars were not erupted. The patient had proclined upper and lower incisors. There were no signs of TMJ problems. Cephalometric analysis indicated dentoalveolar bimaxillary protrusion. The treatment objectives were to reduce the lip protrusion and improve the soft tissue esthetics and correct the axial inclinations of the anterior teeth. These objectives could be achieved by retracting the upper and lower anterior teeth with maximum anchorage after extraction of the four first premolars. Extracting the four first premolars was expected to offer the greatest potential for retraction of the anteriors. Other extraction combinations would not provide as much improvement on the soft tissue profile [9].

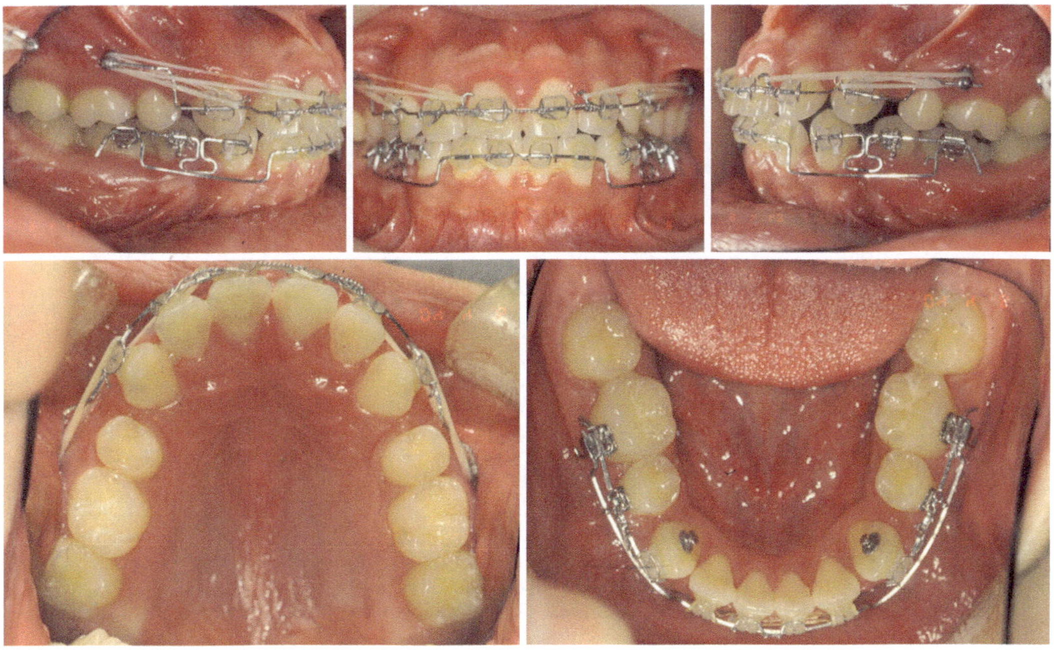

Fig. 2.14 Intraoral photographs of the progression in en masse maxillary retraction demonstrate progression of extraction space closure. Conventional treatment is progressing in the lower arch

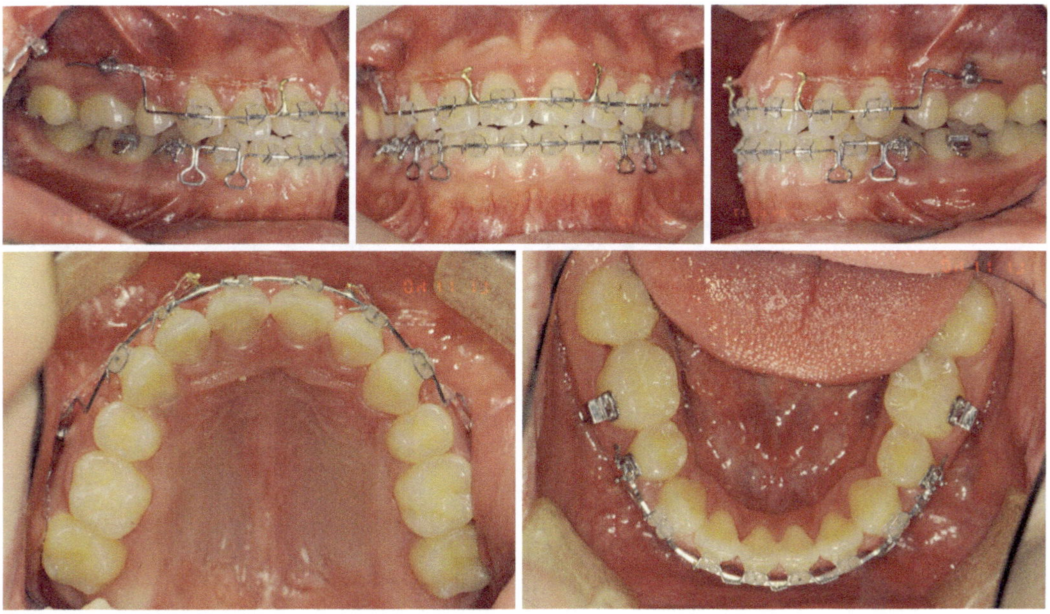

Fig. 2.15 Completed space closure of the extraction space on upper and lower dentition in 9 months

Three treatment options were explained. (1) Use headgear as an extraoral anchorage, (2) use miniscrews as anchorage to reinforce the bonded or banded posterior anchorage teeth during anterior retraction, or (3) use miniscrews as an independent appliance for anterior retraction without placing posterior fixed appliances in the maxilla. The patient and his parents opted

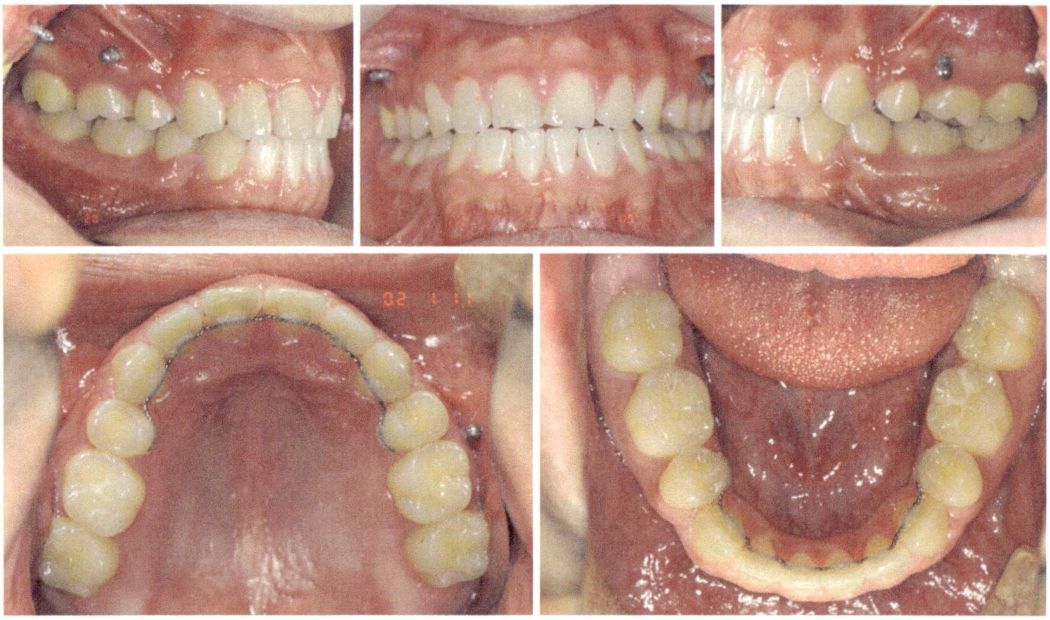

Fig. 2.16 Complete debonding of upper and lower arches and bonding of the fixed lingual retainer in upper and lower arches

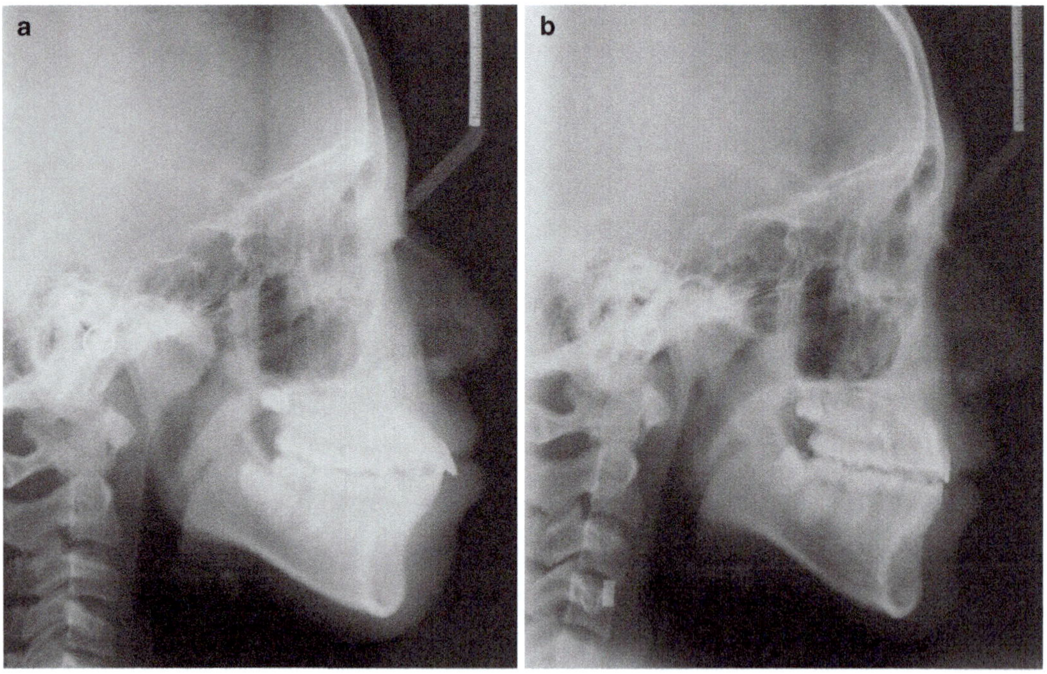

Fig. 2.17 The initial lateral cephalogram (**a**) and the final lateral cephalogram (**b**). Notice the improved facial profile with retruded upper and lower lips

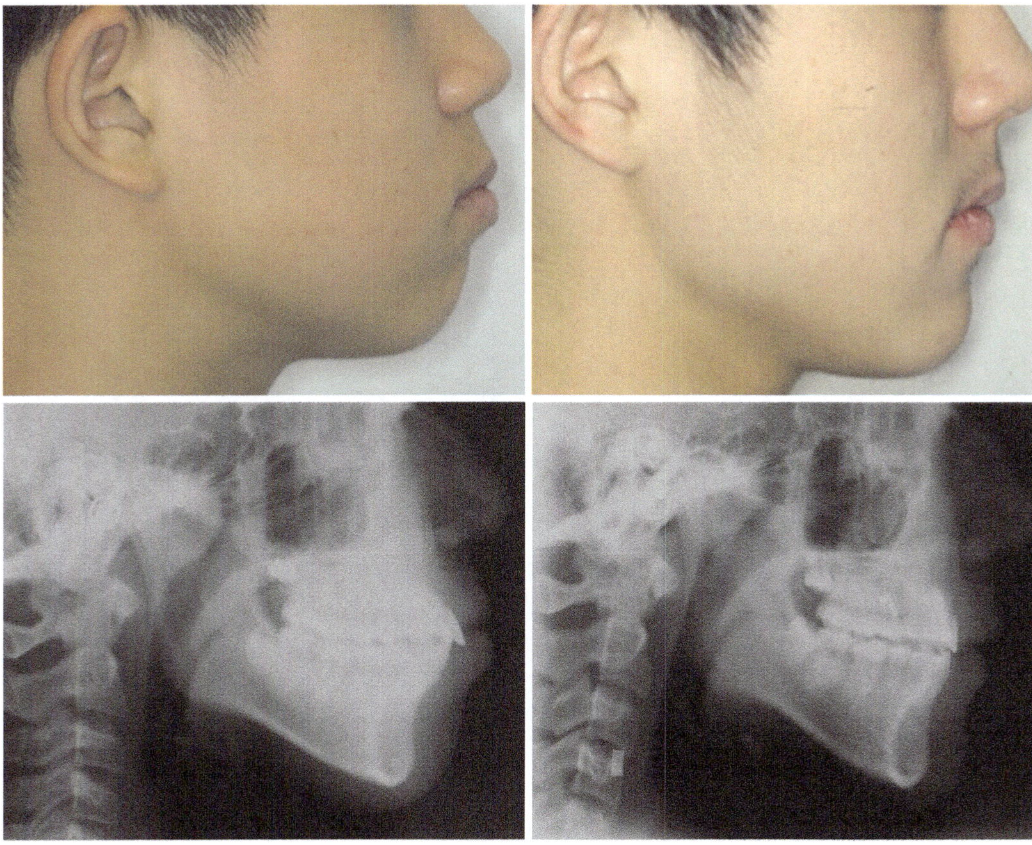

Fig. 2.18 The lateral facial photographs showing the initial (**a**) and final (**b**) profile improvement in lip protrusion, nasolabial angle, and submental sulcus

for the third treatment option. This plan allowed maximum retraction of the upper anterior teeth without disturbing molar occlusal relationships and minimizing stress on the periodontium. This treatment protocol is called "Biocreative Orthodontics," defined as independent en masse retraction of the anterior teeth while avoiding orthodontic appliances on the posterior segments during the retraction period [10, 11]. This alternative approach, which uses partially osseointegrated mini-implants or miniplates to resist multidirectional heavy orthodontic forces, can be beneficial in maximum anchorage cases that present with a poor dental health status such as severe dental caries, advanced periodontal disease, or missing posterior teeth. The aim of Biocreative Orthodontics is to consider this segment as a whole and apply careful torque control during retraction.

Two C-implants were placed in the interradicular space between the upper second premolars and first molars on each side and it was started on the right side first (Fig. 2.13). Four first premolars were extracted. Brackets were bonded on six anterior teeth in the maxilla and from the central incisor to the first molar in the mandible. Upper archwire was bent from distal of canines to pass through the head portion of the C-implant. After preliminary alignment was obtained, 0.018″ stainless steel archwires were placed. Elastics were placed from C-implant to extension hooks of canines and lateral incisors to retract six anterior teeth (Fig. 2.14).

Space closure was completed in 9 months (Fig. 2.15) and brackets were debonded (Fig. 2.16). Posttreatment cephalometric analysis revealed significant amount of incisor retraction by controlled tipping and excellent maintenance of

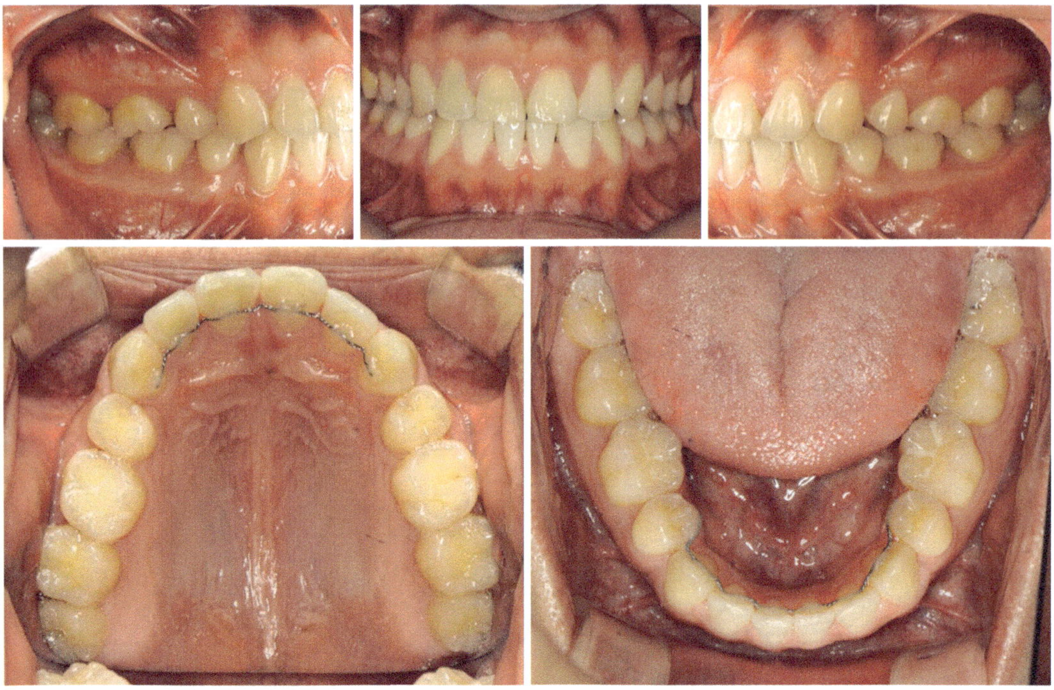

Fig. 2.19 Five-year retention of the same patient shows stable occlusion and ideal overbite and overjet in Class I relationship

molar occlusal relationship (Fig. 2.17). Patient's profile was considerably improved. Soft tissue objectives were met by achieving a significant reduction in the lip protrusion (Fig. 2.18). Treatment result remained stable 5 years after debonding (Fig. 2.19).

Case 2 (Figs. 2.20, 2.21, 2.22, 2.23, 2.24, 2.25, 2.26, and 2.27)

A 30-year-old female visited our department with chief complaint of "crooked front teeth" (Fig. 2.20). Her prior medical and dental history revealed no significant systemic problems and no significant temporomandibular joint disorders. The patient had straight facial profile with long lower facial height and acute nasolabial angle. Intraoral examination showed Class I molar and canine relationship with moderate crowding on both arches. All four wisdom teeth were absent. Cephalometric analysis revealed skeletal Class II with steep mandibular plane (Fig. 2.21). The treatment objectives were to resolve crowding without influencing soft tissue profile. Considering patient's straight facial profile, extraction was excluded. Molar distalization was planned to resolve crowding.

In the maxilla, retraction force was applied by C-palatal plate[1] (temporary skeletal anchorage

[1] <Footnote ID="Fn1"><Para>C-palatal plate: Alternative treatment of choice instead of miniscrews for guarded periodontal health patients. Push and pull mechanics are possible.</Para></Footnote>

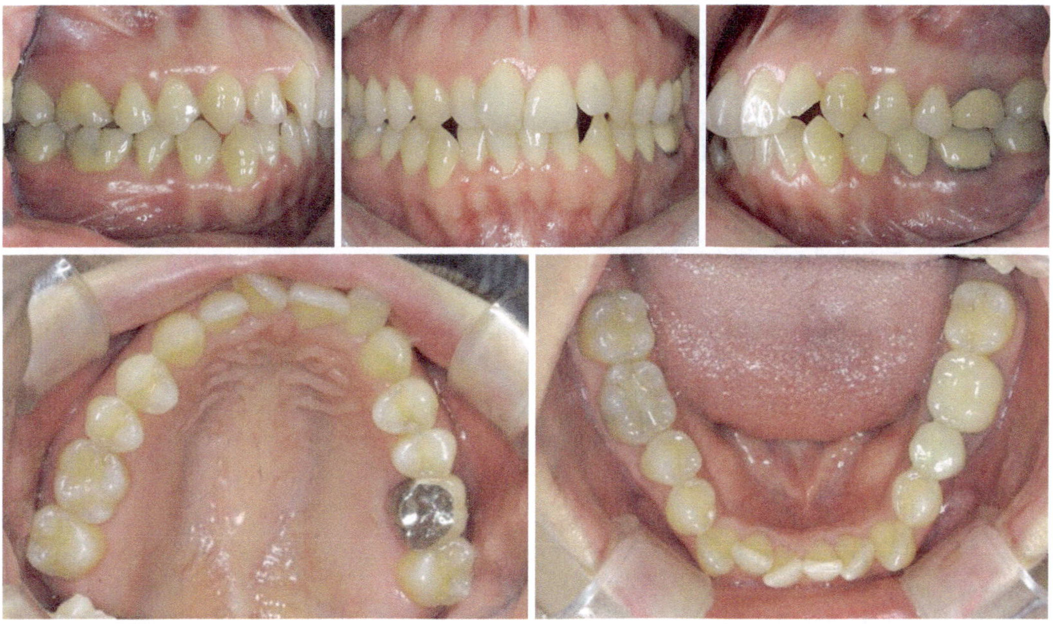

Fig. 2.20 Initial photographs of Case 2 patient showing the anterior crowding and arch length discrepancy but stable posterior occlusion

devices) in the palatal side and open coil spring on the buccal side. In the mandible, distalizing force was applied by open coil spring connected between C-implants and extension hook of the first molar. Two C-implants were placed between the first and second premolars on each side of the mandible (Figs. 2.22 and 2.23). With palatal C-plate and two C-implants, distalization of posterior segments was achieved first, and with gained space, anterior crowding was resolved (Figs. 2.24 and 2.25). After leveling and aligning with conventional brackets on the upper and lower arches, brackets were debonded (Fig. 2.26). Final lateral cephalogram shows no change in soft tissue profile with achievement of the treatment plan, and panoramic radiograph shows satisfying root parallelism (Fig. 2.27).

The C-implants can be further studied in studying the nanoscale examination of bone to implant osseointegrated interface. In the recent study of Kang [8], the implant interface under SEM and TEM analysis, there was intimate surface contact between the bone and implant interface surfaces. Further detailed investigation to find the chemical composition and histotopography of the interface is expected. Also, using the clinical data of C-implants, the failure of dental prosthetic implant can be referred.

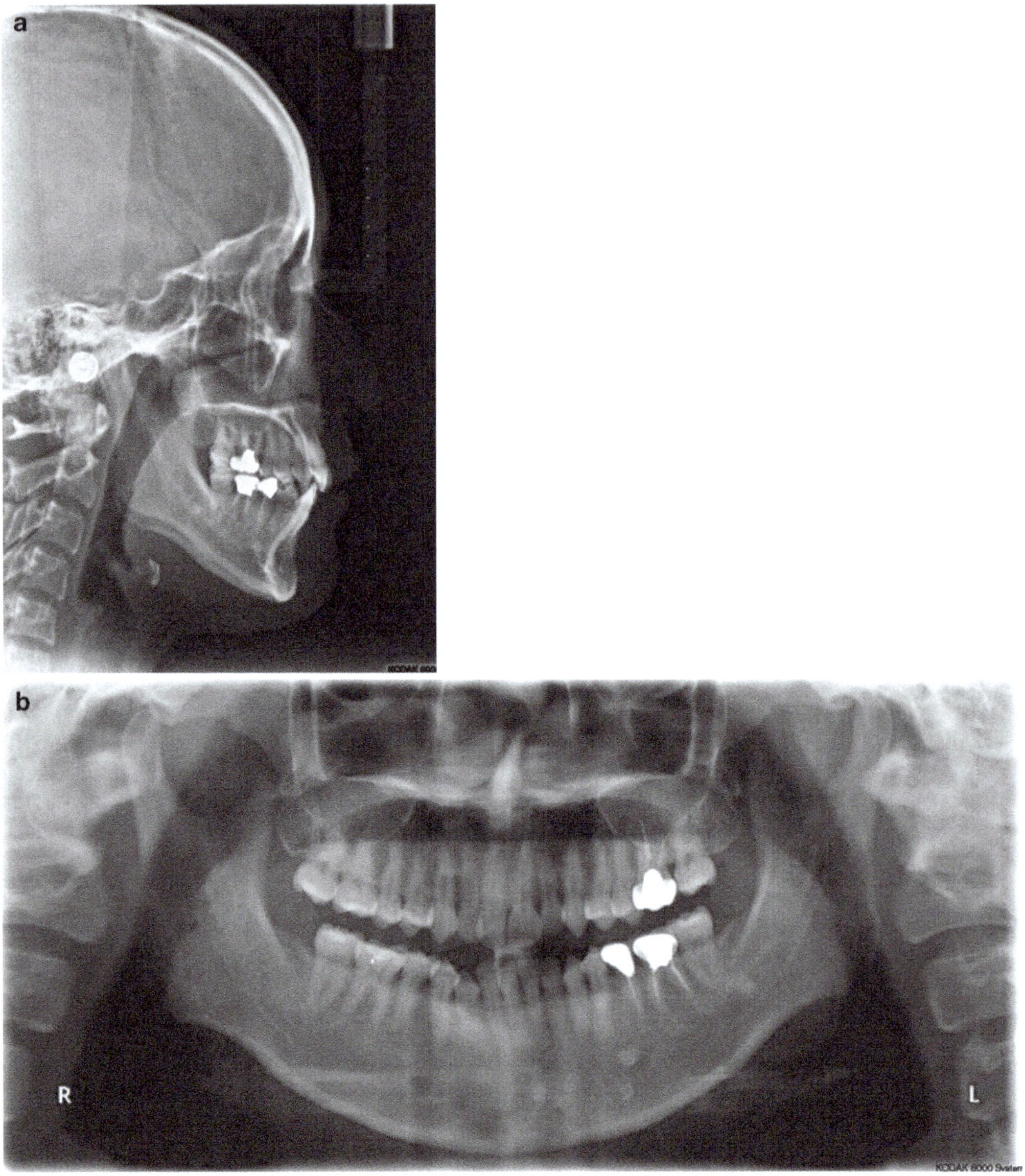

Fig. 2.21 Initial lateral cephalogram (**a**) and panoramic radiograph (**b**)

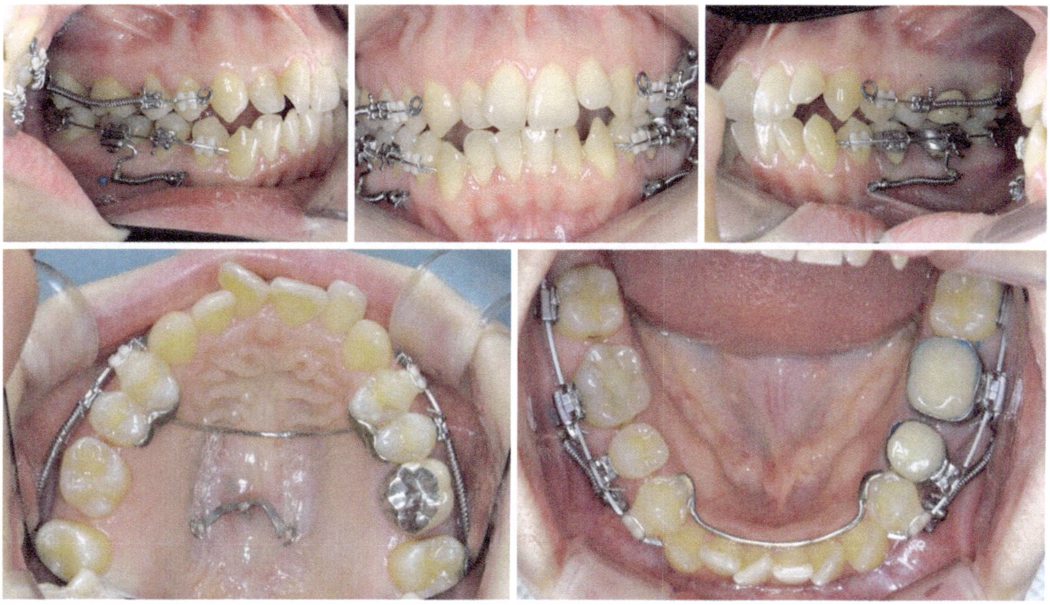

Fig. 2.22 On maxillary arch, palatal C-plate is retracting the transpalatal arch connecting premolars on the palatal side and the open coil springs are pushing the second molars. In the mandible, the C-implants are placed between the first and second premolars and are connected to the posterior segments with extended hook. Open coil springs are pushing the posterior segments with open coil springs from C-implants

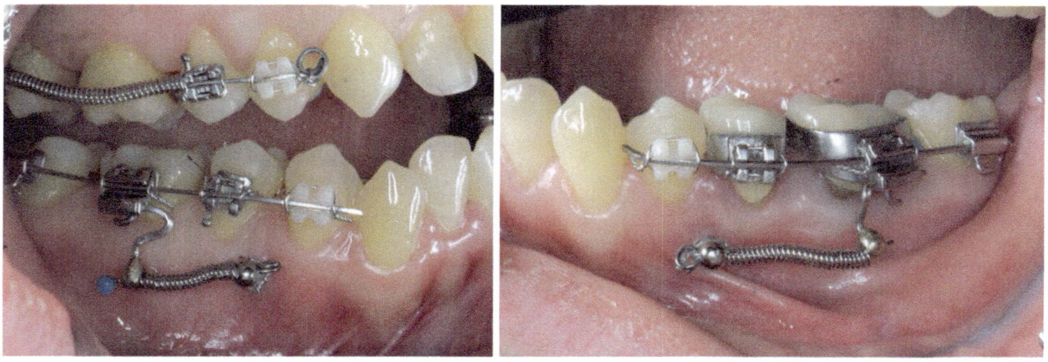

Fig. 2.23 The magnified views of the C-implants demonstrating the pushing mechanics

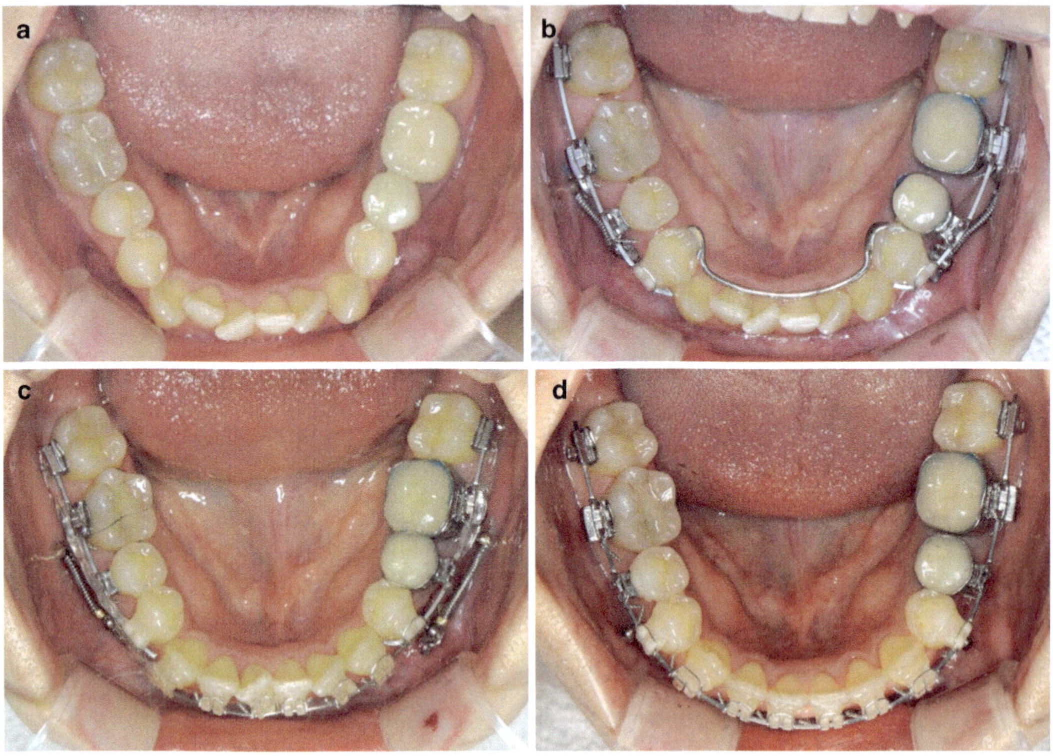

Fig. 2.24 Sequential (**a**–**d**) mandibular intraoral photographs showing the distalization of posterior segments and decrowding of the anterior dentition

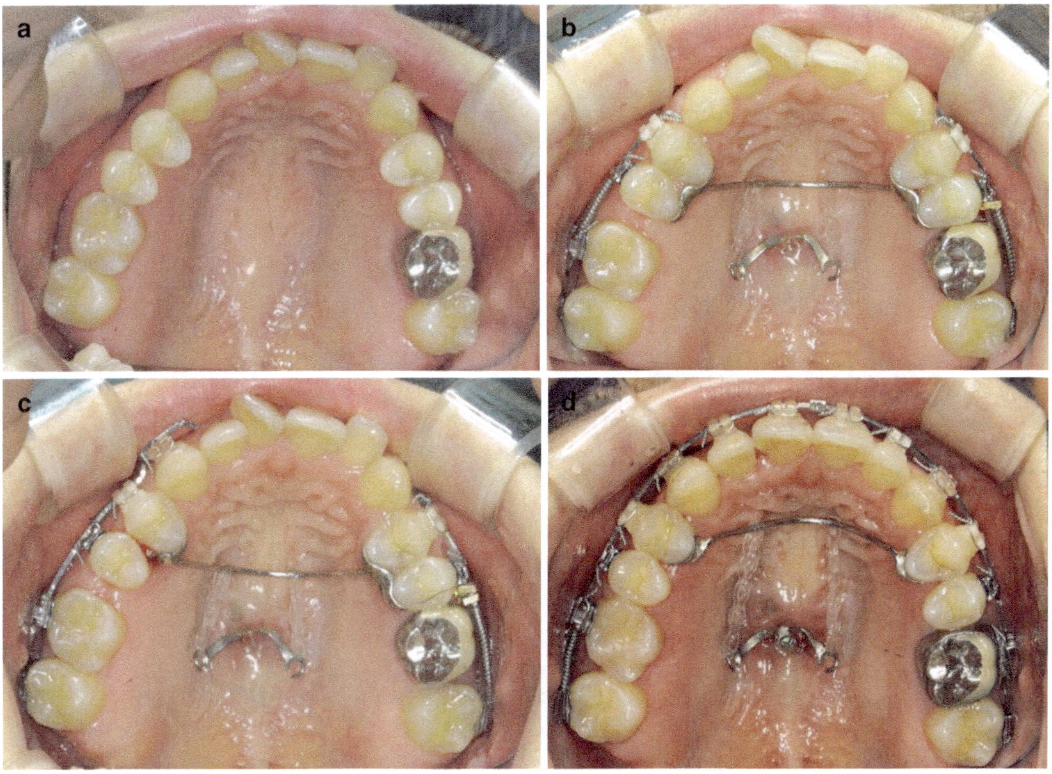

Fig. 2.25 Sequential (**a–d**) maxillary intraoral photographs showing the distalization of posterior segments and decrowding of the anterior dentition

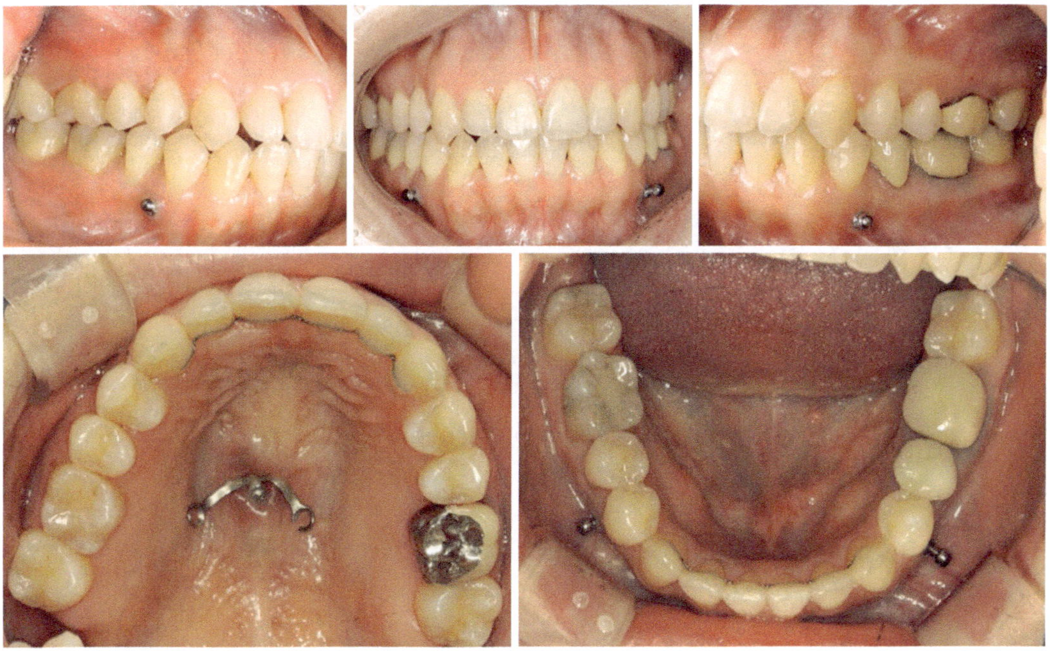

Fig. 2.26 Final intraoral photographs after debonding

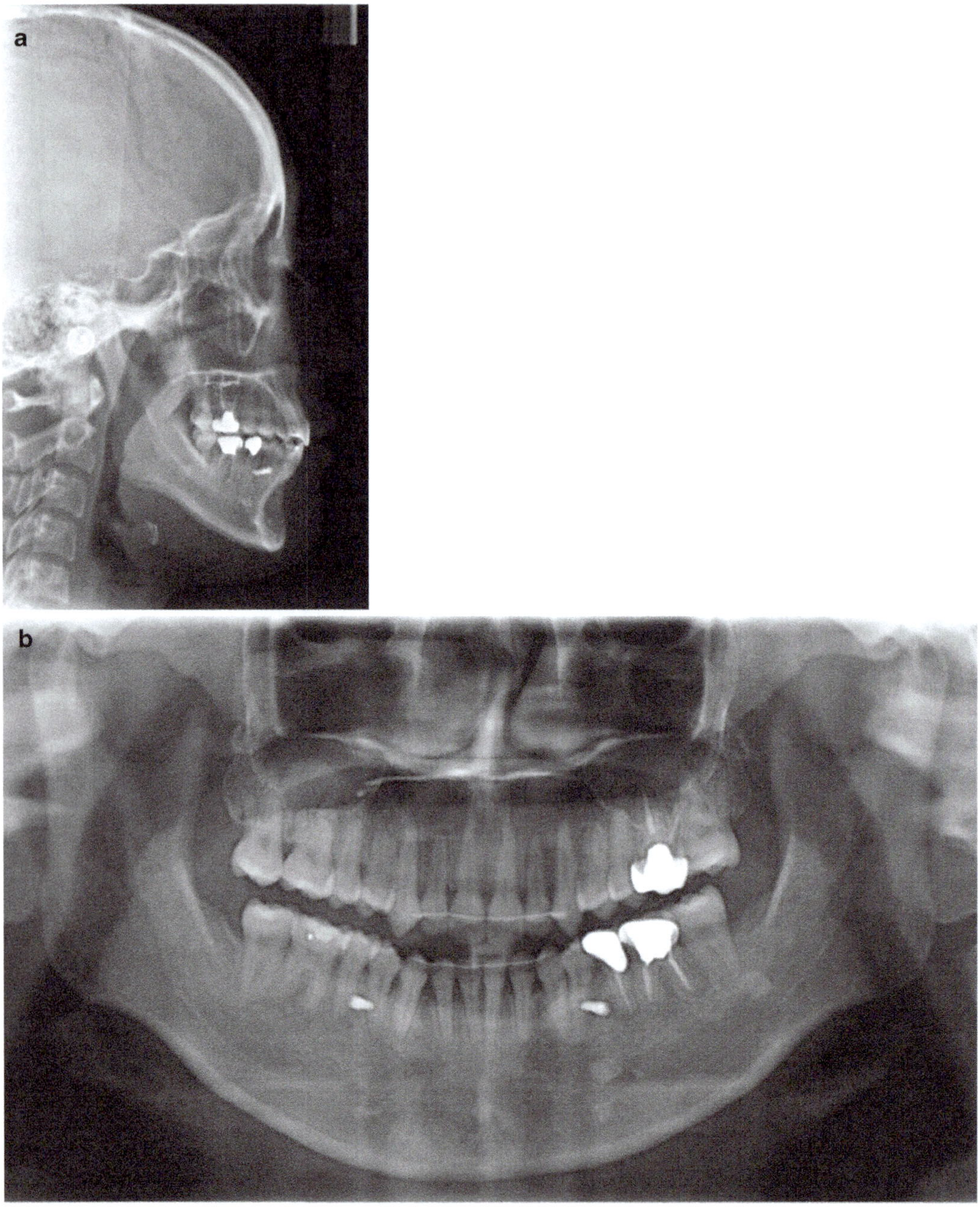

Fig. 2.27 Final lateral cephalogram (**a**) and panoramic radiograph (**b**)

Acknowledgment The authors thank Dr. Kyung Won Seo, postgraduate student of Kyung Hee University School of Dentistry, for manuscript editing.

References

1. Lee S, Chung K. The effect of early loading on the direct bone-to-implant surface contact of the orthodontic osseointegrated titanium implant. Korean J Orthod. 2001;31:173–85.
2. Chung K-R, Kim S-H, Kook Y-A. The C-orthodontic micro-implant. J Clin Orthod. 2004;38(9):478–86, quiz 487–8.
3. Chung K-R, Nelson G, Kim S-H, Kook Y-A. Severe bidentoalveolar protrusion treated with orthodontic microimplant-dependent en-masse retraction. Am J Orthod Dentofacial Orthop. 2007;132(1):105–15.
4. Kim S-H, Lee S-J, Cho I-S, Kim S-K, Kim T-W. Rotational resistance of surface-treated mini-implants. Angle Orthod. 2009;79(5):899–907.
5. Kim S-H, Cho J-H, Chung K-R, Kook Y-A, Nelson G. Removal torque values of surface-treated mini-implants after loading. Am J Orthod Dentofacial Orthop. 2008;134(1):36–43.
6. Kim S-H, Choi J-H, Chung K-R, Nelson G. Do sand blasted with large grit and acid etched surface treated mini-implants remain stationary under orthodontic forces? Angle Orthod. 2012;82(2):304–12.
7. Lee S-J, Lin L, Kim S-H, Chung K-R, Donatelli RE. Survival analysis of a miniplate and tube device designed to provide skeletal anchorage. Am J Orthod Dentofacial Orthop. 2013;144(3):349–56.
8. Kang S-M. Cryo-Transmission electron microscopy evaluation of interface of orthodontic implant surface and cortical bone in human patients [PhD thesis]. Seoul: Kyung Hee University; 2013.
9. Bills DA, Handelman CS, BeGole EA. Bimaxillary dentoalveolar protrusion: traits and orthodontic correction. Angle Orthod. 2005;75(3):333–9.
10. Chung K-R, Kook Y-A, Kim S-H, Mo S-S, Jung J-A. Class II malocclusion treated by combining a lingual retractor and a palatal plate. Am J Orthod Dentofacial Orthop. 2008;133(1):112–23.
11. Kim S-H, Hwang Y-S, Ferreira A, Chung K-R. Analysis of temporary skeletal anchorage devices used for en-masse retraction: a preliminary study. Am J Orthod Dentofacial Orthop. 2009;136(2):268–76.

Contributing Factors to Success Rate of Orthodontic Mini-implants: Important but Ignored Results from Basic Researches

3

Il-Sik Cho and Seung-Hak Baek

Abstract

Among the numerous factors that can affect success or failure rates of orthodontic mini-implants (OMIs), some factors are well studied but others are neglected or ignored in spite of basic and clinical importance. The purpose of this chapter was to describe important but ignored results from basic researches such as shape and microstructure of OMIs, surface treatment of OMIs, predrilling before OMI installation, microdamage in the cortical bone, wobbling of OMIs during manual installation, root contact with OMIs, and fracture properties of OMIs. If more concern about these issues would be given, better clinical results might be obtained.

3.1 Introduction

Orthodontists and other dentists have paid a lot of attention to installation and usage of orthodontic mini-implants (OMIs) in diverse clinical situations. The success rates of OMIs are known as 84–92 % [1–8].

There have been numerous studies about success or failure rates of OMIs including host factors (age, gender, skeletal pattern, oral hygiene, and inflammation), bone quality (thickness and stiffness), design of OMI (shape and diameter), and insertion and loading modality of OMI (implantation location, type of placement surgery, and immediate loading) [5, 6, 9–16]. Among these factors, some factors are well known but others are neglected or ignored despite of basic and clinical importance.

Therefore, the authors would like to describe important but ignored results from basic researches such as shape and microstructure of OMIs, surface treatment of OMIs, predrilling before installation of OMIs, microdamage in the cortical bone during installation of OMIs, wobbling of OMIs during manual installation, root contact with OMIs, and fracture properties of OMIs.

I.-S. Cho, DDS, MSD, PhD (✉)
Department of Dentistry, Korea University Guro Hospital, Gurodong-Ro #148, Guro-Gu, Seoul 152-703, South Korea
e-mail: microphage@naver.com

S.-H. Baek, DDS, MSD, PhD
Department of Orthodontics, School of Dentistry, Seoul National University Dental Hospital, Seoul National University, Daehak-Ro #101, Chongno-Gu, Seoul 110-768, South Korea
e-mail: drwhite@snu.ac.kr

K.B. Kim (ed.), *Temporary Skeletal Anchorage Devices*,
DOI 10.1007/978-3-642-55052-2_3, © Springer-Verlag Berlin Heidelberg 2014

3.2 Shape and Microstructure of OMIs

The conical or tapered OMIs are known to provide tighter contact between the OMI and bone and better initial stability than the cylindrical ones [13, 17, 18]. However, the conical or tapered OMIs are reported to produce higher stress in the cortical bone compared to the cylindrical ones with the same diameters [13, 19].

In the mechanical and histomorphometric analysis of beagle dog, Kim et al. [13] reported that the conical OMIs exhibited significantly higher maximum insertion and removal torque values than the cylindrical ones. However, there was no significant difference in success rate, resonance frequency analysis, and bone-to-implant contact (BIC) ratio between conical and cylindrical OMIs [13]. Therefore, Kim et al. [13] suggested that the conical OMIs might need modification of the thread structure and insertion technique to reduce the excessive insertion torque while maintaining the amounts of removal torque.

The results from several studies about the dental prosthetic implants suggested that the microgroove on the implant surface could play an important role in the proliferation and migration of fibroblasts, formation and adaptation of the connective tissue, and maintenance of the soft tissue around the implant [20–22].

According to the results of histomorphometric analysis of beagle dog by Kim et al. [22], the microgroove OMI exhibited higher success rate and BIC ratio on the pressure side compared to the non-microgroove OMI. In addition, the microgroove OMI revealed no significant differences in BIC between pressure and tension sides [22]. Since the microgroove and non-microgroove OMIs exhibited different alignment of the gingival connective tissue fiber to OMIs (perpendicular or circular in microgroove OMI vs. parallel in non-microgroove OMI), they concluded that the microstructure such as microgrooves might have positive effects on the arrangement of gingival connective tissue fibers and the adaptation of the soft tissue and bony tissue around the OMI [22].

3.3 Surface Treatment of OMIs

The purposes of surface treatment for the dental prosthetic titanium implants are to increase the surface area, to provide a better BIC environment, and to increase the degree of osseointegration between the TiO_2 layer of the implant and the surrounding bony tissue [16, 23–28].

As one of the typical surface treatment methods, sandblasted, large-grit, and acid etching (SLA) method has been commonly used. It involves sandblasting of the implant with 0.25–0.50 μm aluminum particles and acid treatment with HCl and H_2SO_4 [29]. Buser et al. [29] reported that titanium alloy material treated with the SLA method had enhanced BIC ratio and exhibited a higher removal torque than the non-treated material.

Anodic oxidation method is another method that involves the use of 0.1 % phosphoric acid solution at 150–200 V for several minutes [30, 31]. Yamagami et al. [30] reported that titanium alloy treated with a combination of sandblasting and anodic oxidation (SLAO) enhanced active bone formation, resulting in stable fixation in the diaphysis of New Zealand white rabbit femurs.

Similar studies were carried out in the OMIs [16, 32, 33]. Kim et al. [32] reported that the SLA-treated OMIs provided lower maximum insertion torque and higher total removal energy than the machined-surface OMIs. However, the OMIs used in their study were not self-drilling type, and they needed a predrilling procedure for installation. In addition, Karmarker et al. [33] reported that the OMIs with anodic oxidation treatment only (without sandblasting) exhibited the same insertion torque value with the machined-surface OMIs and a higher removal torque value than the machined-surface OMIs.

Comparison of the mechanical properties of SLA- and SLAO-treated OMIs in the tibias of Beagles, Cho et al. [16] reported that both SLA- and SLAO-treated OMIs showed lower maximum insertion torque and total insertion energy than the machined-surface OMIs. They also showed that SLAO-treated OMIs exhibited a higher maximum removal torque than the machined-surface OMIs and SLA-treated OMIs [16]. These results suggested that SLAO treatment might be an effective tool in reducing insertion damage to surrounding tissue and improving the mechanical stability of OMIs [16].

In summary, these studies showed a possibility that the surface treatment of OMI could provide less bone damage and higher mechanical stability.

3.4 Predrilling Before Installation of OMIs

In the area where the cortical bone thickness is thick such as the mandibular posterior area, direct installation using a self-drilling OMI can produce excessive insertion torque, resulting in failure of the OMI [6]. Therefore, it is necessary to predrill the cortical bone and then to install the self-drilling or self-tapping OMI at the mandibular posterior area.

If the entire thickness of the cortical bone is predrilled in the mandibular posterior area, root damage of the posterior teeth and resultant failure of the OMIs can occasionally occur by the predetermined direction of OMI installation [34]. In order to weaken the cortical bone without predetermining the direction of OMI installation, a partial predrilling technique can be used [34].

Cho and Baek [34] performed an in vitro study to investigate the effects of OMI shape (cylindrical and tapered type) and predrilling depth (non-predrilling [control], 1.5 mm predrilling, and 3.0 mm predrilling; predrilled with a drill bit [1 mm in diameter]) on the mechanical properties of OMIs during the insertion procedure. The results were as follows [34]: Within the same shape group, although predrilling groups exhibited shorter total insertion time than control groups, there was no difference in total insertion time between 1.5 and 3.0 mm predrilling groups. Maximum insertion torque and total insertion energy decreased in the order of control, 1.5 mm predrilling, and 3.0 mm predrilling. The maximum insertion torque of the cylindrical shape/non-predrilling group was smaller than the tapered shape/non-predrilling group. In the same predrilling depth, no differences were observed in maximum insertion torque and total insertion energy between cylindrical and tapered groups. Therefore, they concluded that predrilling might be an effective tool for reducing maximum insertion torque, total insertion energy, and microdamage without compromising OMI stability in cases of thick cortical bone [34].

3.5 Microdamage in the Cortical Bone During Installation of OMIs

The self-drilling OMIs with a large diameter and a tapered or conical shape might cause overcompression of the cortical bone by excessive placement torque [13, 35]. This can lead to microdamage, a permanent deformation of the microstructure in loaded cortical bone in the form of fatigue, creep, and eventual cracking [35–37]. Therefore, the accumulation of microdamage can produce local ischemia, bone necrosis, bone remodeling, and premature loss of the OMI [35–38].

Lee and Baek [35] performed the animal study (New Zealand white rabbits) to investigate the effects of the diameter (1.5 and 2.0 mm) and shape of OMIs (cylindrical and tapered) on microdamage to the cortical bone during OMI placement. Experiment methods are as follows [35]: Maximum insertion torque was measured during OMI installation. Immediately after placement of the OMIs, the block of bone with the OMI was harvested. Cortical bone thickness was measured by using microcomputed tomography, and histomorphometric analyses of the number of cracks, accumulated crack length, maximum radius of the crack, and longest crack were performed. Large diameter and tapered shape resulted in increased values of maximum insertion torque, number of cracks, and longest crack [35]. Therefore, they concluded that OMIs with larger diameter and tapered shape might cause greater microdamage to the cortical bone than OMIs with smaller diameter and cylindrical shape [35]. Further studies are needed to investigate how excessive insertion torque and microdamage can affect bone remodeling and the stability of the OMIs.

3.6 Wobbling of OMIs During Manual Installation

There are two methods for OMI installation: the manual insertion method using a hand driver and the motor insertion method using a handpiece.

The motor insertion method can maintain a constant drilling speed and force, prevent excessive insertion torque by the auto-stop or over-limit mechanism during drilling procedure, and approach easily to the palate or the most posterior area of the buccal-attached gingiva in the mouth [39–42]. However, this method requires space for equipment and expensive instruments and is difficult to obtain the proper tactile sensation and to monitor the insertion angle during the insertion procedure [41, 42].

The manual insertion method can provide better tactile sensation when the OMI tip contacts the alveolar bone and allow for confirmation of the insertion orientation [41, 42]. However, it is difficult to obtain the appropriate insertion torque, maintain the proper rotational speed, or access the palate or the most posterior area of the buccal-attached gingiva in the mouth with a hand driver [41, 42].

Lack of experience and improper technique in the manual insertion method may cause the OMI to wobble at the insertion site during the insertion procedure [42]. Wobbling can increase the amount of reduction of the cortical bone, cause microcrack or damage of the cortical bone, and decrease the mechanical retention between the OMI and bone, which might compromise the primary stability of the OMIs [42].

Cho et al. [42] performed an in vitro experiment to investigate the effects of wobbling angle on the stability measures of OMIs during insertion and removal procedures in artificial bone blocks using a driving torque tester with a uniform speed of 28 rpm and wobbling analogs of 2° and 4°. Although the 4° wobbling group showed a 14.5 % (2.9 Ncm) increase in maximum insertion torque compared with the control (0° wobbling) group, there was only a 6 % (1.3 Ncm) decrease in maximum removal torque from the control group to the 4° wobbling group [42]. They suggested that slight wobbling during the OMI insertion procedure might be acceptable in terms of the stability measures of OMIs during insertion and removal procedures [42]. However, it will be necessary to perform an in vivo study to confirm that the same findings will occur in the real bone [42].

3.7 Root Contact with OMIs

Root contact with OMIs is one of the reasons that clinicians hesitate to use this device [43, 44]. The OMI is usually inserted at the buccal-attached gingiva area between the second premolar and first molar for maximum or absolute anchorage [44]. The interdental space between these teeth at 5 mm level below from the alveolar crest is usually about 3.0 mm [44]. Although root contact with OMI can be prevented using a radiograph, computed tomography, or surgical stent, the OMI can be placed close to the periodontal ligament (PDL) or root enough to histologically affect the root and surrounding tissue [44].

There have been numerous opinions about the relationship between root contact or proximity of OMIs to the root and success rate of OMIs [44–47]. Kuroda et al. [46] and Asscherickx et al. [47] suggested that the proximity of OMIs to the root is one of the major risk factors for the failure of screw anchorage. Liou et al. [45] advocated 2 mm of safety clearance between the OMI and dental root. However, Kim et al. [48] proclaimed that root proximity alone is not a major risk factor for OMIs failure.

Lee et al. [44] performed the animal (beagle dog) study to determine the histological reaction of the root and bone as an OMI approaches the root. After the specimens were classified as the near-root group, the PDL-contact group, the root-contact group, and the root-perforation group, resorption of the root (cementum and dentin), repair/growth of the cementum, ankylosis, and cracking/fracture of the root were assessed [44]. They reported that when the distance between the OMI and the root was less than 0.6 mm, the incidence of root resorption increased and that when OMIs came close to root surfaces even without root contact, the incidence of ankylosis was also increased [44]. When an OMI contacts or penetrates the PDL and/or root during installation procedure, tissue damage can induce root resorption or ankylosis [44]. Therefore, it is recommended to use smaller OMI and to check the distance between the OMI and root to reduce the risk of root contact and tissue damage.

3.8 Fracture Properties of OMIs

OMI fracture during installation procedure, which has an incidence of around 4 %, occurs due to the inability of OMIs to resist excessive rotational force [15, 49–51]. In order to reduce the fracture risk of OMIs, their diameter can be increased [51–53]. However, the OMI diameter cannot be increased more than interradicular distance.

Brisceno et al. [54] reported that the insertion torque increased two times in cases of root contact than those without root contact. According to Cho et al. [51], the insertion torque exhibited higher values at the beginning of root contact with OMI. Therefore, abrupt increase in resistance or insertion torque value during the OMI installation can be used as an indicator of possible root contact with the OMI [51].

Cho et al. [51] performed an in vitro study to determine the effects of insertion angle (0°, 8°, 13°, 18°, and 23°) and thread type (dual or single) on the fracture properties of OMIs during insertion. The OMIs were placed into artificial materials simulating human tissues: two-layer bone blocks (Sawbones), root (polymethyl methacrylate stick), and periodontal ligament (Imprint II Garant light body) [51].

According to their results, in the 0°, 8°, and 13° insertion angle groups, none of the OMIs fractured or became deformed. However, dual-thread OMIs exhibited more fracture than deformation compared to single-thread OMIs on the critical insertion angle (18°). In the 23° insertion angle group, all OMIs penetrated the artificial root without fracturing and deformation. Therefore, Cho et al. [51] suggested that the thread type can influence the fracture ratio in the critical insertion angle.

In addition, Cho et al. [51] reported that when the OMI contacts with the artificial root at the critical contact angle, the deformation or fracture of OMIs can occur at lower insertion torque values than those of penetration. Therefore, clinicians should be careful about abrupt increase in the insertion torque value during OMI installation procedure.

Conclusion

If more concern about the issues including shape and microstructure of OMIs, surface treatment of OMIs, predrilling before installation of OMIs, microdamage in the cortical bone during installation of OMIs, wobbling of OMIs during manual installation, root contact with OMIs, and fracture properties of OMIs is given, better clinical results will be obtained.

References

1. Miyawaki S, Koyama I, Inoue M, Mishima K, Sugahara T, Takano-Yamamoto T. Factors associated with the stability of titanium screws placed in the posterior region for orthodontic anchorage. Am J Orthod Dentofac Orthop. 2003;124:373–8.
2. Cheng SJ, Tseng IY, Lee JJ, Kok SH. A prospective study of the risk factors associated with failure of mini-implants used for orthodontic anchorage. Int J Oral Maxillofac Implants. 2004;19:100–6.
3. Park HS, Jeong SH, Kwon OW. Factors affecting the clinical success of screw implants used as orthodontic anchorage. Am J Orthod Dentofac Orthop. 2006;130:18–25.
4. Chen CH, Chang CS, Hsieh CH, Tseng YC, Shen YS, Huang IY, et al. The use of microimplants in orthodontic anchorage. J Oral Maxillofac Surg. 2006;64:1209–13.
5. Kim JW, Cho IS, Lee SJ, Kim TW, Chang YI. Effect of dual pitch mini-implant design and diameter of an orthodontic mini-implant on the insertion and removal torque. Korean J Orthod. 2006;36:275–83.
6. Motoyoshi M, Hirabayashi M, Uemura M, Shimizu N. Recommended placement torque when tightening an orthodontic mini-implant. Clin Oral Implants Res. 2006;17:109–14.

7. Wiechmann D, Meyer U, Büchter A. Success rate of mini- and micro-implants used for orthodontic anchorage: a prospective clinical study. Clin Oral Implants Res. 2007;18:263–7.
8. Moon CH, Lee DG, Lee HS, Im JS, Baek SH. Factors associated with the success rate of orthodontic miniscrews placed in the upper and lower posterior buccal region. Angle Orthod. 2008;78:101–6.
9. Melsen B, Costa A. Immediate loading of implants used for orthodontic anchorage. Clin Orthod Res. 2000;3:23–8.
10. Kim JW, Ahn SJ, Chang YI. Histomorphometric and mechanical analyses of the drill-free screw as orthodontic anchorage. Am J Orthod Dentofac Orthop. 2005;128:190–4.
11. Wilmes B, Rademacher C, Olthoff G, Drescher D. Parameters affecting primary stability of orthodontic mini-implants. J Orofac Orthop. 2006;67:162–74.
12. Motoyoshi M, Yoshida T, Ono A, Shimizu N. Effect of cortical bone thickness and implant placement torque on stability of orthodontic mini-implants. Int J Oral Maxillofac Implants. 2007;22:779–84.
13. Kim JW, Baek SH, Kim TW, Chang YI. Comparison of stability between cylindrical and conical type mini-implants. Mechanical and histological properties. Angle Orthod. 2008;78:692–8.
14. Lim SA, Cha JY, Hwang CJ. Insertion torque of orthodontic miniscrews according to changes in shape, diameter and length. Angle Orthod. 2008;78:234–40.
15. Wilmes B, Ottenstreuer S, Su YY, Drescher D. Impact of implant design on primary stability of orthodontic mini-implants. J Orofac Orthop. 2008;69:42–50.
16. Cho IS, Kim SK, Chang YI, Baek SH. In vitro and in vivo mechanical stability of orthodontic mini-implants. Angle Orthod. 2012;82:611–7.
17. Martinez H, Davarpanah M, Missika P, Celletti R, Lazzara R. Optimal implant stabilization in low density bone. Clin Oral Implants Res. 2001;12:423–32.
18. O'Sullivan D, Sennerby L, Meredith N. Influence of implant taper on the primary and secondary stability of osseointegrated titanium implants. Clin Oral Implants Res. 2004;15:474–80.
19. Siegele D, Soltesz U. Numerical investigation of the influence of implant shape on stress distribution in the jaw bone. Int J Oral Maxillofac Implants. 1989;4: 333–40.
20. Chehroudi B, Gould TR, Brunette DM. Titanium-coated micromachined grooves of different dimensions affect epithelial and connective-tissue cells differently in vivo. J Biomed Mater Res. 1990;24: 1203–19.
21. Chehroudi B, Gould TR, Brunette DM. The role of connective tissue in inhibiting epithelial downgrowth on titanium-coated percutaneous implants. J Biomed Mater Res. 1992;26:493–515.
22. Kim TW, Baek SH, Kim JW, Chang YI. Effects of microgrooves on the success rate and soft tissue adaptation of orthodontic miniscrews. Angle Orthod. 2008;78:1057–64.
23. Klokkevold PR, Nishimura RD, Adachi M, Caputo A. Osseointegration enhanced by chemical etching of the titanium surface: a torque removal study in the rabbit. Clin Oral Implants Res. 1997;8:442–7.
24. Cordioli G, Majzoub Z, Piattelli A, Scarano A. Removal torque and histomorphometric investigation of 4 different titanium surfaces: an experimental study in the rabbit tibia. Int J Oral Maxillofac Implants. 2000;15:668–74.
25. Klokkevold PR, Johnson P, Dadgostari S, Caputo A, Davies JE, Nishimura RD. Early endosseous integration enhanced by dual acid etching of titanium: a torque removal study in the rabbit. Clin Oral Implants Res. 2001;12:350–7.
26. Lim YJ, Oshida Y, Andres CJ, Barco MT. Surface characterizations of variously treated titanium materials. Int J Oral Maxillofac Implants. 2001;16:333–42.
27. Cho SA, Park KT. The removal torque of titanium screw inserted in rabbit tibia treated by dual acid etching. Biomaterials. 2003;24:3611–7.
28. Cho SA, Jung SK. A removal torque of the laser-treated titanium implants in rabbit tibia. Biomaterials. 2003;24:4859–63.
29. Buser D, Schenk RK, Steinemann S, Fiorellini JP, Fox CH, Stich H. Influence of surface characteristics on bone integration of titanium implants: a histomorphometric study in miniature pigs. J Biomed Mater Res. 1991;25:889–902.
30. Yamagami A, Yoshihara Y, Suwa F. Mechanical and histologic examination of titanium alloy material treated by sandblasting and anodic oxidization. Int J Oral Maxillofac Implants. 2005;20:48–53.
31. Aalam AA, Nowzari H. Clinical evaluation of dental implants with surfaces roughened by anodic oxidation, dual acid-etched implants, and machined implants. Int J Oral Maxillofac Implants. 2005;20: 793–8.
32. Kim SH, Lee SJ, Cho IS, Kim SK, Kim TW. Rotational resistance of surface-treated mini-implants. Angle Orthod. 2009;79:899–907.
33. Karmarker S, Yu W, Kyung HM. Effect of surface anodization on stability of orthodontic microimplant. Korean J Orthod. 2012;42:4–10.
34. Cho KC, Baek SH. Effects of predrilling depth and implant shape on the mechanical properties of orthodontic mini-implants during the insertion procedure. Angle Orthod. 2012;82:618–24.
35. Lee NK, Baek SH. Effects of the diameter and shape of orthodontic mini-implants on microdamage to the cortical bone. Am J Orthod Dentofac Orthop. 2010; 138:8.e1–8.
36. Huja SS, Katona TR, Burr DB, Garetto LP, Roberts WE. Micro-damage adjacent to endosseous implants. Bone. 1999;25:217–22.
37. Martin RB. Fatigue microdamage as an essential element of bone mechanics and biology. Calcif Tissue Int. 2003;73:101–7.
38. Wawrzinek C, Sommer T, Fischer-Brandies H. Microdamage in cortical bone due to the overtightening

of orthodontic micro-screws. J Orofac Orthop. 2008; 69:121–34.
39. Gambarini G. Rationale for the use of low-torque endodontic motors in root canal instrumentation. Endod Dent Traumatol. 2000;16:95–100.
40. Yared GM, Bou Dagher FE, Machtou P. Failure of ProFile instruments used with high and low torque motors. Int Endod J. 2001;34:471–5.
41. Kim JS, Choi SH, Cha SK, Kim JH, Lee HJ, Yeom SS, Hwang CJ. Comparison of success rates of orthodontic mini-screws by the insertion method. Korean J Orthod. 2012;42:242–8.
42. Cho IS, Baek SH, Kim YH. Effects of wobbling angle on the stability measures of orthodontic mini-implants during insertion and removal procedures. Angle Orthod. 2013;83:1009–14.
43. Kravitz ND, Kusnoto B. Risks and complications of orthodontic miniscrews. Am J Orthod Dentofac Orthop. 2007;131:S43–51.
44. Lee YK, Kim JW, Baek SH, Kim TW, Chang YI. Root and bone response to the proximity of a mini-implant under orthodontic loading. Angle Orthod. 2010;80: 452–8.
45. Liou EJ, Pai BC, Lin JC. Do miniscrews remain stationary under orthodontic forces? Am J Orthod Dentofac Orthop. 2004;126:42–7.
46. Kuroda S, Sugawara Y, Deguchi T, Kyung HM, Takano-Yamamoto T. Clinical use of miniscrew implants as orthodontic anchorage: success rates and postoperative discomfort. Am J Orthod Dentofac Orthop. 2007;131:9–15.
47. Asscherickx K, Vande Vannet B, Wehrbein H, Sabzevar MM. Success rate of miniscrews relative to their position to adjacent roots. Eur J Orthod. 2008;30:330–5.
48. Kim SH, Kang SM, Choi YS, Kook YA, Chung KR, Huang JC. Cone-beam computed tomography evaluation of mini-implants after placement: is root proximity a major risk factor for failure? Am J Orthod Dentofac Orthop. 2010;138:264–76.
49. Wilmes B, Su YY, Sadigh L, Drescher D. Pre-drilling force and insertion torques during orthodontic mini-implant insertion in relation to root contact. J Orofac Orthop. 2008;69:51–8.
50. Lima GM, Soares MS, Penha SS, Romano MM. Comparison of the fracture torque of different Brazilian mini-implants. Braz Oral Res. 2011;25: 116–21.
51. Cho IS, Kim TW, Ahn SJ, Yang IH, Baek SH. Effects of insertion angle and implant thread type on the fracture properties of orthodontic mini-implants during insertion. Angle Orthod. 2013;83: 698–704.
52. Carano A, Velo S, Incorvati C, Poggio P. Clinical applications of the mini-screw-anchorage-system (M.A.S.) in the maxillary alveolar bone. Prog Orthod. 2004;5:212–35.
53. Barros SE, Janson G, Chiqueto K, Garib DG, Janson M. Effect of mini-implant diameter on fracture risk and self-drilling efficacy. Am J Orthod Dentofac Orthop. 2011;140:e181–92.
54. Brisceno CE, Rossouw PE, Carrillo R, Spears R, Buschang PH. Healing of the roots and surrounding structures after intentional damage with miniscrew implants. Am J Orthod Dentofac Orthop. 2009;135: 292–301.

4 Settling the Score with Class IIs Using Miniscrews

S. Jay Bowman

Abstract

Class IIs have been one of the most prevalent malocclusions treated in orthodontic practice. Throughout the history of the specialty, all manner of methods and devices have been employed to resolve these bad bites. Yet, after decades, there is still no consensus on the best technique or approach. In fact, we seemingly cannot even agree on the etiology nor the correct jaw to address with our mechanics. It does appear that we might find common ground regarding the most common issues with any of our treatment approaches, namely, that we are constrained by two major limitations: the requirements of patient compliance and anchorage control. It is this interminable battle for compliance and anchorage that has led us to employ skeletal anchorage for the management of Class IIs.

4.1 How Are Class IIs Corrected?

Despite the fact that Class IIs have presumably been the second most common malocclusion sign that patients present with to orthodontic practices, there has been no consensus over the past century as to when and how to correct them. In fact, there is still misunderstanding in regard to how the correction actually occurs. As a result, the multitude of philosophies and associated devices for the resolution of Class IIs remain staggering, even though substantial amounts of research have been published on the effects and effectiveness of nearly all approaches.

S.J. Bowman, DMD, MSD
Kalamazoo Orthodontics,
1314 West Milham Avenue, Portage, MI 49024, USA
e-mail: drjwyred@aol.com

From an examination of the wide range of different types of investigations of Class II treatments, there seem to be little demonstrable differences among the results produced by the menagerie of methods [1–8]. Whether addressing maxilla or mandible [2], early or late treatment timing [8], results are virtually the same. This is especially true in terms of the magnitude of mandibular growth contributing to the overall correction: it's also nearly identical [2].

Although some Class II mechanisms are intended to modify skeletal growth (i.e., orthopedics) or move teeth (i.e., orthodontics) or even both, the actual effects are, on average, mostly found in the midface and not so much in the mandible [1–8]. Moreover, it seems that the key to Class II correction in the growing patient is primarily due to the interruption of dentoalveolar compensation—no matter the treatment method chosen [3, 9].

K.B. Kim (ed.), *Temporary Skeletal Anchorage Devices*,
DOI 10.1007/978-3-642-55052-2_4, © Springer-Verlag Berlin Heidelberg 2014

Consequently, it is simple to say that the selection of an orthodontic method to correct Class II is primarily a practice management decision; however, there are some factors that may sway that selection, especially if miniscrews are added to the equation.

4.2 The Role of Miniscrews in the Battle over Patient Compliance and Anchorage Loss

The most enduring orthodontic treatment challenges have been that of (1) battling patient compliance and (2) controlling anchorage loss. Newton's third law places limits on the effectiveness of our biomechanics. We are simultaneously attempting to elicit patient adherence for prescribed wear and care of different appliances and devices that we've devised to correct malocclusions (and negate Sir Isaac). It is this balancing act between what a patient will do and the compromises limiting our biomechanics that continues to plaque the practitioners of our art and science. For example, the use of headgear has been long celebrated as it significantly improves the stakes in the battle of anchorage loss, not only in the correction of Class II but also during space closure. Unfortunately, the headgear frequently fails in the other struggle: the battle for patient compliance.

In the past quarter century, there has been an increased focus upon more predictable treatment outcomes, especially for methods that are less reliant upon patient cooperation. It seems, however, in the rush to adopt all manner of noncompliance approaches, the conflict with anchorage loss was often overlooked. Few paid attention to anchorage loss in the lower anterior teeth resulting from functionals or in the upper anterior with molar distalization. Since the Class IIs were corrected, we either lived with or found ways to reverse some of those iatrogenic effects. In other words, the adverse consequences, or additional treatments to correct them, were tolerated because the Class IIs were more consistently addressed. As more practitioners grew aware of the limitations of their newfound mechanisms to reduce reliance upon compliance, the introduction of skeletal anchorage came at the right time to give new hope in balancing the books. What could be more ideal than a mildly invasive method of providing absolute anchorage by incorporating miniscrews? It was almost too good to be true and in some ways led to a false sense of "anchorage" security.

Unfortunately, miniscrews move—they tip [10–14]. When employed as direct anchorage (i.e., retraction or pushing forces are applied directly to the head of a miniscrew and then to the tooth or group of teeth that are to be acted upon), it matters not if the miniscrew tips. If, however, the force is applied indirectly through a tooth or group of teeth with the intent that the miniscrew will provide absolute support, there is the possibility that as the screws tip, so shall some of the anchorage be lost. The orthodontist must then determine if the presumed amount of potential anchorage loss is enough to make a significant difference in the treatment outcome. Depending upon miniscrews for absolute indirect anchorage support may, consequently, be a fool's errand in some circumstances. The decision process for introducing miniscrews into Class II scenarios will be described with that disconcerting factor in mind.

4.3 Intervening in the Mixed Dentition

Early intervention for Class IIs was certainly the growth industry of the 1980s in orthodontics. The siren's call to address small mandibles early and often was once purported to be the epitome of patient care. It would seem logical that the sooner that a growth discrepancy could be corrected, the better. Unfortunately, treatments for patients with all manner of methods came before the understanding of the actual mechanisms and their effects.

Fortunately, substantial amounts of research were conducted during the rise in popularity of early treatment with functional appliances [2–9, 15, 16]. Prospective and retrospective studies have both demonstrated that earlier is not necessarily better. In fact, for the most part, dual-phase treatments cost patients more and often take longer than one-stage methods, and, most importantly, the results are no better or worse [17]. In addition, the battle for patient compliance is at odds with many of the methods chosen for prosecution of early treatment (e.g., headgear, Class II elastic-powered distalizers, removable functionals, etc.) or unintended anchorage loss resulted (e.g., functionals). In addition, attempting to wear many of these obtrusive appliances was hardly "functional," and long periods of "retention-between-phases" with other obturating devices were often recommended.

If early treatment for Class II is desired for patients with severe overjets, diminished chins, or air-cooled incisors (especially if the child is subject to ridicule by classmates), then, certainly, the issues of compliance and anchorage loss must be included in the cost/benefit analysis. However, it appears that the majority of mild-to-moderate Class IIs *can* wait for shorter, more conservative, less obtrusive, one-stage treatments. In fact, ideal timing of treatment, especially for many female patients, may be best initiated in the late mixed dentition [3, 18].

Mellion et al. [18] have reported that statural growth measures are more reliable predictors for a preadolescent's growth spurt than other methods requiring ionizing radiation evaluation. In the course of their investigation, it was confirmed that the female growth spurt is occurring at younger ages, prior to the typical complete eruption of the adult dentition. Therefore, to maximize the contribution of mandibular growth in the correction of Class II, treatment might be optimized in some instances before the loss of the last of the primary molars. If treatment is initiated prior to the loss of the leeway or "e" space, there is an added bonus for patients that have mild-to-moderate dental arch discrepancies accompanying their Class II [19, 20], and miniscrews can improve the predictability of this process [21, 22].

In Fig. 4.1, a female in late mixed dentition presented with sufficient leeway space to resolve her dental crowding if the residual space from the exchange of the primary second molars for permanent second premolars was maintained. Orthodontic treatment was initiated just prior to the loss of the primary molars with indirect anchorage derived from two miniscrews inserted interradicularly between the lower lateral incisors and canines. Sectional supporting wires were bonded using flowable composite into the slotted heads of the miniscrews and extended posteriorly into auxiliary tubes on standard molar orthodontic bands. These sectional square wires were intended to provide anchorage support to the first molars, preventing them from migrating forward as light retraction forces were applied to the first premolars. Teeth were retracted distally into residual leeway space as the second premolars were erupting and the anterior crowding was dispersed without intercanine expansion.

In this scenario, the leeway space was not violated by mesially moving molars and, as a result, the Class II molar relationship would not spontaneously improve. Class II intermaxillary elastics were added, and the lower incisors were controlled anteriorly and vertically by means of the miniscrew-supported sectional "arms" (i.e., assisted in preventing untoward flaring of incisors and maintaining some vertical control). Consequently, preservation of leeway space (to correct dental crowding without intercanine expansion) and simultaneously counteracting the negative effects of Class II elastics (e.g., maintaining mandibular incisors upright over the bone and reducing extrusion of mandibular molars) are certainly laudable goals for miniscrews, especially when they are accomplished in a single phase of treatment. Caution is warranted in regard to the potential for unintended impaction of permanent second molars in some cases when preserving leeway space and especially during unstable 2-phase mandibular expansive treatments [23, 24].

4.4 En Masse Retraction in the Permanent Dentition

If Class II correction is not initiated until the eruption of the permanent dentition, this does not necessarily mean that we have missed our golden

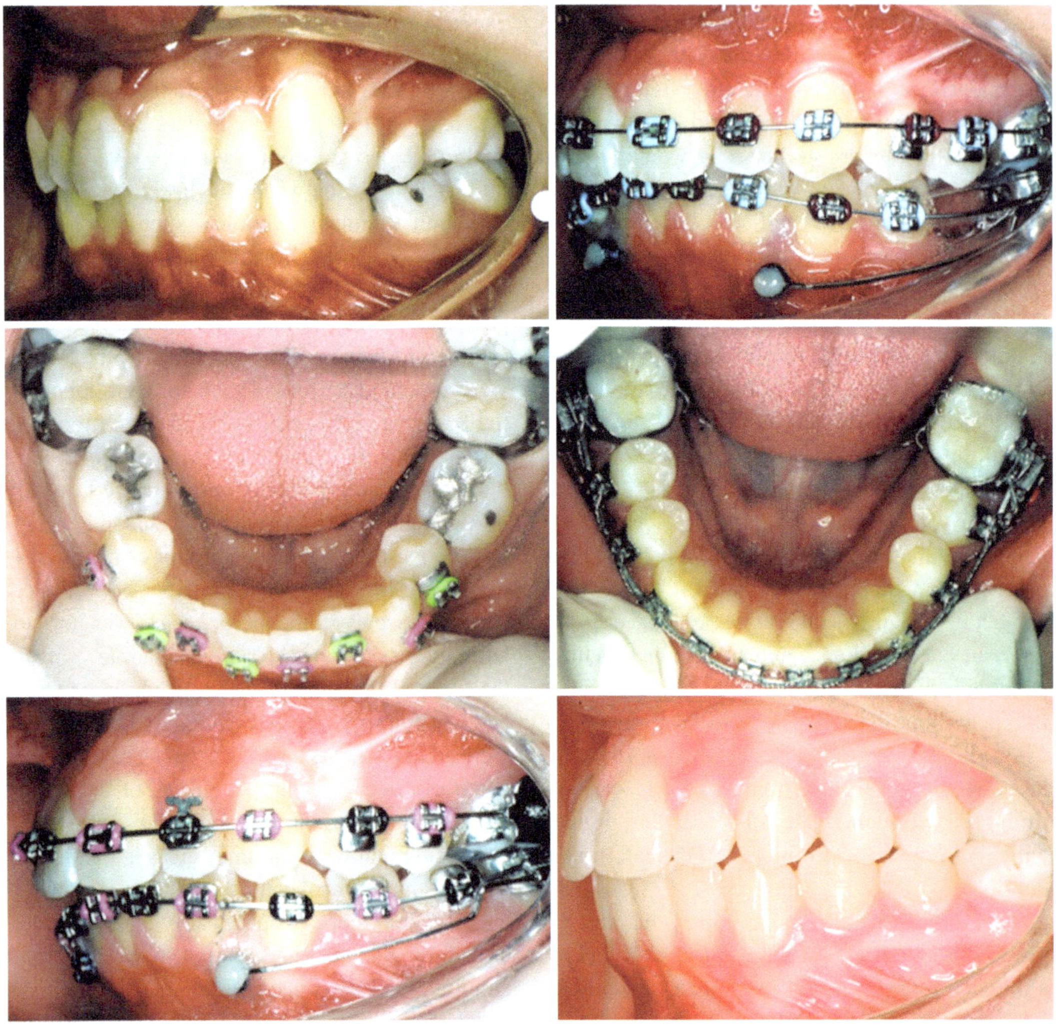

Fig. 4.1 Indirect anchorage from bonded segmental wires bonded to miniscrews inserted in the anterior mandibular alveolus was used to support several aspects of treatment: (1) effective maintenance of the leeway space as second premolars erupted, (2) preventing mesial molar movement (i.e., anchorage loss) as teeth were retracted using elastic thread into the residual leeway space to resolve crowding, (3) support for Class II elastics; (4) direct anchorage for intrusion of lower anterior teeth with elastic thread. This scenario offered a one-stage approach to resolving mild-to-moderate dental crowding without introducing the instability of mandibular expansion. Note: It would have been preferable to avoid the application of orthodontic brackets on the anterior teeth until after the retraction of premolars had created space

opportunity, especially if miniscrews are to be employed to assist in the battle over compliance and anchorage issues. Miniscrew success rates are certainly poorer and less predictable with preadolescent patients as they exhibit less mature alveolar bone and fewer reliable insertion sites (i.e., favorable interradicular sites are virtually nonexistent between primary teeth). As an upshot, most miniscrew-supported Class II correction methods are designed to begin after the eruption of the adult dentition and include:

1. En masse retraction
2. Fixed functional appliances
3. Molar distalization
4. Support for retraction after extraction (not discussed in this chapter)

It would seem obvious in a non-growing patient with a protrusive maxilla that the en masse retraction of the maxillary dentition could be incredibly beneficial. But can we really retract the entire maxillary dentition?

What are the effects for the growing patient, especially if they are deemed to be deprived of a sufficient mandible? Wouldn't addressing the maxilla with retraction be *prima facie* evidence of treating the wrong jaw?

We previously noted that whether forces are directed to the maxilla or the mandible in a growing patient, the majority of correction comes from the interruption of the dentoalveolar compensation mechanism [3, 25]. No matter what, the biomechanics of en masse maxillary retraction are identical for adolescent and adult patients. Meanwhile, growth will do what it does for the adolescent, but in the background [2]. The arrangement of the occlusion is adjusted by orthodontic treatment while growth benefits a grower [9, 26]. Without growth, obviously more dentoalveolar correction is required (additional miniscrews have been suggested) [27] or alternatives involving extractions or surgery may be considered for more significant discrepancies.

Figure 4.2 demonstrates an adolescent with a mild Class II Division 1 malocclusion treated with full-fixed orthodontic brackets. Distal en masse retraction was accomplished using simple, direct anchorage derived from miniscrews inserted into the buccal alveolus between the maxillary first molars and second premolars [28]. Typical elastic orthodontic "chain" was regularly re-applied from the miniscrews to T-pin hooks inserted in vertical slot canine brackets. Interruption of dentoalveolar compensation accompanied mild retraction of the entire maxillary dentition, accounting for the predictable correction. No patient compliance with headgear/elastics was required, nor were untoward side effects from those devices (i.e., lower incisor tipping, extrusion of molars, change in vertical dimension and occlusal plane) possible.

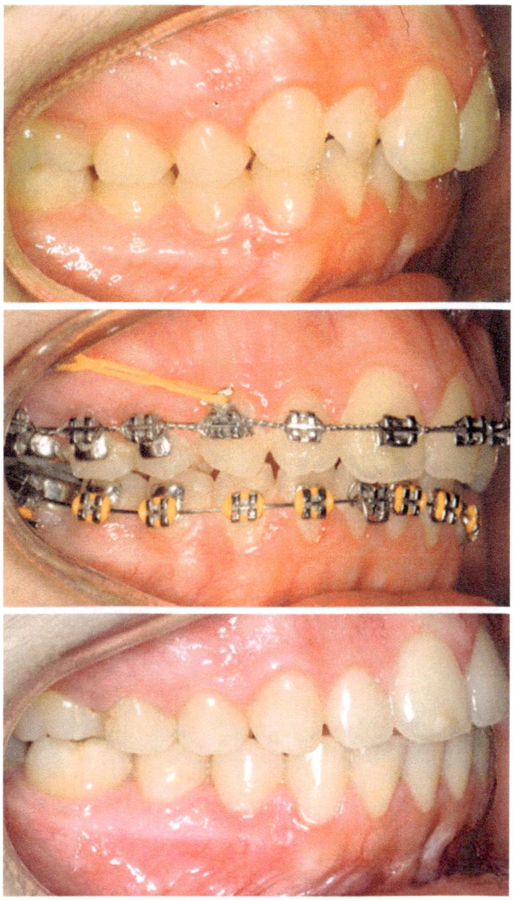

Fig. 4.2 Distal en masse retraction applied using elastic chain stretched from miniscrews in the maxillary buccal alveolus to full-fixed appliances. No compliance was required nor anchorage loss experienced during the resolution of this Class II relationship for an adolescent patient

Adult en masse maxillary retraction is depicted for two patients in Fig. 4.3. The left-side images show a male with a Class II malocclusion featuring a deep overbite. Miniscrews inserted between the lower lateral incisors and canines were employed as direct anchorage for elastic chain to intrude the mandibular anterior teeth to resolve the overbite. Miniscrews were also placed between the upper first molars and second premolars to provide direct anchorage support for distal en masse retraction of the maxillary dentition to Class I. The right-side photographs illustrate an adult female who transferred into care with an unresolved left-side Class II relationship and midline deviation. Simple en masse retraction biomechanics were successful using a single miniscrew for direct anchorage.

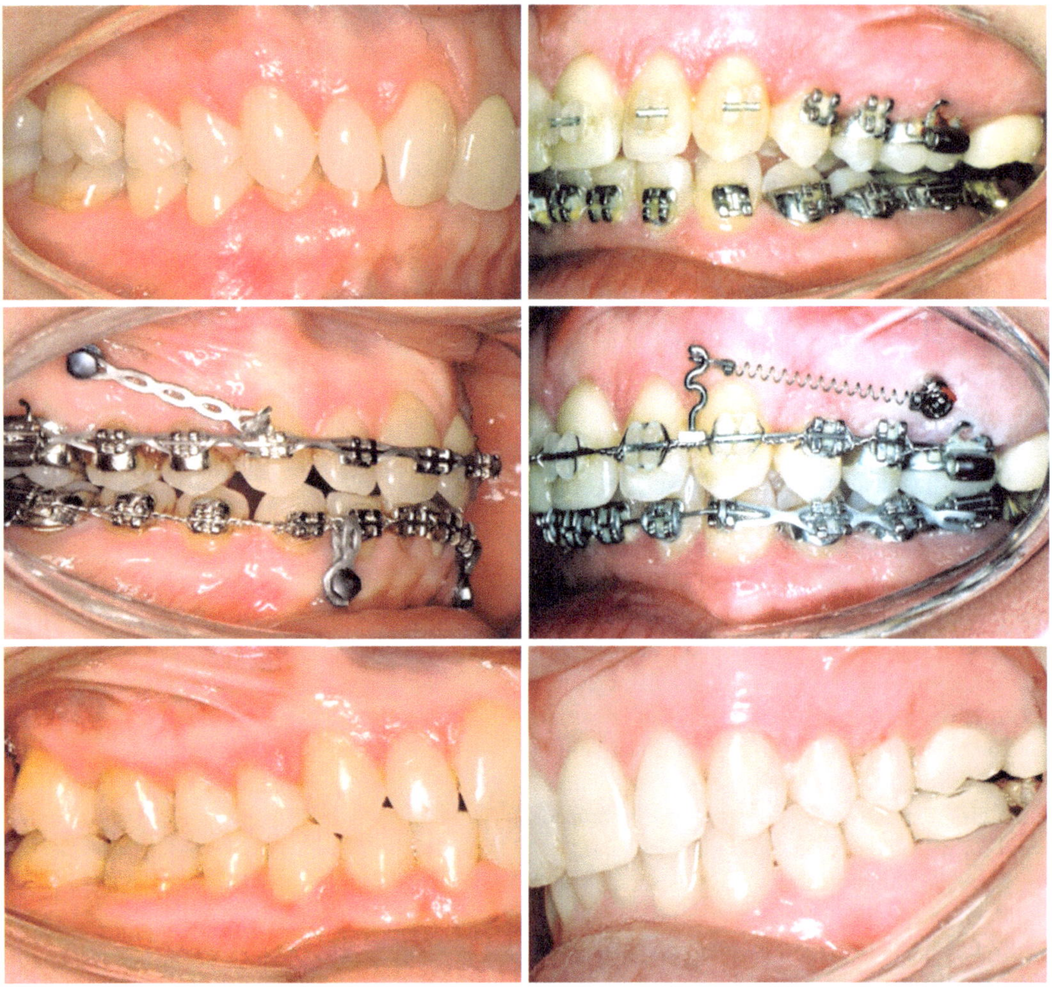

Fig. 4.3 Simple, direct anchorage support for Class II en masse retraction forces applied from miniscrews to the dentition with elastic chain for an adult male in the left-side photos and with coil springs for the female on the right side

4.5 Miniscrew-Supported Fixed Functionals: Addressing the Mandible

If one accepts the notion that Class IIs are primarily an issue of deficient mandibles, then it would seem a small leap to focus efforts on treating mandibles. This premise presumes that a particular type of orthodontic therapy will actually address the assumed primus inter pares cause of Class IIs: altering mandibular development. In the late 1800s, multiple methods of holding the mandible forward (i.e., devices to produce bite-jumping or treat "tongue-swallowing" (apnea)) were introduced, and they continued to evolve into today's family of fixed and removable functional appliances.

In the battle of anchorage loss and compliance, removable functional appliances fail on both accounts, so we will address only the fixed varieties of mandibular-focused treatments. There are perhaps hundreds of proprietary devices in the orthodontic marketplace that are designed to hold the mandible forward into a protrusive position with hopes that subsequent

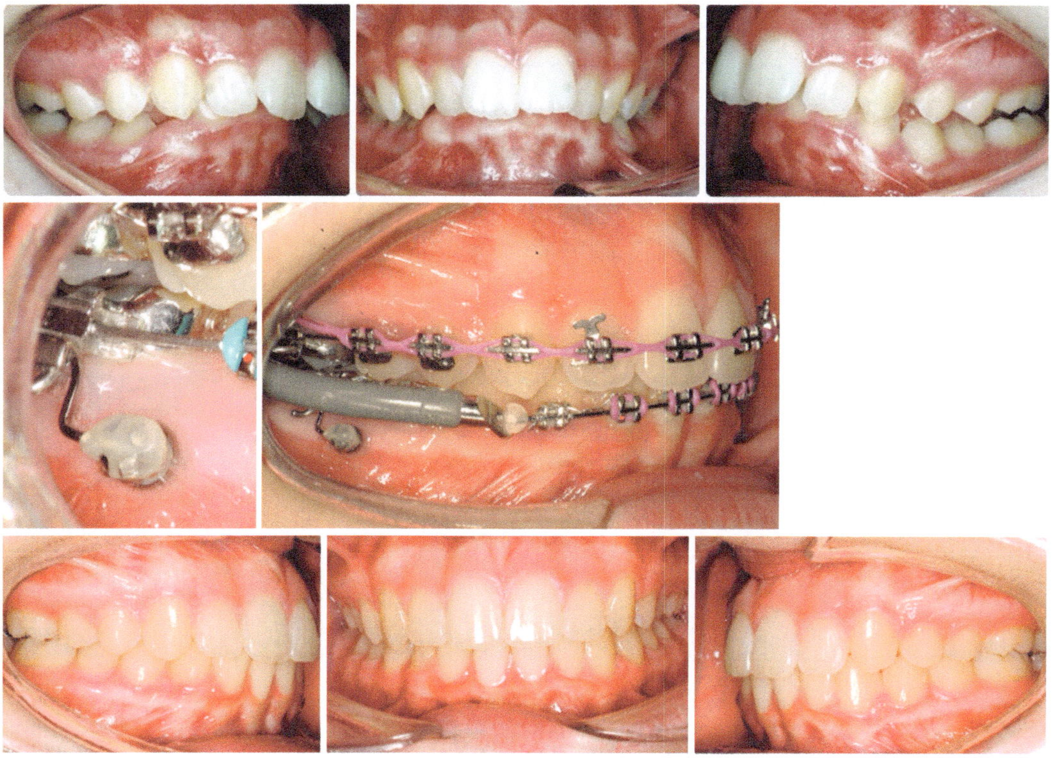

Fig. 4.4 Fixed functional correction of Class II supported by miniscrews inserted in the buccal alveolus between molars and premolars. Sectional supporting wires are bonded into the screw heads and used as support for the molars to counteract the mesial forces from the functionals

growth will stabilize that correction. A substantial amount of orthodontic research has been conducted to determine the effects of these approaches and compare them to other methods of Class II correction. As noted previously, there appear to be many more similarities than differences among the menagerie of methods available to the orthodontist.

In the crusade for patient compliance while limiting anchorage loss, fixed functionals have adequately addressed the first issue, as long as wearing a somewhat obtrusive jaw-protruding device does not elicit adverse patient cooperation. Unfortunately, all functionals suffer from the same unintended consequences of losing anchorage in the mandible (i.e., "flaring" or labial movement of lower anterior teeth) [29–31]. Not only could this affect long-term stability (as incisors are likely to upright later), but, more importantly, the tipped lower incisors can limit the amount of correction. In other words, more jaw or dental correction may have been desired at the outset of treatment [32], but less correction may be achieved as overjet is prematurely reduced [33]. Consequently, methods to control anchorage loss of the lower anteriors have been recommended when using functional devices. Employing lingual crown torque in lower incisor orthodontic brackets, inserting uprighting springs in vertical slot canine brackets, or even concurrent lip bumpers may help to resist the protrusive forces of fixed functionals [34]. Recently, the addition of miniscrews to provide anchorage support to counteract the mesial component force on the dentition has also been evaluated [22, 35].

In Fig. 4.4, a 12-year-old female with a Class II Division 1 malocclusion with mild crowding, deep overbite, and severe overjet was treated by first leveling and alignment, followed by intrusion of the lower anteriors. Only then were fixed

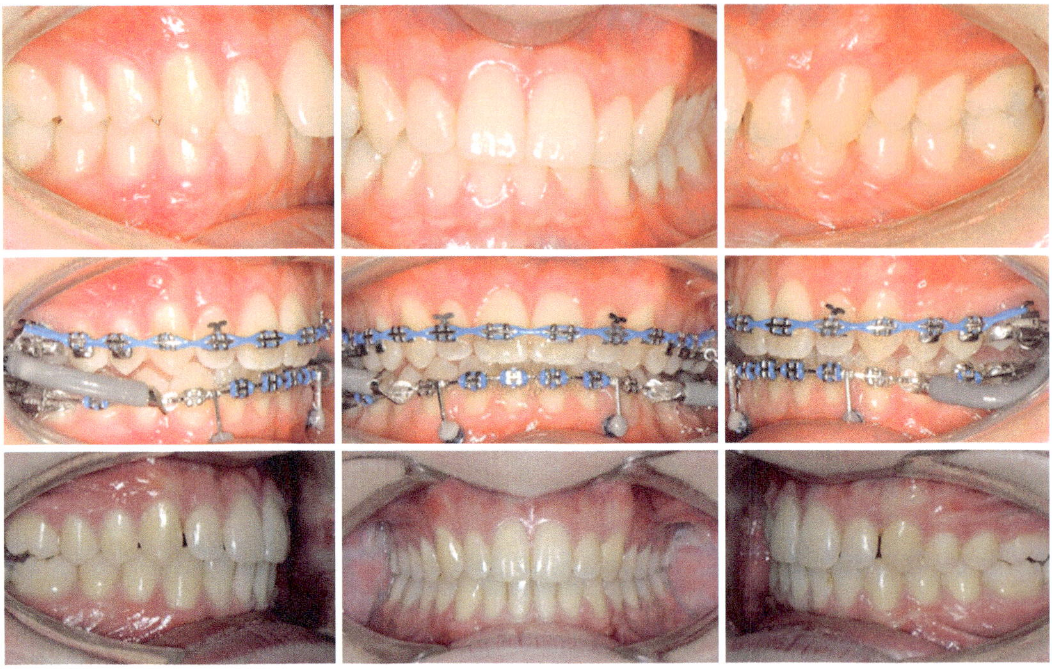

Fig. 4.5 Indirect miniscrew anchorage applied to a mandibular rectangular steel arch wire was used to support fixed functional appliances. The intent was to reduce the iatrogenic loss of anchorage resulting from labial tipping of lower incisors attending the anterior component of force from functionals (and/or Class II elastics). Note: A mild Bolton tooth-size discrepancy necessitated residual space adjacent to maxillary laterals that will be "filled" by esthetic bonding

functional, bite-jumping devices applied to affect interruption of dentoalveolar compensation. Two miniscrews were inserted between the mandibular first molars and second premolars. Sectional square wires were bonded with light-cured adhesive into the slotted heads of the screws to serve as "stops" to resist mesial forces on the dentition (maximizing the mandibular response while limiting anchorage loss). In addition, mandibular anterior brackets featuring 10° of lingual crown torque were employed.

An alternative approach for indirect anchorage support for fixed functionals is demonstrated in Fig. 4.5. Cast tubes with soldered sectional wires were slid onto a stainless steel rectangular arch wire. Next, fixed functionals were added to the arch wire inserted into the patient's orthodontic brackets. The sectional, square wire segments were seated into the slotted heads of the miniscrews and bonded in place with light-cured adhesive. Indirect anchorage from the screws to the base arch wire prevented tipping and intrusion of the lower incisors (to avoid alteration of the occlusal plane).

4.6 Miniscrew-Supported Distalization: Addressing the Maxilla

Molar distalization is simply the first step in an overall process of maxillary retraction. Distalization may be applied to either growing or non-growing, mild-to-moderate Class II patients. Moving the molars back is not the intended goal, but rather a means to the real end—the correction of the Class II relationship. Since moving molars posteriorly has always been challenging, presumably due to the molars' substantial root surface areas within the alveolar crest, attention to pushing them posteriorly, prior to addressing any of the other maxillary teeth, became the focus. Consequently, the distalization process might seem a contradiction to the proponents of simultaneous distal en masse retraction of *all* maxillary teeth. As clinical experience continued to meld with research results, it appeared that these treatments might be interchangeable, but perhaps in only certain circumstances. In any event, distalization contributes to the interruption of dentoalveolar compensation, and the amount of mandibular response during the process is the same as was found when forces were directed to the mandible with fixed functionals [2].

Patients with overjets featuring flared, but normally angulated (i.e., "torqued"), and/or "spaced" maxillary incisors may be better candidates for en masse maxillary retraction (or perhaps even fixed functionals or a Class II combination approach 34). In contrast, those exhibiting lingually inclined maxillary incisors with deep overbites would be better served by moving the maxillary molars before retracting the remaining upper teeth. Within this concept are two distinct strategies: (1) opening the bite and tipping the incisors labially (i.e., decompensating the Class II Division 2 into a Class II Division 1 malocclusion), prior to either en masse retraction or molar distalization, and (2) molar distalization followed by bite opening and applying appropriate anterior retraction and torque (i.e., avoiding the "round-trip" for the anteriors) [34, 36].

The first scenario necessitates some degree of "round-tripping" of the maxillary incisors by flaring them during leveling, later followed by their retraction. In the second scenario, no orthodontic brackets are placed on the maxillary anterior teeth until after space has been created by distalization to resolve crowding and permit retraction. Only then are the incisors intruded and torque added simultaneously during that retraction [34, 36].

Some limited molar distalization was recognized as resulting from cervical headgear or Class II elastic-supported sectionals or "jigs," so strategies for noncompliance-dependent treatment options began to gain popularity in the 1980s. This gave rise to a number of different devices designed to push molars posteriorly without requirements for patient adherence to prescribed wear of headgears or elastics. Unfortunately, these devices exhibited their own set of problems resulting from reciprocal anchorage loss (e.g., increasing overjet, flaring incisors, tipping molars, increasing vertical). So, in the balance between battling patient compliance and anchorage loss, it appears that distalization methods gained an advantage over the former, but at some detriment to the latter. Even the initial introduction of miniscrews into the distalization scenario to balance the books on anchorage loss can be seen as failure.

When miniscrews first appeared on the orthodontic scene, there was little thought that they could actually move or tip as they were touted to provide for "absolute anchorage." For instance, they were introduced as support for almost every imaginable molar distalization gadget with an expectation that they would prevent the unpredictable amounts of anterior anchorage loss attending these devices [14, 21, 37–43]. Unfortunately, most of these applications involved indirect anchorage from miniscrews to the appliance frameworks that are, in turn, attached to premolars (e.g., tying or bonding the screws to premolar supporting wires, keying screws into holes in acrylic palatal "buttons," or using screws "locked" into abutment caps connected to supporting teeth). As miniscrews can tip mesially [10–14] in response to the reciprocal traction from the molar pushing forces that they were intended to counteract, the teeth within the appliance framework could also move mesially, negating the purpose of using screws [14]. Consequently, changing the designs to apply pure skeletal anchorage appeared to be the only mechanism to consistently avoid untoward anchorage loss resulting from reciprocal forces.

On another front, if miniscrews are bonded to or locked into an appliance framework, the integrity of the screws cannot be checked for failure (the clinician or patient is unlikely to detect a loose or infected screw). In addition, if a screw

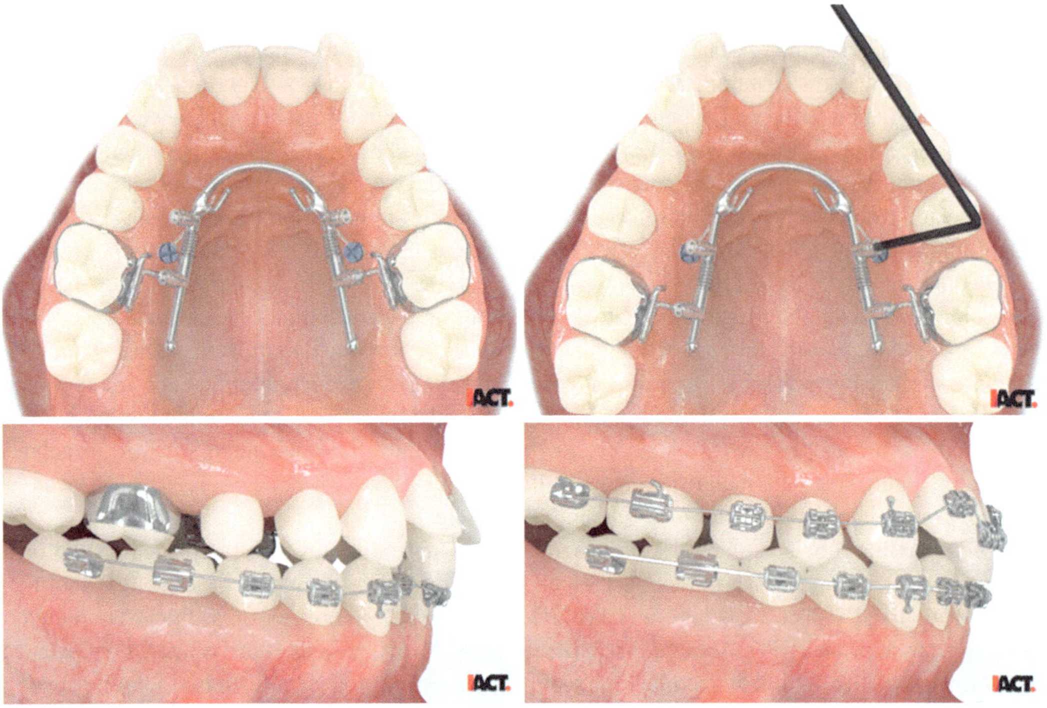

Fig. 4.6 Horseshoe Jet distalizer. Stainless ligatures are secured from miniscrews (inserted between the first molars and second premolars in the palatal alveolus) to hooks on the anterior part of the tracking wire. The mesial setscrews are moved distally to compress coil springs and then locked in place using the hex wrench. The distal setscrews are then unlocked one-fourth turn to permit distalization. At the completion of distal molar movement, the setscrews are all locked, creating a miniscrew-supported transpalatal arch for retraction of the remaining maxillary dentition. Orthodontic brackets do not need to be applied to the maxillary teeth until space is created by distalization, thereby precluding "round-tripping" (Images used by permission of InterActive Communication & Training IACT, Birmingham, AL)

that is locked to an appliance fails, the appliance would need to be re-fabricated as the miniscrew should be inserted into a new location. Using abutment "caps" in the construction of "locked-in" appliance also necessitates extra procedures including precision, parallel miniscrew insertion, and "pick-up" impressions to insure a proper line-of-draw of the device.

The Horseshoe Jet [22, 34, 36] is a modification of the Distal Jet that derives support from pure skeletal anchorage (i.e., no indirect dental anchorage) using nearly any type of miniscrew (Figs. 4.6, 4.7, and 4.8). These screws may be inserted into a variety of locations in the palate and may be connected by securing them with steel ligatures, bonded into or abutted against screws, or the devices may be constructed with locking abutments in the anterior palate if so desired. This versatile appliance can also be adjusted anteroposteriorly by unlocking the setscrews and moving the tracking wire back to avoid impingement of the palate or to increase the working length of distalization. Upon the completion of distalization, the setscrews are locked to provide rigid support for retraction of the rest of the maxillary dentition (i.e., the appliance is converted into a miniscrew-supported transpalatal arch). As a result, the Horseshoe Jet serves two distinct purposes in the correction of Class II and succeeds in struggles in both the arenas of patient compliance *and* eliminating anchorage loss during distalization.

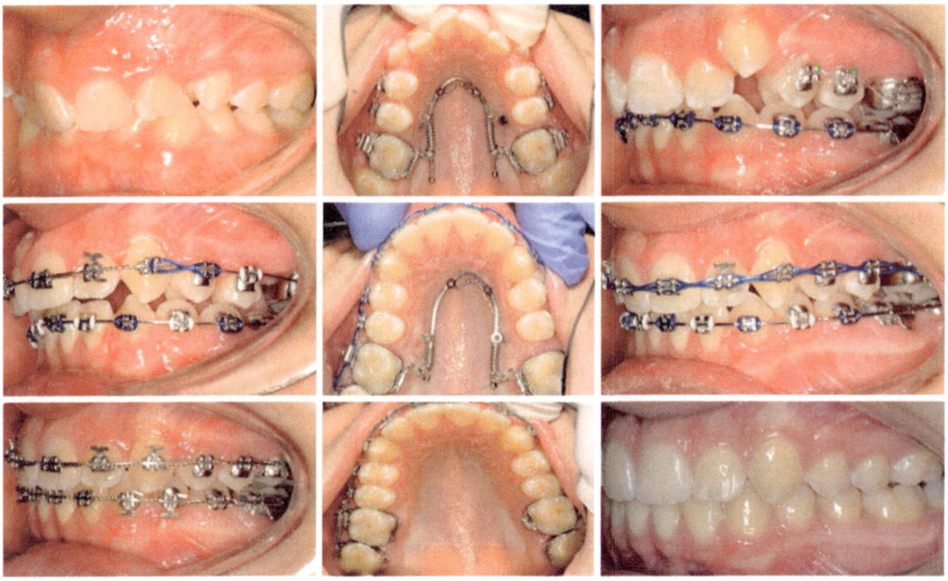

Fig. 4.7 A 13-year-old male with Class II molars and significant maxillary arch length discrepancy was treated using a miniscrew-supported Horseshoe Jet. As the molars were distalized, elastic thread was applied to the premolars to retract them and create space for the eruption of canines. Lower fixed appliances were employed to level and align, but the remaining upper brackets were not applied until the completion of distalization. Then the appliance was locked to serve as indirect anchorage for retraction and support for torque applied to the anterior teeth. No anterior anchorage loss can occur with distalization when pure skeletal anchorage is employed

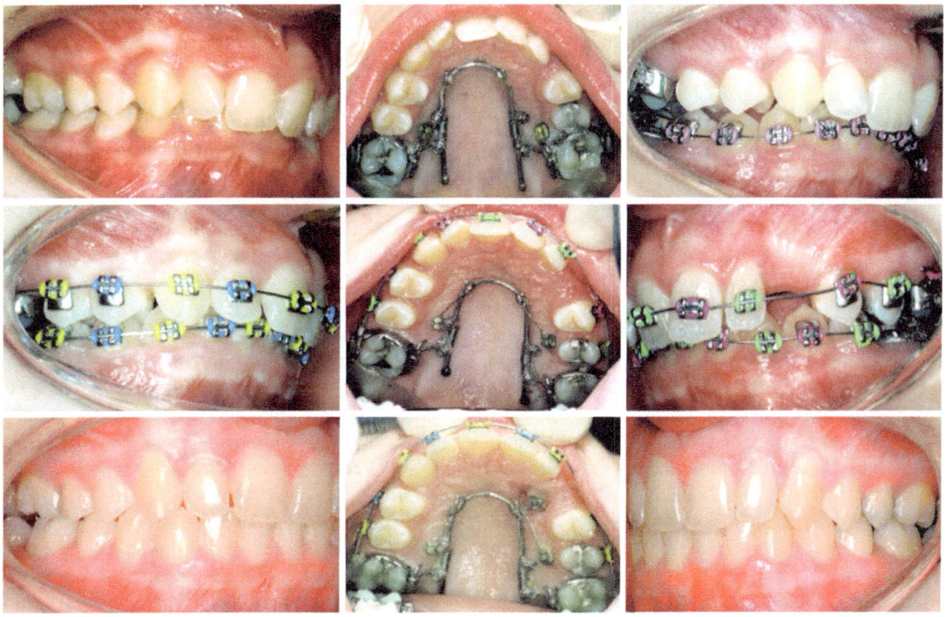

Fig. 4.8 A 13-year-old female's Class II relationship was corrected using a Horseshoe Jet with miniscrew anchorage. The molars were pushed posteriorly without anterior anchorage loss, premolars were pulled distally by transseptal fibers, and the lower dentition was leveled and aligned. At the conclusion of distalization, not only were molars positioned in Class I, but space was created to direct the eruption of an impacted canine. Elimination of the overbite, appropriate anterior torque, retraction of canines to Class I, and space closure were all supported by the miniscrew-supported transpalatal arch (Created when the Horseshoe Jet setscrews were locked down at the completion of distal molar movement)

4.7 Summary

The application of miniscrew anchorage in the treatment of Class II malocclusions has offered improved predictability for the correction, whether using either direct anchorage retraction or creative indirect anchorage support for traditional biomechanics.

References

1. Johnston Jr LE. A comparative analysis of Class II treatment methods. In: McNamara Jr JA, Carlson DS, Vig PS, Ribbens KA, editors. Science and clinical judgment in orthodontics, Craniofacial growth series. Ann Arbor: The University of Michigan; 1986. p. 103–48.
2. Burkhardt DR, McNamara Jr JA, Baccetti T. Maxillary molar distalization or mandibular enhancement: a cephalometric comparison of comprehensive orthodontic treatment including the pendulum and the Herbst appliances. Am J Orthod Dentofacial Orthop. 2003;123:108–16.
3. Tsourakis AK, Johnston Jr LE. Class II malocclusion: the aftermath of a "perfect storm." Semin Orthod. 2014;20:59–73.
4. O'Brien K, Sandler J. The treatment of Class II malocclusion-have we the evidence to make decisions? In: Huang GJ, Richmond S, Vig KWL, editors. Evidence-based orthodontics. Singapore: Wiley-Blackwell; 2011. p. 49–62.
5. Ghafari JG, Haddad RV, Saadeh ME. Class III malocclusion-the evidence on diagnosis and treatment. In: Huang GJ, Richmond S, Vig KWL, editors. Evidence-based orthodontics. Singapore: Wiley-Blackwell; 2011. p. 247–80.
6. Vig KWL, O'Brien K, Harrison J. Early orthodontic and orthopedic treatment: the search for evidence: will it influence clinical practice? In: Early orthodontic treatment: is the benefit worth the burden? Craniofacial growth series, vol. 44. Ann Arbor: Center for Human Growth and Development, The University of Michigan; 2007. p. 13–38.
7. Johnston Jr LE. If wishes were horses. In: McNamara Jr JA, editor. Early orthodontic treatment: is the benefit worth the burden, Craniofacial growth series, vol. 44. Ann Arbor: Center for Human Growth and Development, The University of Michigan; 2007. p. 39–51.
8. Livieratos FA, Johnston Jr LE. A comparison of one-stage and two-stage nonextraction alternatives in matched Class II samples. Am J Orthod Dentofacial Orthop. 1995;108(2):118–31.
9. Johnston Jr LE. Growth and the Class II patient: rendering unto Caesar. Semin Orthod. 1998;4(1):59–62.
10. Chatzigianni A, Keilig L, Reimann S, Eliades T, Bourauel C. Effect of mini-implant length and diameter on primary stability under loading with two force levels. Eur J Orthod. 2011;33:381–7.
11. Liou EJ, Pai BC, Lin JC. Do miniscrews remain stationary under orthodontic forces? Am J Orthod Dentofacial Orthop. 2004;126:42–7.
12. El-Beialy AR, Abou-El-Ezz AM, Attia KH, El-Bialy AM, Mostafa YA. Loss of anchorage of miniscrews: a 3-dimensional assessment. Am J Dentofac Orthop. 2009;136(5):700–7.
13. Alves Jr M, Baratieri C, Nojima LI. Assessment of mini-implant displacement using cone beam computed tomography. Clin Oral Implants Res. 2011;22(10):1151–6.
14. Kinzinger GSM, Diedrich PR, Bowman SJ. Upper molar distalization with a miniscrew-supported Distal Jet. J Clin Orthod. 2006;40:672–8.
15. Pangrazio MNK, Pangrazio-Kulbersh V, Berger JL, Bayirli B, Movahhedian A. Treatment effects of the mandibular repositioning appliance in patients with Class II skeletal malocclusions. Angle Orthod. 2012;82:971–7.
16. Franchi L, Pavoni C, Kaltin Jr K, McNamara Jr JA, Cozza P. Long-term skeletal and dental effects and treatment timing for functional appliances in Class II malocclusion. Angle Orthod. 2013;83:334–40.
17. Johnston Jr LE. Functional appliances: a mortgage on mandibular position. Aust Orthod J. 1996;14: 154–6.
18. Mellion ZJ, Behrents RG, Johnston Jr LE. The pattern of facial skeletal growth and its relationship to various common indexes of maturation. Am J Orthod Dentofacial Orthop. 2013;143(6):845–54. doi:10.1016/j.ajodo.2013.01.019.
19. Dugoni SA, Lee JS, Varela J, Dugoni AA. Early mixed dentition treatment: post retention evaluation of stability and relapse. Angle Orthod. 1995;65:311–20.
20. Gianelly AA. A strategy for nonextraction Class II treatment. Semin Orthod. 1998;4:26–32.
21. Bowman SJ. Thinking outside the box with miniscrews. In: McNamara Jr JA, Ribbens KA, editors. Microimplants as temporary anchorage in orthodontics, Craniofacial growth series. Ann Arbor: The University of Michigan; 2008. p. 327–90.
22. Ludwig B, Baumgartel S, Bowman SJ, editors. Mini-implants in orthodontics: innovative anchorage concepts. Berlin: Quintessence; 2008.
23. Sonis A, Ackerman M. E-space preservation. Angle Orthod. 2011;81(6):1045–9. doi:10.2319/030711-165.1. Epub 2011 May 25.
24. Rubin RL, Baccetti T, McNamara Jr JA. Mandibular second molar eruption difficulties related to the maintenance of arch perimeter in the mixed dentition. Am J Orthod Dentofacial Orthop. 2012;141(2):146–52. doi:10.1016/j.ajodo.2011.06.040.
25. Lundström A, McWilliam JS. Dento-alveolar compensation for antero-posterior variations between the upper and lower apical bases. Eur J Orthod. 1984;6:116–22.

26. Baccetti T, Franchi L, Kim LH. Effect of timing on the outcome of 1-phase nonextraction therapy of Class II malocclusion. Am J Orthod Dentofacial Orthop. 2009;136(4):501–9. doi:10.1016/j.ajodo.2007.08.029.
27. Bechtold TE, Kim JW, Choi TH, Park YC, Lee KJ. Distalization pattern of the maxillary arch depending on the number of orthodontic miniscrews. Angle Orthod. 2013;83:266–73.
28. Jeon JM, Yu HS, Baik HS, Lee JS. En-masse distalization with miniscrew anchorage in Class II nonextraction treatment. J Clin Orthod. 2006;40(8):472–6.
29. Hansen K, Koutsonas TG, Pancherz H. Long-term effects of Herbst treatment on the mandibular incisor segment: a cephalometric and biometric investigation. Am J Orthod Dentofacial Orthop. 1997;112: 92–103.
30. Nalbantgil D, Arun T, Sayinsu K, Isik F. Skeletal, dental and soft-tissue changes induced by the Jasper Jumper appliance in late adolescence. Angle Orthod. 2005;75:426–36.
31. Rothenberg J, Campbelll ES, Nanda R. Class II correction with the twin force bite corrector. J Clin Orthod. 2004;38:232–40.
32. LeHaye MB, Buschang PH, Alexander RG, Boley JC. Orthodontic treatment changes of chin position in Class II Division 1 patients. Am J Orthod Dentofacial Orthop. 2006;130(6):732–41.
33. Ye C, Du X, Zhao Q, Tan Z. Dentoskeletal effects of 2-phase treatment versus 1-phase treatment with extraction of 4 first premolars in nonhypodivergent class II patients. J Craniofac Surg. 2012;23(5):1544–7. doi:10.1097/SCS.0b013e31824f6454.
34. Bowman SJ. Class II combination therapy: molar distalization and fixed functionals. In: Nanda R, Kapila S, editors. Current therapy in orthodontics. St. Louis: Elsevier/Mosby; 2009. p. 115–36.
35. Luzi C, Luzi V, Carletti P, Melsen B. The miniscrew-anchored Herbst. J Clin Orthod. 2012;46(7): 399–405.
36. Bowman SJ. Miniscrew molar distalization: evolution of the Horseshoe Jet. In: Papadopoulos MS, editor. Skeletal anchorage in orthodontic treatment of Class II malocclusion: contemporary applications of orthodontic implants, miniscrew implants and miniplates. Mosby (in press).
37. Fudalej P, Antoszewska J. Are orthodontic distalizers reinforced with the temporary anchorage devices effective? Am J Orthod Dentofacial Orthop. 2011;139:722–9.
38. Kinzinger G, Wehrbein H, Byloff FK, Yildizhan F, Didrich P. Innovative anchorage alternatives for molar distalization: an overview. J Orofac Orthop. 2005;66:397–413.
39. Chang H, Hsiao H, Tsai C, Roberts WE. Bone-screw anchorage for Pendulum appliances and other fixed mechanics. Semin Orthod. 2006;12:284–93.
40. Velo S, Rotunno E, Cozzani M. The implant Distal Jet. J Clin Orthod. 2007;41:88–93.
41. Gelgör IE, Büyükyilmaz T, Karaman AIY, Dolanmaz D, Kalayci A. Intraosseous screw-supported upper molar distalization. Angle Orthod. 2004;74:838–50.
42. Carano A, Velo S. The miniscrew anchorage system. In: Cope J, editor. OrthoTADs: the clinical guide and atlas. Dallas: Under Dog Media; 2007. p. 231–43.
43. Papadopoulos MA. Orthodontic treatment of Class II malocclusion with miniscrew implants. Am J Orthod Dentofacial Orthop. 2008;134(5):604.e1–16. doi:10.1016/j.ajodo.2008.03.013; discussion 604–5.

Modified Palatal Plate

5

Yoon-Ah Kook, Mohamed Bayome, Sung-Seo Mo, Yoonji Kim, and Kyu-Rhim Chung

Abstract

Distalization appliances supported by temporary skeletal anchorage devices (TSADs) have been proposed. In this chapter, we have introduced the modified palatal anchorage plate (MPAP) appliance for maxillary arch distalization, its clinical relevance, indications, complications, and treatment outcome. The quality and the quantity of the paramedian palatal bony structure can mechanically support several mini-implants in both adults and adolescents. The design of the palatal plate has been modified for easier and more accurate placement and less inflammation to the tissues. Clinically successful distalization was achieved in 11.6 ± 4.3 months. The maxillary first molar showed 3.70 mm of distalization, 3.29° of distal tipping, and 2.40 mm of intrusion. Therefore, the palatal plate might be recommended for maxillary molar distalization in adults and adolescents.

Y.-A. Kook, DDS, PhD (✉) • S.-S. Mo, DDS, PhD
Y. Kim, DDS, PhD
Department of Orthodontics, Seoul Saint Mary's Hospital, The Catholic University of Korea, 222, Banpodaero, Seocho-gu, Seoul 137-701, South Korea
e-mail: kook2002@catholic.ac.kr; dmoss1@hanmail.net; juice@catholic.ac.kr

M. Bayome, BDS, MMS, PhD
Department of Orthodontics, Graduate School, The Catholic University of Korea, 222, Banpodaero, Seocho-gu, Seoul, South Korea
e-mail: mac_kral@hotmail.com

K.-R. Chung, DMD, MSD, PhD
Department of Orthodontics, School of Medicine, Ajou University, Wonchun-dong 5, Yeongtong-gu, Suwon 443-380, South Korea
e-mail: speedor@hotmail.com

5.1 Introduction

Distalization of the maxillary posterior teeth is one of the viable treatment strategies for Class II and bimaxillary protrusion patients. Extraoral appliances have been prescribed for such treatment over decades. However, patient cooperation is an essential factor required for these devices [1]. To effectively overcome this problem, intraoral noncompliance appliances have been developed [2–6]. Nevertheless, the undesirable side effects of these appliances include anchorage loss at the reactive part, distal tipping, extrusion of molars, clockwise rotation of the mandible, and an increase in lower facial height [7–9].

Recently, distalization appliances supported by temporary skeletal anchorage devices (TSADs) have been proposed [10–15]. The skeletal

K.B. Kim (ed.), *Temporary Skeletal Anchorage Devices*,
DOI 10.1007/978-3-642-55052-2_5, © Springer-Verlag Berlin Heidelberg 2014

anchorage has overcome the undesirable reaction on the anterior segment and allowed for better vertical control. However, the application of TSADs on the buccal side might be complicated especially in adolescents with narrow interradicular widths. In addition, the placement of the miniplate on the zygoma requires invasive surgical procedures. Therefore, the palatal anchorage might be the most convenient for supporting distalization appliances.

In this chapter, we have introduced the modified palatal anchorage plate (MPAP) appliance for maxillary arch distalization, its clinical relevance, indications, complications, and treatment outcome.

5.2 The Pertinence of the Palate

The palate has become a popular site for placement of TSADs. Anatomically, there is no vital structure in the area of interest; therefore, the risks of complications are decreased substantially. Also, the quality and the quantity of its bony structure can mechanically support several mini-implants.

5.2.1 Palatal Bone Density

The density of the bone is a determinant factor for the initial stability of TSADs. Several studies have evaluated the bone density through cone beam CT [16–19]. Moon et al. [20] showed that the palatal bone density in adults decreased laterally and posteriorly. Han et al. [21] reported that although palatal bone densities were significantly higher in adults than in adolescents, the anterior area of adolescents were of similar values to those at the posterior palate of adults. The means of the cortical bone density in the adult group of their study ranged between 1,059 and 573 HU, corresponding to the D2 (850–1,250 HU) and the upper range of the D3 (350–850 HU) categories in Misch [22] classification of bone tissue. Likewise, the cortical bone density in the adolescent group fell into the D3 category, ranging between 743 and 476 HU (Fig 5.1).

In addition, Bernhart et al. [23] reported that the most suitable area in adults for implant placement in the palate was located 6–9 mm posterior to the incisive foramen and 3–6 mm paramedian to the suture. However, other study indicated that the area of high density in the cortical bone

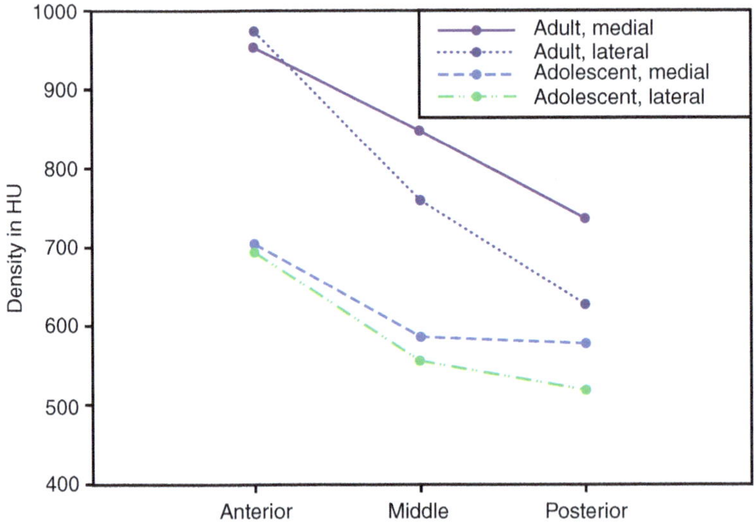

Fig. 5.1 Palatal cortical bone density in adults and adolescents according to palatal area (From Han et al. [21])

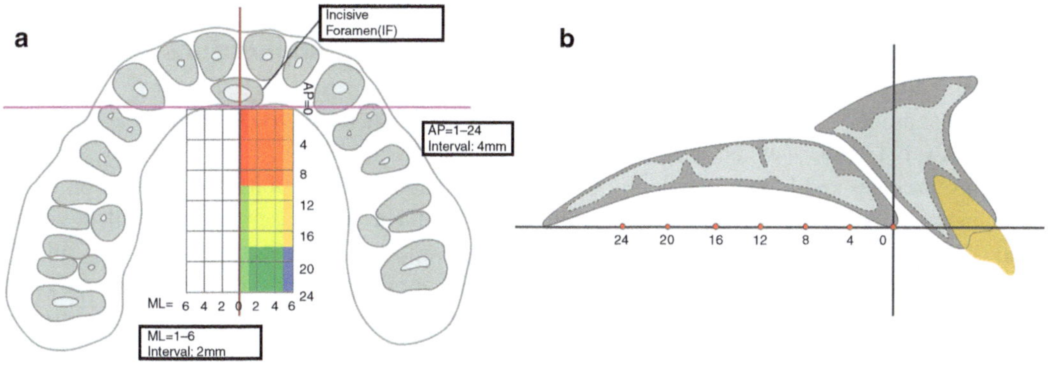

Fig. 5.2 Reference lines for evaluation of palatal bone thickness according to palatal area (From Ryu et al. [32])

extended 15 mm posterior to the incisive foramen at the medial half of the measured area and 6 mm in the lateral half [21].

These studies supported Wehrbein's [24] conclusion that the density of the median palate was high enough to support mini-implants. He also suggested that the reported 10 % failed micro-implants inserted in the palatal area [25, 26] may be attributed to factors other than bone density.

5.2.2 Palatal Bone Thickness

Several authors considered the palatal bone thickness a key factor of successful placement of TSADs [27–30]. King et al. [29] evaluated the palatal bone volume for placement of implants in adolescents (mean age: 14.0 years) using computed tomography. Gracco et al. [31] also compared bone thickness in adults to that of adolescents using cone beam computed tomography (CBCT) and reported insignificant differences. Ryu et al. [32] compared the bone thickness of various palatal areas among early and late mixed dentition and permanent dentition using CBCT (Fig. 5.2).

The palatal bone might be significantly thin in the midsagittal area due to incomplete ossification of the midpalatal suture. Therefore, placement of TSADs in the paramedian palatal area has been recommended because of its thin keratinized soft tissue and sufficient cortical bone [28, 31, 33–39].

The bone thickness decreased laterally and posteriorly in the paramedian area in adults [28, 32]. For adolescents, the anterior medial and lateral areas had the thickest palatal bone [32]. King et al. [29] demonstrated a sufficient vertical bone depth at 4 mm distal and 3 mm lateral to the incisive foramen to install a 3-mm-long implant in adolescents. In contrast, Gracco et al. [31] found no significant differences in the palatal bone thickness between adults and adolescents. However, their youngest group was over 10 years old, while Ryu et al. [32] focused on the adolescents and subdivided them into early mixed dentition (EMD) (mean age: 8.0 years) and late mixed dentition (LMD) groups (mean age: 11.5 years). The EMD group had significantly lower bone thickness than the two other groups, mainly in the anterior area. This inconsistency may be due to differences in methodology. Nevertheless, the bone thickness was greater in the anterior paramedian area than in the posterior one in all three groups of their study. This might be due to the difference in amounts of remodeling growth between the posterior and anterior parts [40].

5.2.3 Palatal Soft Tissue Thickness

The thickness of the palatal soft tissue has a great influence on the length of the miniscrew embedded in the bone. Therefore, it might be important to evaluate the soft tissue thickness of the palate before the installation of TSADs. Several methods have been applied to measure soft tissue thickness: direct measurement using a needle or periodontal probe [41, 42]; indirect measurement using CBCT [43–46], which has a radiation exposure problem and limited resolution due to slice thickness; and direct measurement via ultrasonic device which is a noninvasive method that showed acceptable repeatability, reliability, and accuracy [47–54].

Recently, the soft tissue thickness of midpalatal suture has been evaluated in cadavers [55]. It was thickest at a point 4 mm posterior from the incisive papilla (mean 2.93 mm) and decreased in more posterior areas, ranging from 0.90 to 1.01 mm. Lee et al. [56] showed thicker soft tissue thickness medially (1.80–2.21 mm) than that previous study [55] in the midpalatal region of the permanent dentition group. This difference may be due to shrinkage during the processing of the specimens [57, 58]. Table 5.1 shows comparison of palatal soft tissue thickness in different age groups according to their dental stage: late mixed, early permanent, and permanent dentitions (adopted from Lee et al. [56]).

Vu et al. [59] have evaluated the soft tissue thickness on CBCT images and showed that the thinnest was over the midpalatal suture (1.22–1.27 mm), while the lateral area was the thickest (2.71–2.93 mm). Barriviera et al. [44] reported that the mucosal thickness of the higher region of the palate ranged from 3.13 to 4.51 mm. Song et al. [45] reported an increase in the soft tissue thickness of the area over the palatal slope from the anterior to the posterior (3.13–3.81 mm). These differences might be due to the different measurement sites and the ethnicity of the patients.

Wara-aswapati et al. [41] showed that the older (30–59 years old) population had thicker palatal masticatory mucosa than the younger (14–21 years old). However, this was not the case in other studies [49, 59]. Gender dimorphism was also controversial. Several studies reported no significant differences in the mucosal thickness between males and females [41, 59, 60]. Others found thinner palatal mucosal tissue in females [45, 53].

5.3 Clinical Application and Complications

5.3.1 Application of MPAP

The clinical applications and installation of the MPAP have been described in detail in several case reports [12, 13]. The MPAP should be adjusted on the dental cast to fit the shape of the patient's palate. To achieve the best positioning of the MPAP, its arms should extend in the area between the first molar and second premolar or second deciduous molar. Enough space should be left between the arms and the palatal slopes.

Then, a silicon jig extending on the occlusal surfaces of the first molar and second premolar is fabricated to hold the plate firmly during placement and to keep even space between the arms and palatal soft tissue bilaterally.

At the placement appointment, local anesthesia is administrated; the jig-MPAP assembly should be placed by fitting the jig to the occlusal surfaces of the molars and premolars. And then, self-drilling mini-implants should be inserted through the screw tubes with an implant engine (30 RPM and less than 30 Ncm). After placement of three mini-implants, the jig is removed using a utility plier. Tightening of the mini-implant may be required after removal of the jig, as well as fine adjustment of the position of the arms. Then, a palatal bar with hooks is bonded to the first molars (Fig. 5.3). Immediately after placement, distalization can be initiated with elastics or NiTi closed coil springs.

5.3.2 Complications

Altered Pronunciation

Recently, the speech perturbation and adaptation related to MPAP appliance over time has been evaluated [61]. A speech recording session of the alveolar, alveopalatal, and palatal sounds [t], [d], [s], [z], [n], [r], and [j] was made five times throughout treatment: T0, prior to PP placement; T1, just after the PP placement; T2, T3, T4, and T5, 1, 2, 3, and 4 weeks after MPAP placement, respectively. Acoustic analysis was

Table 5.1 Comparison of palatal soft tissue thickness among late mixed, early permanent, and permanent dentitions (unit: mm)

	Late mixed dentition (n=42)							Early permanent dentition (n=41)							Permanent dentition (n=38)							
	Median		Middle		Lateral			Median		Middle		Lateral			Median		Middle		Lateral			
	Mean	SE	Mean	SE	Mean	SE	p-value[b]	Mean	SE	Mean	SE	Mean	SE	p-value[b]	Mean	SE	Mean	SE	Mean	SE	p-value[b]	p-value[c]
Anterior	1.79	0.41	2.05	0.40	2.39	0.39	< 0.0001	1.94	0.42	2.25	0.46	2.49	0.54	<0.0001	2.21	0.56	2.50	0.42	2.93	0.51	<0.0001	<0.001
Middle	1.83	0.69	2.04	0.66	2.38	0.61		1.83	0.70	2.20	0.72	2.47	0.67		1.80	0.69	2.70	0.84	3.19	0.75		
Posterior	2.32	0.99	2.95	1.09	3.04	1.20		2.08	0.96	2.97	0.98	3.18	1.16		2.15	0.93	3.18	1.04	3.92	1.21		
p-value[a]	<0.0001							<0.0001							<0.0001							

From Lee et al. [56]
Repeated measures ANOVA
Median represents the area between lines 0 and 4 mm lateral to the midpalatal suture; middle, between lines 4 and 8 mm; lateral, between lines 8 and 12 mm
Anterior represents the areas between lines 0–4, 4–8, and 8–12 mm posterior to lingual interdental papilla of incisors
Middle represents the areas between lines 12–16, 16–20, and 20–24 mm posterior to lingual interdental papilla of incisors
Posterior represents the areas between lines 24–28, 28–32, and 32–36 mm posterior to lingual interdental papilla of incisors
SE standard error
[a]The significance level of the effect of the anteroposterior position in late mixed, early permanent, and permanent dentition groups
[b]The significance level of the effect of the mediolateral position in late mixed, early permanent, and permanent dentition groups
[c]The significance level of the comparison of the three groups

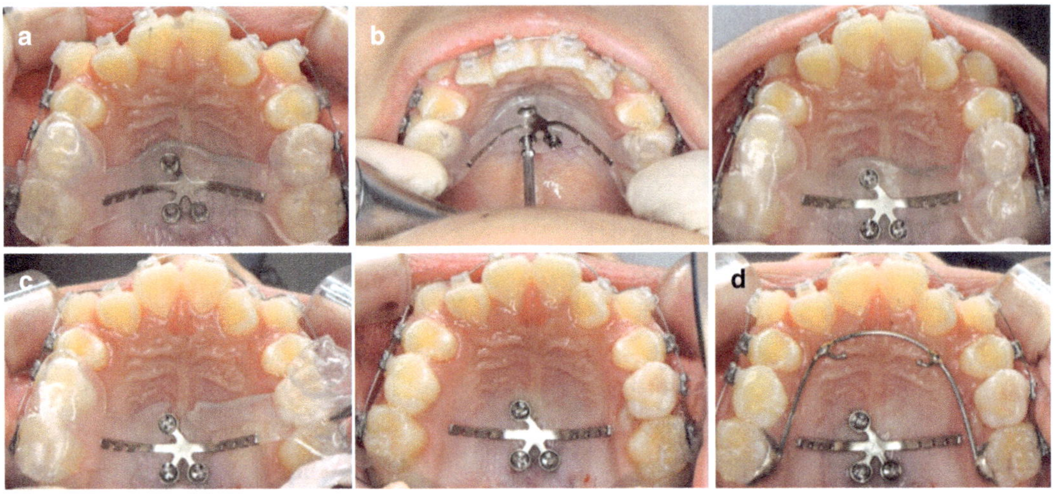

Fig. 5.3 (**a**) The Jig-MPAP assembly is placed in the patient's mouth; (**b**) the assistant is holding the jig while the operator is inserting the miniscrews; (**c**) removal of the jig using a utility plier; (**d**) a palatal bar is bonded to the first molars to start distalization (From Kook et al. [13])

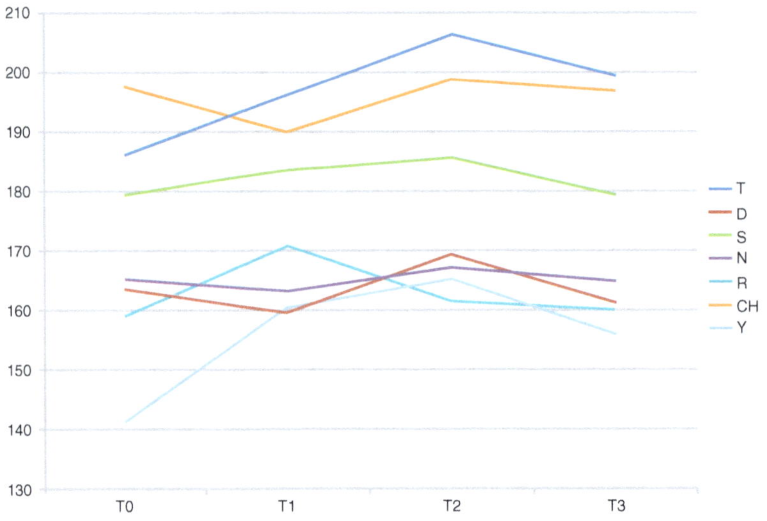

Fig. 5.4 Pitch of different sounds over time

performed using the Praat software (Paul Boersma and David Weenink, University of Amsterdam, Amsterdam, the Netherlands) to assess the pitch and the voice onset time (VOT) for each sound.

There were no significant changes in the pitch except for [r]; however, it changed back to normal after 1 week (Fig. 5.4). The sounds [t], [n], and [j] showed an increase in the VOT after MPAP placement followed by a decrease 1 week later. The VOT of [s] and [r] also increased after MPAP placement but decreased back to normal after 2 weeks (Fig. 5.5).

It was concluded that MPAP might cause speech alteration in some patients. However, adaptation to the placement of MPAP appliance occurs within 1–2 weeks. Therefore, the clinician should advice patient and/or parents regarding

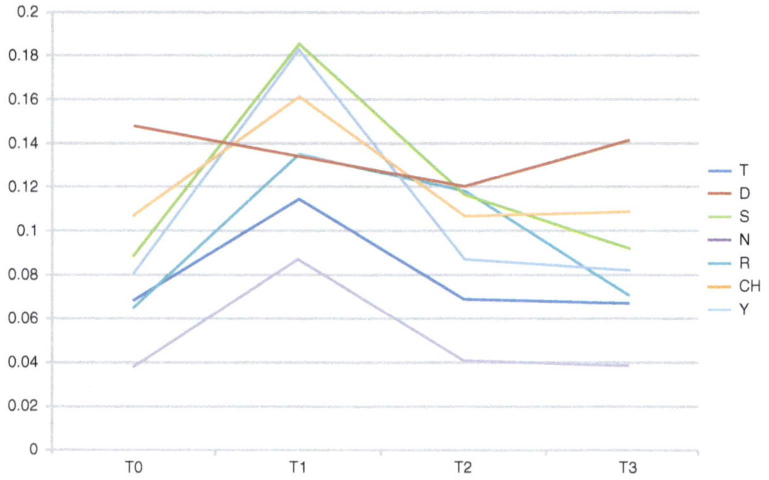

Fig. 5.5 VOT of different sounds over time

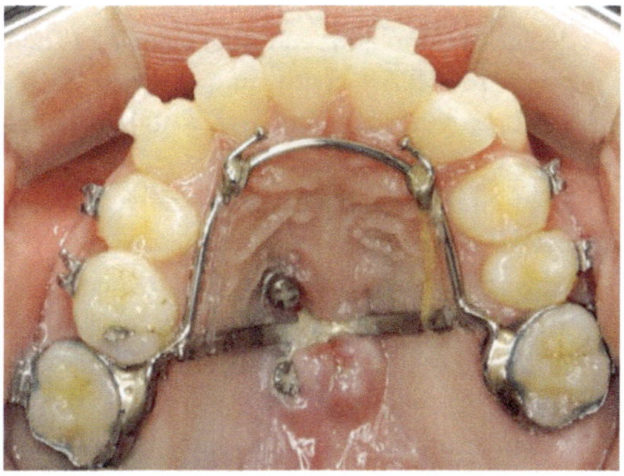

Fig. 5.6 Palatal soft tissue inflammation after placement of the early designs of the MPAP (From Kook et al. [13])

the possible temporary effect of the MPAP appliance on speech prior to its placement.

Inflammation

Inflammation of the palatal soft tissue was commonly encountered in the early designs of the MPAP. This might have been due to the uneven positioning of the palatal arms during placement, the close contact between the plate and palatal soft tissue which results in impingement on the soft tissues due to micro-movement of the plate, and the difficulty in the maintenance of oral hygiene (Fig. 5.6).

5.4 The Design Improvements of the MPAP

The design of the palatal plate has been modified several times to cope with the needs of the patient and the operator for easier and more accurate placement and less irritation to the tissues.

5.4.1 Screw Tubes

Tubes have been added to the screw holes to prevent or decrease soft tissue inflammation and overgrowth that might result from tissue impingement under the prototype of the MPAP. These tubes encountered the micro-movements of the plate under the distalization forces especially the torquing element. In addition, it might provide a plate-bone contact, which leads to reduction of the possibility of inducing inflammation on the soft tissue around the MPAP (Fig. 5.7).

5.4.2 Angulated Arms

In some of the cases treated by the early design of the MPAP, the palatal bar becomes too close to the arms of the MPAP, and consequently, the distalization forces were decreased due to a very small range of action. This was corrected by

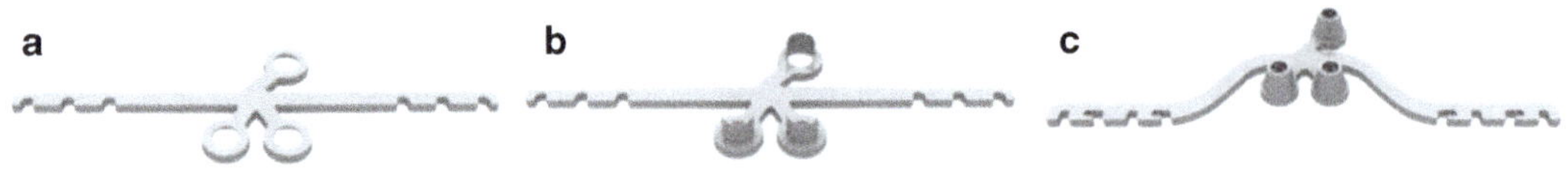

Fig. 5.7 Design improvement of the MPAP. (a) Prototype; (b) half tube extensions on the screw holes; (c) final design: screw tubes, angulated arms, and modified notches (From Kook et al. [13])

manufacturing of a new palatal bar and in fewer cases by replacing the MPAP more posteriorly. However, this was perceived as undue waste of time and cost. Therefore, instead of having straight arms as in the prototype of the MPAP, the final design has been modified to have posteriorly angulated arms to increase the range of action (Fig. 5.7).

5.4.3 Modified Hooks (Notches)

The notches on the prototype were difficult to engage due to its shape and size that made it difficult for the clinician to place the elastic chain or the coil spring. Also, the elastic chain and coil spring were liable for easy disengagement during patients' activities such as teeth brushing or flossing. Therefore, the shape of the notch was modified by adding a vertical extension at its opening to prevent the slippage of the elastic chain (Fig. 5.7). In addition, this has allowed for the use of the plate for intrusion of the posterior teeth. Moreover, a fourth notch has been added to have better control over the force vector especially in patients with deep palatal vault.

5.4.4 Jig

The installation of the palatal plate has been a difficult procedure in which the assistant has to hold the plate accurately in place while the operator is placing the miniscrews. It was difficult to prevent the rotation of the MPAP during the miniscrew placement and to ensure the evenness and consistency of the space between the MPAP arms and the palatal soft tissue. Therefore, to facilitate the installation procedures and ensure the symmetry of the placement, a silicone jig was applied to hold the MPAP in position during the placement of the miniscrews.

The jig fabrication procedure is as follows:

1. Stabilize the MPAP in its appropriate location on the working cast by making shallow indentations for the screw tubes. Adapt the plate and arms to the contour of the palate (Fig. 5.8a).
2. Place a layer of silicone material across the palate and extending over the occlusal surfaces of the second premolars (or second deciduous molars) and first molars. Then, press the MPAP gently into position on the silicone, guided by the screw-tube indentations on the cast (Fig. 5.8b).
3. Heat-cure the silicone and remove the jig-MPAP assembly from the cast.
4. Clear the screw tubes from the silicone plugs. To facilitate the removal of the jig after MPAP installation, slice diagonally through the silicone (Fig. 5.8c).
5. Sterilize the jig-MPAP assembly in ethylene oxide gas for 24 h.

5.5 Treatment Outcome of the MPAP

The amount of distalization and the dental effect of the MPAP appliance have been evaluated on 46 sets of pre- and posttreatment lateral cephalograms created from CBCT images of consecutively treated Class II adult patients [62].

Clinically successful distalization was achieved in 11.6±4.3 months. The maxillary first molar showed a mean of 3.70±1.81 mm of distalization, 3.29°±7.01° of distal tipping, and 2.40±2.78 mm of intrusion. The maxillary central incisors showed 3.56±3.58 mm of retraction, with a retroclination angle of 8.92°±6.81° and no significant change in the vertical position (Fig. 5.9).

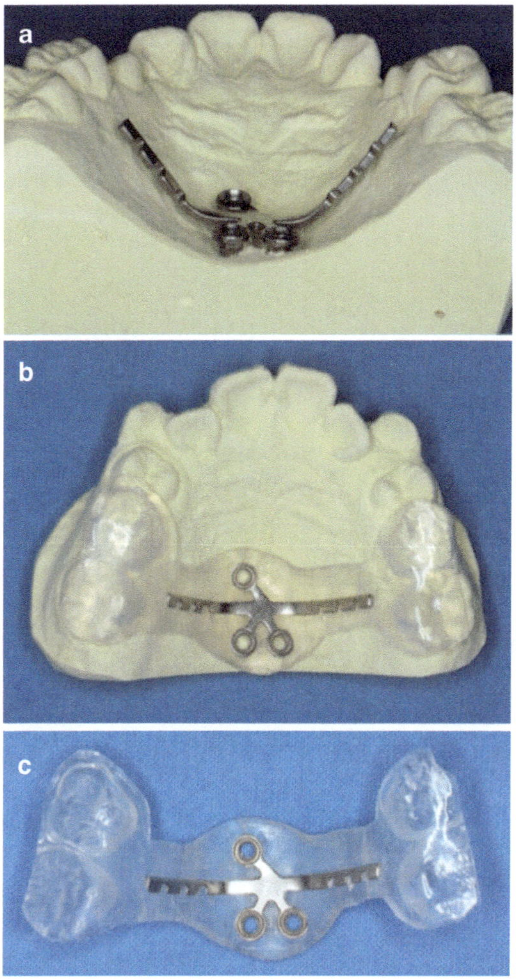

Fig. 5.8 (**a**) MPAP adapted to the contour of the palate leaving approximately 2 mm between the arms and the palatal soft tissue; (**b**) MPAP positioned into a silicon layer placed across the palate; (**c**) the Jig after being heat-cured and diagonally sliced (*dashed line*) (From Kook et al. [13])

Regarding mandibular central incisor and first molar, the amount of distalization was 2.57±2.97 and 1.41±2.95 mm, respectively. There was no significant change in the vertical position of the central incisors. The first molar showed about 1-mm intrusion. There were no significant differences in the angulation of the mandibular dentition.

The upper and lower lips were retracted about 2 mm. The nasolabial angle was significantly increased to be 103.8°. There was a clockwise rotation of the occlusal plane angle. However, the palatal plane angle was not changed.

5.6 Case Presentation

A 12-year-old girl was presented with a chief complaint of protrusive upper lip. She had skeletal Class II, Class I molar, and Class II canine relationships, a retruded chin, a convex facial profile, a mild crowding in both arches, and a 5-mm overjet (Fig. 5.10). Her parents denied extraction treatment. Therefore, full-arch distalization using MPAP was decided.

After leveling of the upper dentition, the second-generation MPAP was installed in the patient's mouth using a silicone jig. Then, a palatal bar made of stainless steel wire (1 mm in diameter) was soldered to the upper first molar bands. A distalizing force of about 250 g was applied on each side through a power chain connecting the palatal bar hook and the MPAP arm. After 14 months of treatment, upper and lower 0.019″×0.025″ stainless steel archwires were

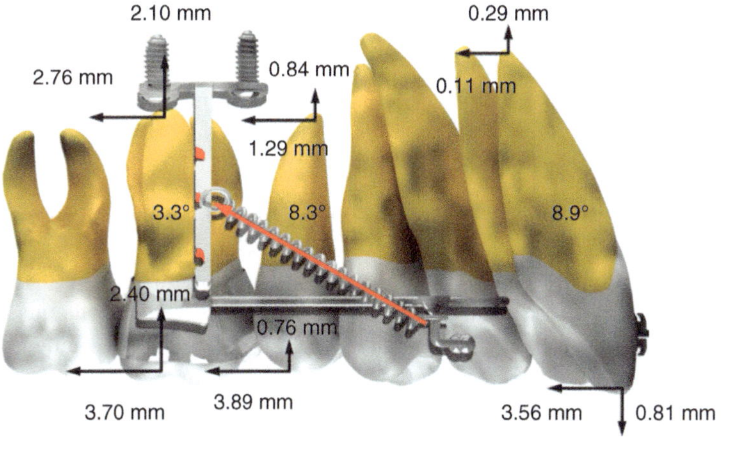

Fig. 5.9 Amount and direction of dental movement after distalization using MPAP appliance (Kook et al. [62])

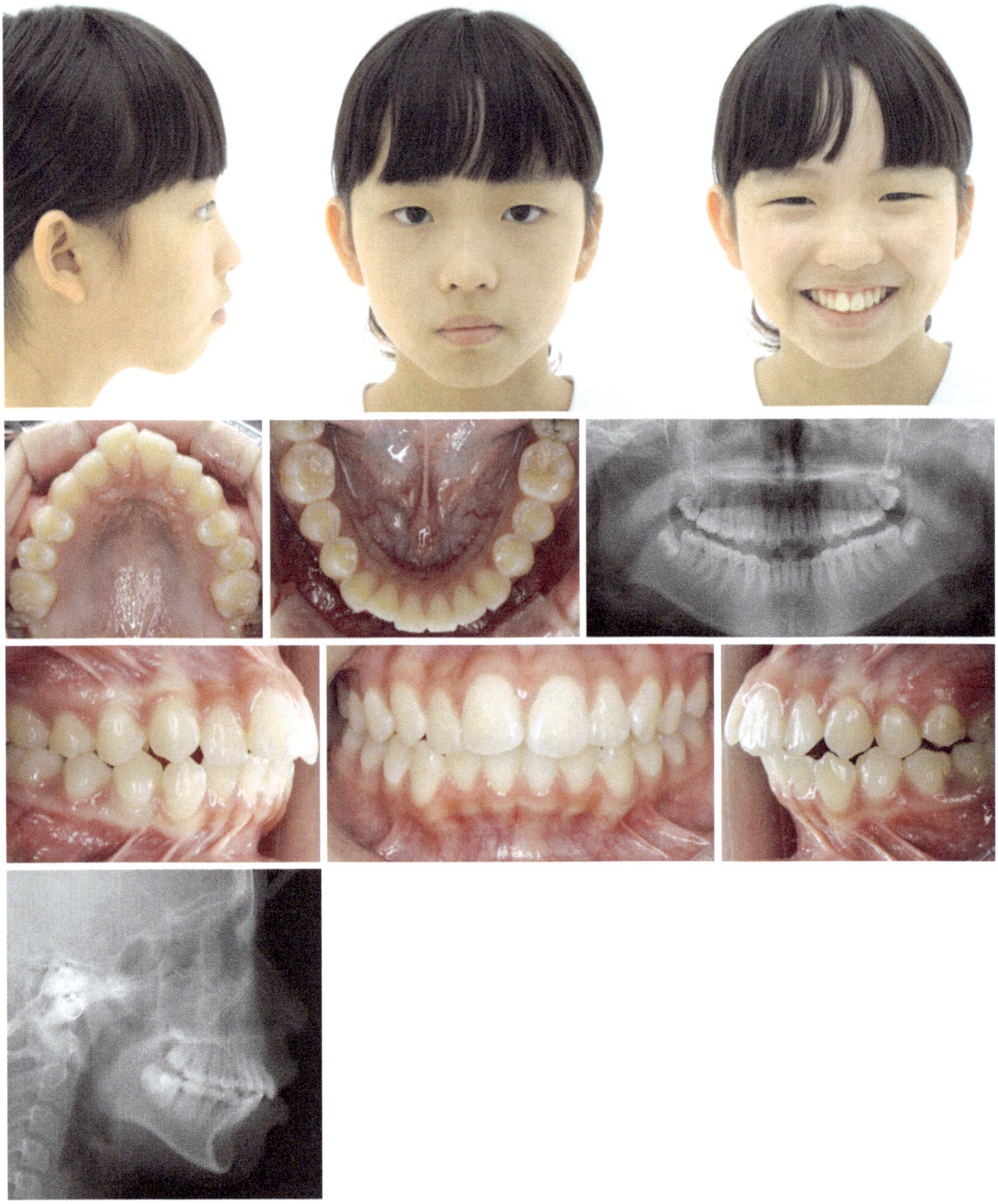

Fig. 5.10 Pretreatment records of a 12-year-old girl with convex facial profile, skeletal Class II relationship, and vertical growth pattern (From Kook et al. [12])

placed (Fig. 5.11). Class III elastics were then used for retraction of the lower dentition.

There were no noticeable signs of inflammation of the palatal soft tissue during active treatment. After removal of the MPAP, the mucosal tissue of the palate regenerated quickly, and healing by secondary intention occurred within a few days.

After 33 months of treatment, the protrusion of the upper lip had been resolved, and adequate overjet and overbite have been achieved (Fig. 5.12). The upper molars demonstrated

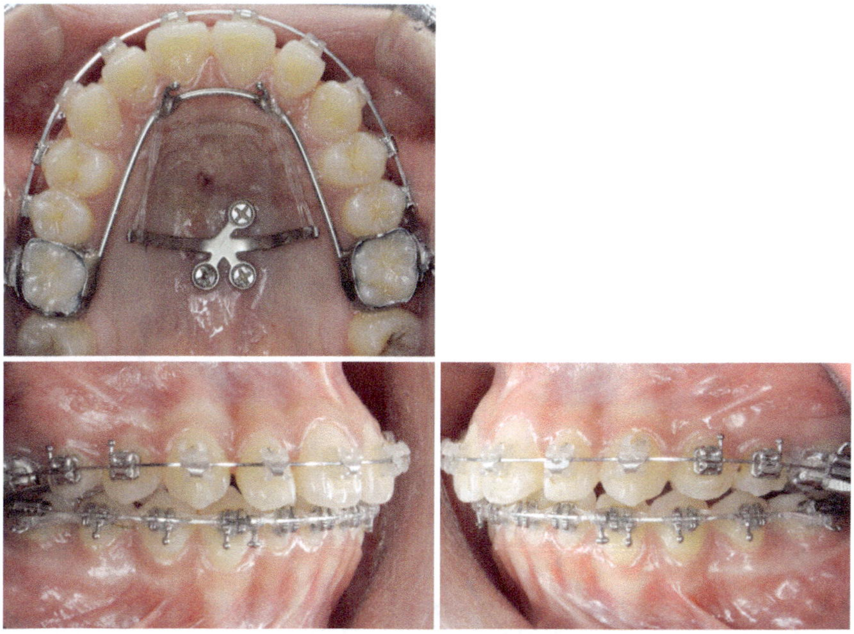

Fig. 5.11 After 14 months of treatment, *upper* and *lower* 0.019″ × 0.025″ stainless steel archwires were placed (From Kook et al. [12])

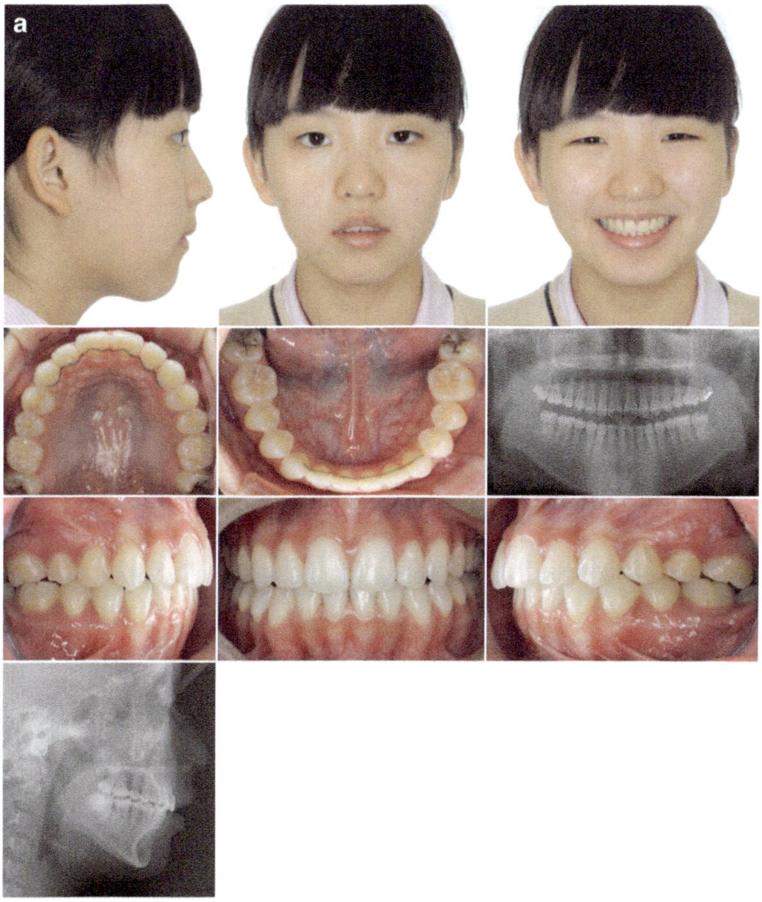

Fig. 5.12 (**a**) Debonding records after 33 months of treatment; (**b**) superimposition of pre- and posttreatment lateral cephalometric tracings; (**c**) 3D superimposition of CBCT images showing an axial section passing through the CEJ of the maxillary first molars (*left*) and a sagittal section passing through the left (From Kook et al. [12])

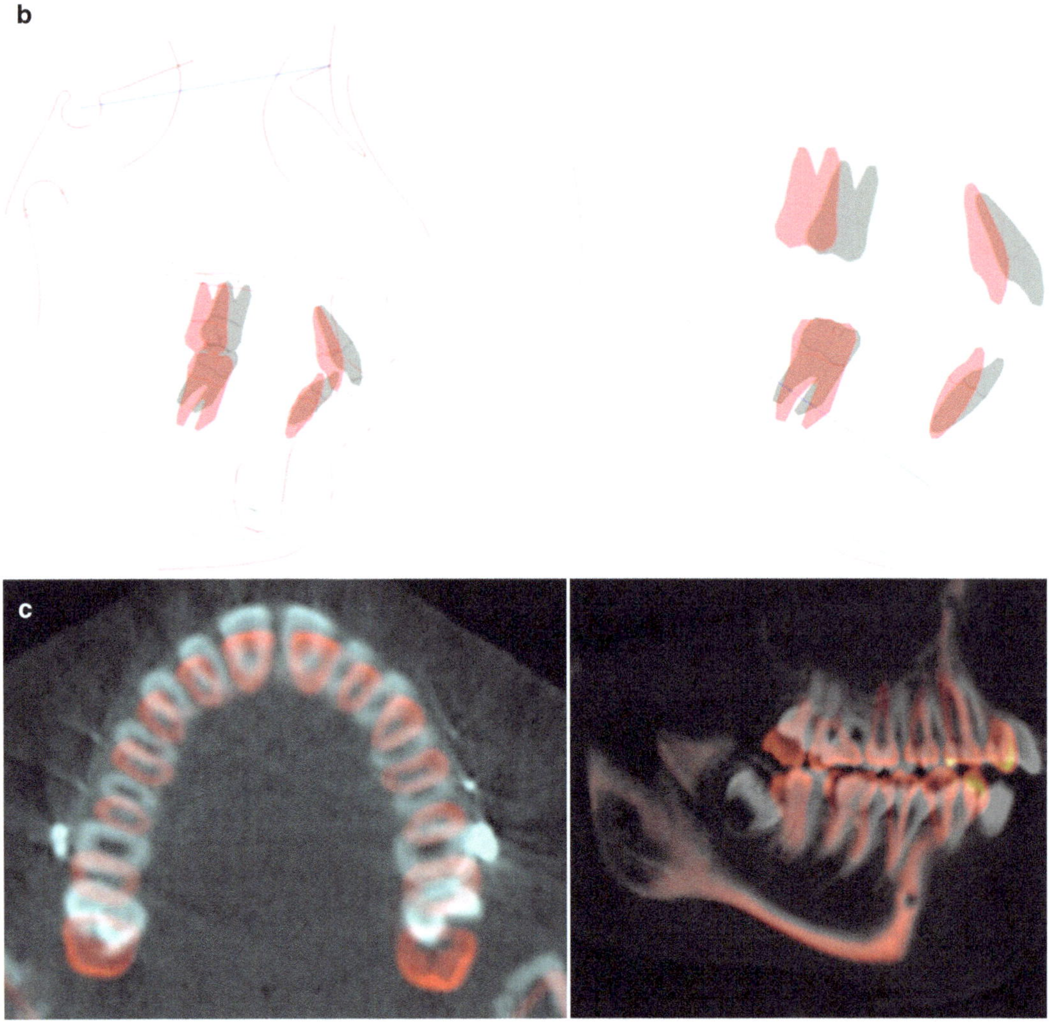

Fig. 5.12 (continued)

more root than crown movement. The patient's three remaining third molars were extracted after debonding. Ten months posttreatment, records showed a stable occlusion with good molar positions and a pleasant profile (Fig. 5.13).

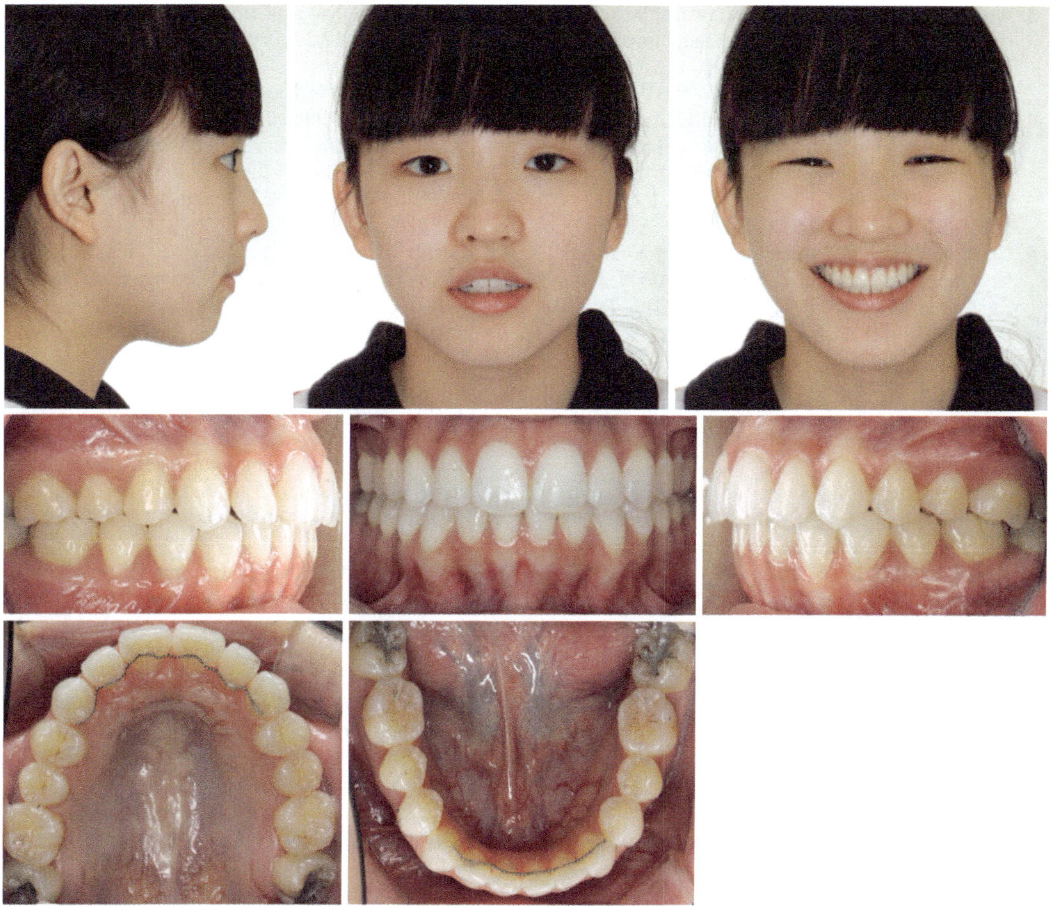

Fig. 5.13 Ten months posttreatment records (From Kook et al. [12])

Conclusion

The paramedian area of the palate provides a safe site for TSADs installation with sufficient bone quantity and quality and acceptable soft tissue thickness. The MPAP offers a simple and effective nonextraction approach for distalization of the maxillary dentition with a relatively true bodily movement of the maxillary first molars. The new features of the MPAP made the system more versatile, easier to install, and comfortable for the patients. The MPAP may result in alteration of the pronunciation of few sounds; however, this effect disappears within 2 weeks. The MPAP is our appliance of choice for chin retrusion and moderate skeletal discrepancies requiring more than 3 mm of distalization, in both adults and adolescents.

References

1. Fields HW, Proffit WR. Treatment of skeletal problems in children and preadolescents. In: Proffit WR, Fields HW, Sarver DM, editors. Contemporary orthodontics. 5th ed. St. Louis: Mosby Elsevier; 2013. p. 507.
2. Bolla E, Muratore F, Carano A, Bowman SJ. Evaluation of maxillary molar distalization with the distal jet: a comparison with other contemporary methods. Angle Orthod. 2002;72(5):481–94. PubMed PMID: 12401059. Epub 2002/10/29. eng.

3. Bussick TJ, McNamara Jr JA. Dentoalveolar and skeletal changes associated with the pendulum appliance. Am J Orthod Dentofacial Orthop. 2000;117(3):333–43. PubMed PMID: 10715093. Epub 2000/03/14. eng.
4. Chiu PP, McNamara Jr JA, Franchi L. A comparison of two intraoral molar distalization appliances: distal jet versus pendulum. Am J Orthod Dentofacial Orthop. 2005;128(3):353–65. PubMed PMID: 16168332. Epub 2005/09/20. eng.
5. Ghosh J, Nanda RS. Evaluation of an intraoral maxillary molar distalization technique. Am J Orthod Dentofacial Orthop. 1996;110(6):639–46. PubMed PMID: 8972811. Epub 1996/12/01. eng.
6. Muse DS, Fillman MJ, Emmerson WJ, Mitchell RD. Molar and incisor changes with Wilson rapid molar distalization. Am J Orthod Dentofacial Orthop. 1993;104(6):556–65. PubMed PMID: 8249931. Epub 1993/12/01. eng.
7. Keles A, Sayinsu K. A new approach in maxillary molar distalization: intraoral bodily molar distalizer. Am J Orthod Dentofacial Orthop. 2000;117(1):39–48. PubMed PMID: 10629518.
8. Kinzinger GS, Eren M, Diedrich PR. Treatment effects of intraoral appliances with conventional anchorage designs for non-compliance maxillary molar distalization: a literature review. Eur J Orthod. 2008;30(6):558–71. PubMed PMID: 18820306.
9. Fontana M, Cozzani M, Caprioglio A. Soft tissue, skeletal and dentoalveolar changes following conventional anchorage molar distalization therapy in class II non-growing subjects: a multicentric retrospective study. Prog Orthod. 2012;13(1):30–41. PubMed PMID: 22583585.
10. Ishida T, Yoon HS, Ono T. Asymmetrical distalization of maxillary molars with zygomatic anchorage, improved superelastic nickel-titanium alloy wires, and open-coil springs. Am J Orthod Dentofacial Orthop. 2013;144(4):583–93. PubMed PMID: 24075667.
11. Kaya B, Sar C, Arman-Ozcirpici A, Polat-Ozsoy O. Palatal implant versus zygoma plate anchorage for distalization of maxillary posterior teeth. Eur J Orthod. 2013;35(4):507–14. PubMed PMID: 22968670.
12. Kook YA, Kim SH, Chung KR. A modified palatal anchorage plate for simple and efficient distalization. J Clin Orthod. 2010;44(12):719–30, quiz 43. PubMed PMID: 21591548.
13. Kook YA, Lee DH, Kim SH, Chung KR. Design improvements in the modified C-palatal plate for molar distalization. J Clin Orthod. 2013;47(4):241–8, quiz 67–8. PubMed PMID: 23660818.
14. Ludwig B, Glasl B, Kinzinger GS, Walde KC, Lisson JA. The skeletal frog appliance for maxillary molar distalization. J Clin Orthod. 2011;45(2):77–84, quiz 91. PubMed PMID: 21710878.
15. Sar C, Kaya B, Ozsoy O, Ozcirpici AA. Comparison of two implant-supported molar distalization systems. Angle Orthod. 2013;83(3):460–7. PubMed PMID: 23106546.
16. Valiyaparambil JV, Yamany I, Ortiz D, Shafer DM, Pendrys D, Freilich M, et al. Bone quality evaluation: comparison of cone beam computed tomography and subjective surgical assessment. Int J Oral Maxillofac Implants. 2012;27(5):1271–7. PubMed PMID: 23057044.
17. Parsa A, Ibrahim N, Hassan B, Motroni A, van der Stelt P, Wismeijer D. Influence of cone beam CT scanning parameters on grey value measurements at an implant site. Dentomaxillofac Radiol. 2013;42(3):79884780. PubMed PMID: 22933535. Pubmed Central PMCID: 3667541.
18. Kaya S, Yavuz I, Uysal I, Akkus Z. Measuring bone density in healing periapical lesions by using cone beam computed tomography: a clinical investigation. J Endod. 2012;38(1):28–31. PubMed PMID: 22152615.
19. Fuster-Torres MA, Penarrocha-Diago M, Penarrocha-Oltra D, Penarrocha-Diago M. Relationships between bone density values from cone beam computed tomography, maximum insertion torque, and resonance frequency analysis at implant placement: a pilot study. Int J Oral Maxillofac Implants. 2011;26(5):1051–6. PubMed PMID: 22010089.
20. Moon SH, Park SH, Lim WH, Chun YS. Palatal bone density in adult subjects: implications for mini-implant placement. Angle Orthod. 2010;80(1):137–44. PubMed PMID: 19852653. Epub 2009/10/27. eng.
21. Han S, Bayome M, Lee J, Lee YJ, Song HH, Kook YA. Evaluation of palatal bone density in adults and adolescents for application of skeletal anchorage devices. Angle Orthod. 2012;82(4):625–31. PubMed PMID: 22077190.
22. Misch CE. Density of bone: effect on treatment plans, surgical approach, healing, and progressive boen loading. Int J Oral Implantol. 1990;6(2):23–31. PubMed PMID: 2073394. Epub 1990/01/01. eng.
23. Bernhart T, Vollgruber A, Gahleitner A, Dortbudak O, Haas R. Alternative to the median region of the palate for placement of an orthodontic implant. Clin Oral Implants Res. 2000;11(6):595–601. PubMed PMID: 11168253. Epub 2001/02/13. eng.
24. Wehrbein H. Bone quality in the midpalate for temporary anchorage devices. Clin Oral Implants Res. 2009;20(1):45–9. PubMed PMID: 19126107. Epub 2009/01/08. eng.
25. Crismani AG, Bernhart T, Schwarz K, Celar AG, Bantleon HP, Watzek G. Ninety percent success in palatal implants loaded 1 week after placement: a clinical evaluation by resonance frequency analysis. Clin Oral Implants Res. 2006;17(4):445–50. PubMed PMID: 16907777. Epub 2006/08/16. eng.
26. Wehrbein H, Feifel H, Diedrich P. Palatal implant anchorage reinforcement of posterior teeth: a prospective study. Am J Orthod Dentofacial Orthop. 1999;116(6):678–86. PubMed PMID: 10587603. Epub 1999/12/10. eng.
27. Deguchi T, Nasu M, Murakami K, Yabuuchi T, Kamioka H, Takano-Yamamoto T. Quantitative evaluation of cortical bone thickness with computed tomographic scanning for orthodontic implants. Am J Orthod Dentofacial Orthop. 2006;129(6):721.e7–12. PubMed PMID: 16769488. Epub 2006/06/14. eng.

28. Kang S, Lee SJ, Ahn SJ, Heo MS, Kim TW. Bone thickness of the palate for orthodontic mini-implant anchorage in adults. Am J Orthod Dentofacial Orthop. 2007;131(4 Suppl):S74–81. PubMed PMID: 17448390. Epub 2007/04/24. eng.
29. King KS, Lam EW, Faulkner MG, Heo G, Major PW. Vertical bone volume in the paramedian palate of adolescents: a computed tomography study. Am J Orthod Dentofacial Orthop. 2007;132(6):783–8. PubMed PMID: 18068597. Epub 2007/12/11. eng.
30. Stockmann P, Schlegel KA, Srour S, Neukam FW, Fenner M, Felszeghy E. Which region of the median palate is a suitable location of temporary orthodontic anchorage devices? A histomorphometric study on human cadavers aged 15–20 years. Clin Oral Implants Res. 2009;20(3):306–12. PubMed PMID: 19397643. Epub 2009/04/29. eng.
31. Gracco A, Lombardo L, Cozzani M, Siciliani G. Quantitative cone-beam computed tomography evaluation of palatal bone thickness for orthodontic miniscrew placement. Am J Orthod Dentofacial Orthop. 2008;134(3):361–9. PubMed PMID: 18774082. Epub 2008/09/09. eng.
32. Ryu JH, Park JH, Vu Thi Thu T, Bayome M, Kim Y, Kook YA. Palatal bone thickness compared with cone-beam computed tomography in adolescents and adults for mini-implant placement. Am J Orthod Dentofacial Orthop. 2012;142(2):207–12. PubMed PMID: 22858330.
33. Melsen B. Palatal growth studied on human autopsy material. A histologic microradiographic study. Am J Orthod. 1975;68(1):42–54. PubMed PMID: 1056143. Epub 1975/07/01. eng.
34. Revelo B, Fishman LS. Maturational evaluation of ossification of the midpalatal suture. Am J Orthod Dentofacial Orthop. 1994;105(3):288–92. PubMed PMID: 8135215. Epub 1994/03/01. eng.
35. Schlegel KA, Kinner F, Schlegel KD. The anatomic basis for palatal implants in orthodontics. Int J Adult Orthodon Orthognath Surg. 2002;17(2):133–9. PubMed PMID: 12099317. Epub 2002/07/09. eng.
36. Wehrbein H, Merz BR, Diedrich P, Glatzmaier J. The use of palatal implants for orthodontic anchorage. Design and clinical application of the orthosystem. Clin Oral Implants Res. 1996;7:410–6.
37. Bernhart T, Freudenthaler J, Dortbudak O, Bantleon HP, Watzek G. Short epithetic implants for orthodontic anchorage in the paramedian region of the palate. A clinical study. Clin Oral Implants Res. 2001;12(6):624–31. PubMed PMID: 11737107. Epub 2001/12/12. eng.
38. Gracco A, Lombardo L, Cozzani M, Siciliani G. Quantitative evaluation with CBCT of palatal bone thickness in growing patients. Prog Orthod. 2006;7(2):164–74. PubMed PMID: 17143344. Epub 2006/12/05. Eng. ita.
39. Tosun T, Keles A, Erverdi N. Method for the placement of palatal implants. Int J Oral Maxillofac Implants. 2002;17(1):95–100. PubMed PMID: 11858579. Epub 2002/02/23. eng.
40. Enlow DH, Hans MG. Essentials of facial growth. Philadelphia: Saunders; 1996. p. 79–98.
41. Wara-aswapati N, Pitiphat W, Chandrapho N, Rattanayatikul C, Karimbux N. Thickness of palatal masticatory mucosa associated with age. J Periodontol. 2001;72(10):1407–12. PubMed PMID: 11699483.
42. Poggio PM, Incorvati C, Velo S, Carano A. "Safe zones": a guide for miniscrew positioning in the maxillary and mandibular arch. Angle Orthod. 2006;76(2): 191–7. PubMed PMID: 16539541.
43. Januario AL, Barriviera M, Duarte WR. Soft tissue cone-beam computed tomography: a novel method for the measurement of gingival tissue and the dimensions of the dentogingival unit. J Esthet Restor Dent. 2008;20(6):366–73; discussion 74. PubMed PMID: 19120781.
44. Barriviera M, Duarte WR, Januario AL, Faber J, Bezerra AC. A new method to assess and measure palatal masticatory mucosa by cone-beam computerized tomography. J Clin Periodontol. 2009;36(7):564–8. PubMed PMID: 19538329.
45. Song JE, Um YJ, Kim CS, Choi SH, Cho KS, Kim CK, et al. Thickness of posterior palatal masticatory mucosa: the use of computerized tomography. J Periodontol. 2008;79(3):406–12. PubMed PMID: 18315422.
46. Ueno D, Sato J, Igarashi C, Ikeda S, Morita M, Shimoda S, et al. Accuracy of oral mucosal thickness measurements using spiral computed tomography. J Periodontol. 2011;82(6):829–36. PubMed PMID: 21073331.
47. Lost C, Irion KM, Nussle W. Ultrasonic B-scans of the facial/oral periodontium in pigs. J Clin Periodontol. 1989;16(8):534–8. PubMed PMID: 2674205.
48. Uchida H, Kobayashi K, Nagao M. Measurement in vivo of masticatory mucosal thickness with 20 MHz B-mode ultrasonic diagnostic equipment. J Dent Res. 1989;68(2):95–100. PubMed PMID: 2645334.
49. Eger T, Muller HP, Heinecke A. Ultrasonic determination of gingival thickness. Subject variation and influence of tooth type and clinical features. J Clin Periodontol. 1996;23(9):839–45. PubMed PMID: 8891935.
50. Studer SP, Allen EP, Rees TC, Kouba A. The thickness of masticatory mucosa in the human hard palate and tuberosity as potential donor sites for ridge augmentation procedures. J Periodontol. 1997;68(2):145–51. PubMed PMID: 9058332.
51. Muller HP, Schaller N, Eger T. Ultrasonic determination of thickness of masticatory mucosa: a methodologic study. Oral Surg Oral Med Oral Pathol Oral Radiol Endod. 1999;88(2):248–53. PubMed PMID: 10468471.
52. Muller HP, Heinecke A, Schaller N, Eger T. Masticatory mucosa in subjects with different periodontal phenotypes. J Clin Periodontol. 2000;27(9): 621–6. PubMed PMID: 10983595.
53. Muller HP, Schaller N, Eger T, Heinecke A. Thickness of masticatory mucosa. J Clin Periodontol. 2000;27(6):431–6. PubMed PMID: 10883873.
54. Schulze RK, Curic D, D'Hoedt B. B-mode versus A-mode ultrasonographic measurements of mucosal thickness in vivo. Oral Surg Oral Med Oral Pathol

Oral Radiol Endod. 2002;93(1):110–7. PubMed PMID: 11805786.
55. Kim HJ, Yun HS, Park HD, Kim DH, Park YC. Soft-tissue and cortical-bone thickness at orthodontic implant sites. Am J Orthod Dentofacial Orthop. 2006;130(2):177–82. PubMed PMID: 16905061.
56. Lee SM, Park JH, Bayome M, Kim HS, Mo SS, Kook YA. Palatal soft tissue thickness at different ages using an ultrasonic device. J Clin Pediatr Dent. 2012;36(4):405–9. PubMed PMID: 23019841.
57. Gedrange T, Mai R, Mack F, Zietek M, Borsos G, Vegh A, et al. Evaluation of shape and size changes of bone and remodelled bone substitute after different fixation methods. J Physiol Pharmacol. 2008;59 Suppl 5:87–94. PubMed PMID: 19075329.
58. Moelans CB, ter Hoeve N, van Ginkel JW, ten Kate FJ, van Diest PJ. Formaldehyde substitute fixatives. Analysis of macroscopy, morphologic analysis, and immunohistochemical analysis. Am J Clin Pathol. 2011;136(4):548–56.
59. Vu T, Bayome M, Kook YA, Han SH. Evaluation of the palatal soft tissue thickness by cone-beam computed tomography. Korean J Orthod. 2012;42(6):291–6. PubMed PMID: 23323243. Pubmed Central PMCID: 3542449.
60. Cha BK, Lee YH, Lee NK, Choi DS, Baek SH. Soft tissue thickness for placement of an orthodontic mini-screw using an ultrasonic device. Angle Orthod. 2008;78(3):403–8. PubMed PMID: 18416626.
61. Joo MC. Evaluation of palatal plate effects on the speech articulation using acoustic analysis [Master]. Seoul: The Catholic University of Korea; 2012.
62. Kook YA, Bayome M, Trang VT, Kim HJ, Park JH, Kim KB, et al. Evaluation of treatment effects of a modified palatal anchorage plate for distalization using CBCT. Am J Orthod Dentofacial Orthop. In press.

6 The Temporary Skeletal Anchorage Device-Supported Frog Appliance

Kevin C. Walde and Eustaquio A. Araujo

Abstract

In an effort to deal with the compliance issue required of most systems developed for Class II correction, a number of noncompliance appliances have been developed. This chapter focuses on the fabrication, delivery, and use of the TSAD-supported Simplified Molar Distalizer or Frog appliance. Case selection is discussed and two examples of treated cases are presented. The TSAD-supported Frog appliance is an excellent appliance for correcting Class II molars and/or for opening space in the maxillary arch to alleviate a maxillary arch length discrepancy.

For years, the Class II malocclusion has been quite a challenge in deciding upon an orthodontic treatment plan. Because of this challenge, many methods have been devised to successfully manage this problem. The systems that have been developed include various headgears, many types of functional appliances, the use of coil springs, and perhaps the most widely used – elastics. All of the above work quite well. Yet, the majority of these systems depend on the most important ingredient of successful orthodontics – *compliance*. Without compliance treatment is often doomed to failure, particularly with adolescents [1].

In recent years, various noncompliance appliances have been developed to drive maxillary molars distally, including repelling magnets, the Jones Jig, the Pendulum appliance, the Distal Jet, and the Simplified Molar Distalizer, also known as the "Frog" (Forestadent USA) [2–6].

This chapter will focus on the temporary skeletal anchorage device (TSAD)-supported version of the "Frog" appliance. The Frog was originally developed as a tooth-borne appliance and can still be used in this fashion. The introduction of the mini-implant or "TSAD" to provide anchorage has dramatically improved the efficiency of the "Frog."

The appliance includes an expansion screw and a removable transpalatal arch (TPA) that connects the expansion screw to the maxillary first molars. The TPA is fabricated from 0.032-in. stainless steel or TMA wire with adjustment

K.C. Walde, DDS, MS (✉)
Walde Orthodontics,
1507 Heritage Hills Drive, Washington,
MO 63090, USA
e-mail: kwalde@sbcglobal.net

E.A. Araujo, DDS, MDS
Department of Orthodontics,
Center for Advanced Dental Education,
Saint Louis University, 3320 Rutger Street,
St. Louis, MO 63104, USA
e-mail: araujoea@slu.edu

K.B. Kim (ed.), *Temporary Skeletal Anchorage Devices*,
DOI 10.1007/978-3-642-55052-2_6, © Springer-Verlag Berlin Heidelberg 2014

loops used for fine-tuning and double back bends for insertion into the lingual sheaths of the upper first molar bands [6]. This combination is anchored to a pair of TSADs placed on either side of the midline of the anterior palate. It is attached to the TSADs using either a small, modified, acrylic Nance button or by soldering it to transfer abutments (OrthoEasy, Forestadent USA) that attach to the TSADs.

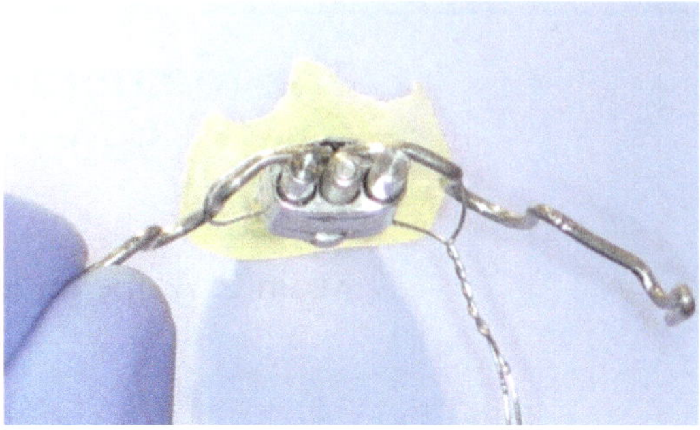

Fig. 6.1 The Frog appliance with trenching on the palatal side of the Nance button to allow insertion past the TSADs

6.1 Fabrication of the TSAD-Supported Frog with Nance Button Anchorage

Maxillary first molar bands with lingual sheaths are fitted and cemented. Place the TSADs in the anterior palate as close to the midline as possible for improved bony support [7]. An accurate maxillary impression is obtained including the palatal surface with the TSADs and the lingual sheaths of the molars. The body of the appliance is located at approximately the mesial edges of the lingual sheaths and 10–12 mm from the occlusal surface. It is sometimes necessary to move the appliance distally to provide better access for activation. It is important to keep it located approximately 10–12 mm from the occlusal surface so that it is near the center of resistance of the maxillary first molars. This helps maintain bodily movement of the molars rather than tipping. An acrylic button is fabricated from a light-cured acrylic gel (Triad). The palatal surface of the button is "trenched" to allow insertion of the appliance over the TSADs intraorally (Fig. 6.1). (Earlier versions used a "salt and pepper" acrylic button fixed to the TSADs with a fast-set self-curing acrylic.) The spring is adjusted so that the double back bends fit into the lingual sheaths of the molar bands. Five to ten degrees of "toe-in" can help prevent undesirable rotation of the molars. If slight expansion is desired, the spring can be adjusted laterally using adjustment loops on either side of the midline. The spring is generally "pre-activated" before initial insertion. The completed appliance is ready for delivery to the patient (Fig. 6.2).

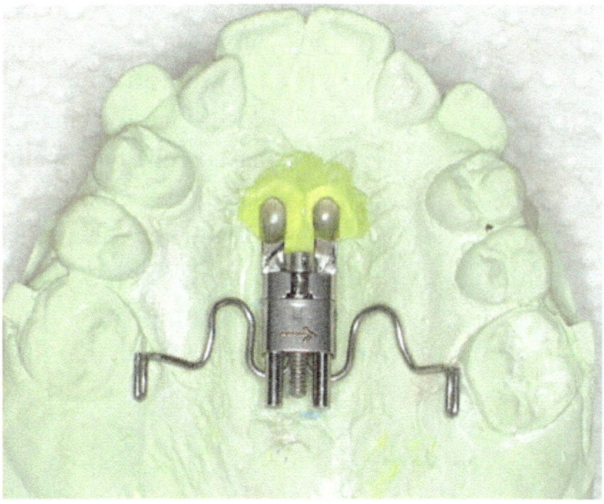

Fig. 6.2 The Nance button version of the Frog using Triad gel

6.2 Fabrication of the TSAD-Supported Frog with OrthoEasy Abutments

The "Skeletal Frog" was introduced in 2011 [7]. There are some modifications necessary when using OrthoEasy abutments to attach to the TSAD anchors. First of all, the TSADs are placed slightly farther apart (but still near the midline) to allow placement of the abutments without interference. If the TSADs are too close together, it becomes necessary to modify the abutments so they can be in place simultaneously. Also, the TSADs should be as parallel as possible for easier insertion of the finished appliance. After the bands are cemented and the TSADs are in place, the abutments are placed on the TSADs. A light

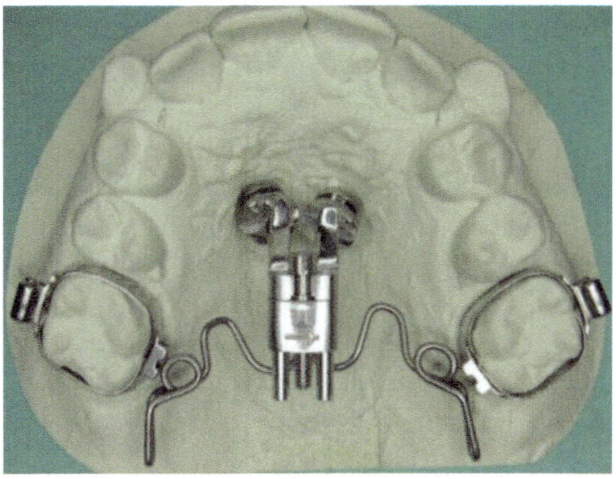

Fig. 6.3 The "Skeletal Frog" using OrthoEasy abutments (Photo courtesy of Dr. Bjorn Ludwig)

coating of petroleum jelly inside the abutments will prevent them from slipping off the TSADs before taking the impression. The abutments should come off with the impression as it is removed from the mouth. Analog TSADs are placed in the abutments that are now in the impression. The analogs and abutments are secured in the impression using a small amount of sticky wax. Care should be used when pouring the stone model to prevent the abutments and analog TSADs from dislodging from the impression. After the model has hardened, the abutments are removed from the impression and placed on the analogs. The body of the appliance is then positioned on the model and soldered to the abutments. The spring is adjusted as described earlier and the appliance is ready to deliver to the patient (Fig. 6.3). An advantage of the OrthoEasy abutments is the elimination of accumulating plaque and debris from under the acrylic Nance button [7].

6.3 Appliance Delivery

Delivering the appliance is relatively simple. The Nance button Frog appliance is tried in initially to be certain that the appliance will seat properly over the TSADs. If the appliance does not insert and seat smoothly, the "trenching" on the palatal surface may require modification. Once the appliance is in place, the Nance button can be lifted slightly off the palate with a scaler or explorer. A small amount of light-cured acrylic gel is placed over the TSADs, and the Nance button is then held in place over the TSADs using light pressure. Any excess acrylic can be wiped off with a cotton roll before light curing the appliance to fix it in place. The appliance is now ready for activation (Fig. 6.4).

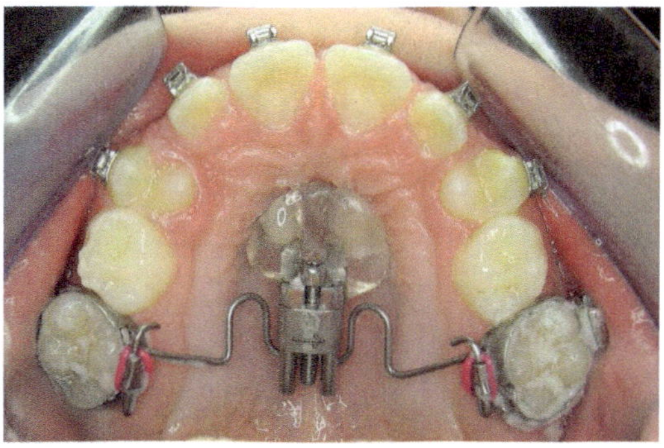

Fig. 6.4 The Triad gel version delivered and ready to be activated

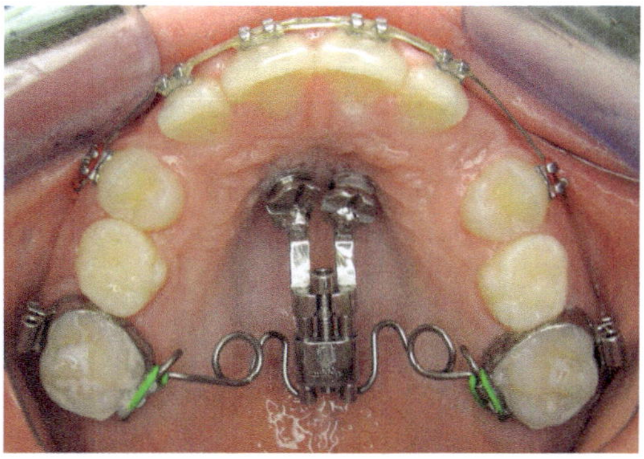

Fig. 6.5 The "Skeletal Frog" delivered and ready for activation (Photo courtesy of Dr. Bjorn Ludwig)

The OrthoEasy Frog appliance is also tried in to be certain that it seats properly. Depending on how parallel the TSADs are, it may be necessary to adjust the heads of the TSADs to allow parallel insertion of the abutments. When the appliance is ready for insertion, a small amount of *self-curing* composite is placed inside the abutments and placed over the TSADs. Any excess should be removed immediately. Once the composite is fully cured, the appliance is ready for activation (Fig. 6.5).

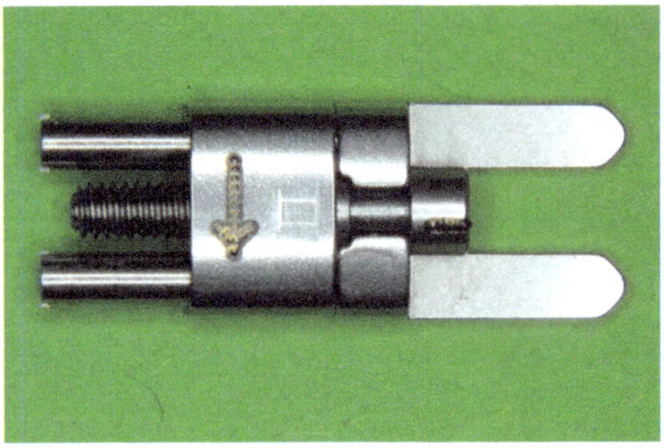

Fig. 6.6 Laser etching on the head of the screw is used to confirm activation. The laser etched *arrow* indicates the proper direction of activation (Photo courtesy of Dr. Bjorn Ludwig)

6.4 Activating the Appliance

A laser-etched marking on the head of the activation screw aids the clinician in confirming activation (Fig. 6.6). Each 360° turn of the screw provides 0.4 mm of activation. Typical activation is 3 turns (1.2 mm) per month or 5 turns (2 mm) per 2 months. If desired, the spring can be removed and adjusted.

6.5 Case Selection

Maxillary molar distalizers are indicated for a variety of conditions. Some of the conditions include malocclusions that have the following characteristics:

1. Class II molar relationship.
2. Maxillary crowding with a non-extraction mandibular arch and non-extraction treatment is desirable.
3. Normal or low mandibular plane angle.
4. Straight or flat profile.

Contraindications include:

1. A high mandibular plane angle
2. Anterior open bite
3. Mandibular arch that requires extractions
4. A protrusive profile where anterior retraction is desirable
5. Excessive overjet (this is less important or possibly not important with a TSAD-supported appliance)

The ideal treatment time is in the late mixed or early permanent dentition before the eruption of the maxillary second molars. However, the presence of erupted maxillary second molars does not preclude the use of the Frog appliance. Simultaneous distalization of the maxillary first and second molars may take slightly longer but is effective.

6.6 Treated Cases

Case 1

A completed case illustrates the effectiveness of the TSAD-supported Frog. An 11-year-old female presented for treatment to the orthodontic clinic at the Saint Louis University Center for Advanced Dental Education. The chief complaint was that "My canines are sticking out too much."

Facial evaluation showed harmony, competent lips, and appropriate gingival display. The profile was straight with adequate nasolabial angle.

Intra-arch dental evaluation presented ovoid symmetrical arch forms with minimal crowding of the mandibular arch and 11 mm of crowding of the maxillary arch resulting in blocked out maxillary canines. Second molars were already present in the oral cavity. Inter-arch examination showed Class II molars with overjet and overbite within normal limits. Cephalometric evaluation confirmed a Class II skeletal relationship.

The treatment plan consisted of a non-extraction approach with a TSAD-supported Frog distalizer, bonding of both arches, correction of the midlines and retention with a maxillary wraparound Hawley retainer, and a lower canine to canine fixed retainer.

Treatment was initiated as planned and the Frog was supported by two mini-screw implants.

In less than 2 years, treatment objectives were achieved and the final result shows a Class I occlusion in a well-balanced and harmonic face (Figs. 6.7, 6.8, 6.9, and 6.10).

Case 2

A 10-year-old female presented to private practice with a Class II malocclusion. The chief complaint was "crowded teeth and overbite."

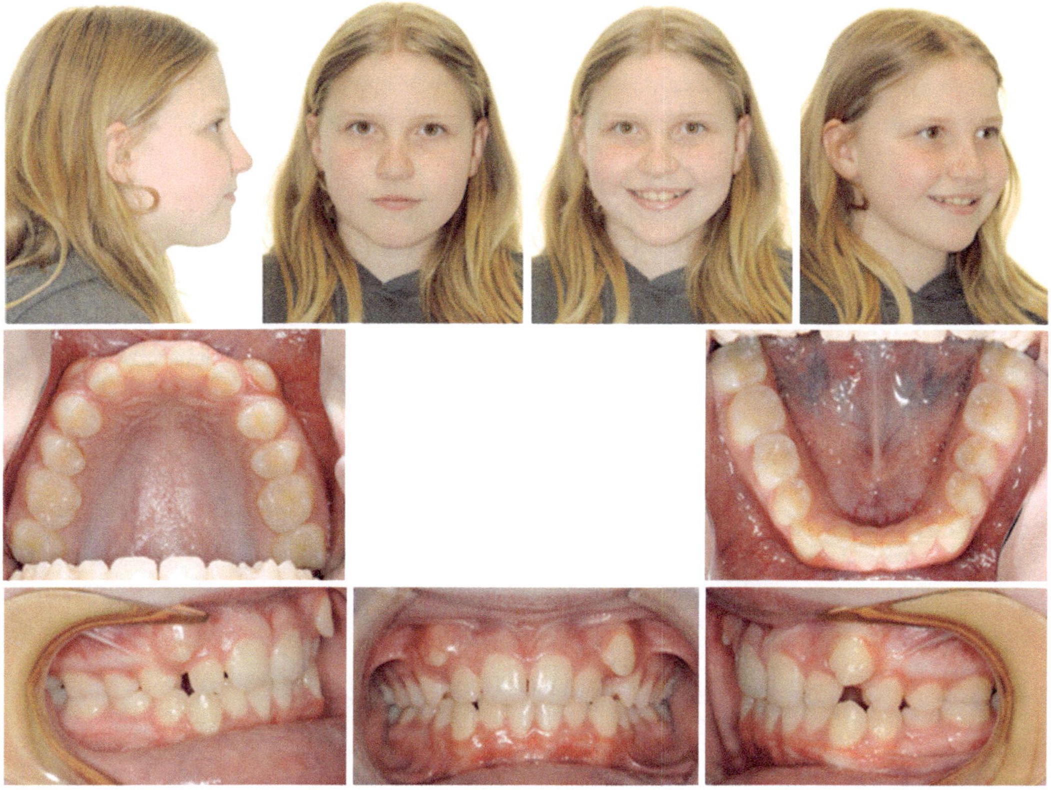

Fig. 6.7 Initial composite of Case 1

Facial evaluation demonstrated a retruded chin and slight lip incompetence with normal gingival display. The profile was convex with an obtuse nasolabial angle and prominent lower lip curl.

The dental arches were ovoid and symmetrical with minimal mandibular crowding. There was approximately 10 mm of crowding in the maxillary arch with moderate incisor protrusion. The maxillary and mandibular second molars were unerupted. Cephalometric evaluation confirmed a Class II skeletal relationship.

The Frog distalizer anchored against two TSADs placed in the anterior palate was placed. Molar distalization to a "super" Class I was accomplished in approximately 7.5 months (Fig. 6.11a–c). The patient's parents were then given the option of fixed appliances or aligners to complete the treatment. Fixed appliances were chosen and the maxillary and mandibular arches were bonded. The Frog appliance was left in place for 6 months to preserve the maxillary molar position, while initial leveling, alignment, and retraction of the anterior teeth were accomplished. Total treatment time was 27 months. Vacuum-formed slipcover retainers were used for retention (Fig. 6.12a–c).

A lateral superimposition of Case 2 (Fig. 6.13) demonstrates the distalization achieved utilizing the TSAD-supported Frog appliance. Note the relatively unchanged position of the maxillary incisors prior to placement of any other fixed appliances.

Previously, when using a tooth-borne Frog appliance, the presence of protruded maxillary incisors would have been a contraindication for its use. With the use of TSAD anchorage, the Frog can be used effectively without the risk of pushing the incisors anteriorly.

The lateral superimposition comparing initial, post-distalization, and posttreatment cephalometric

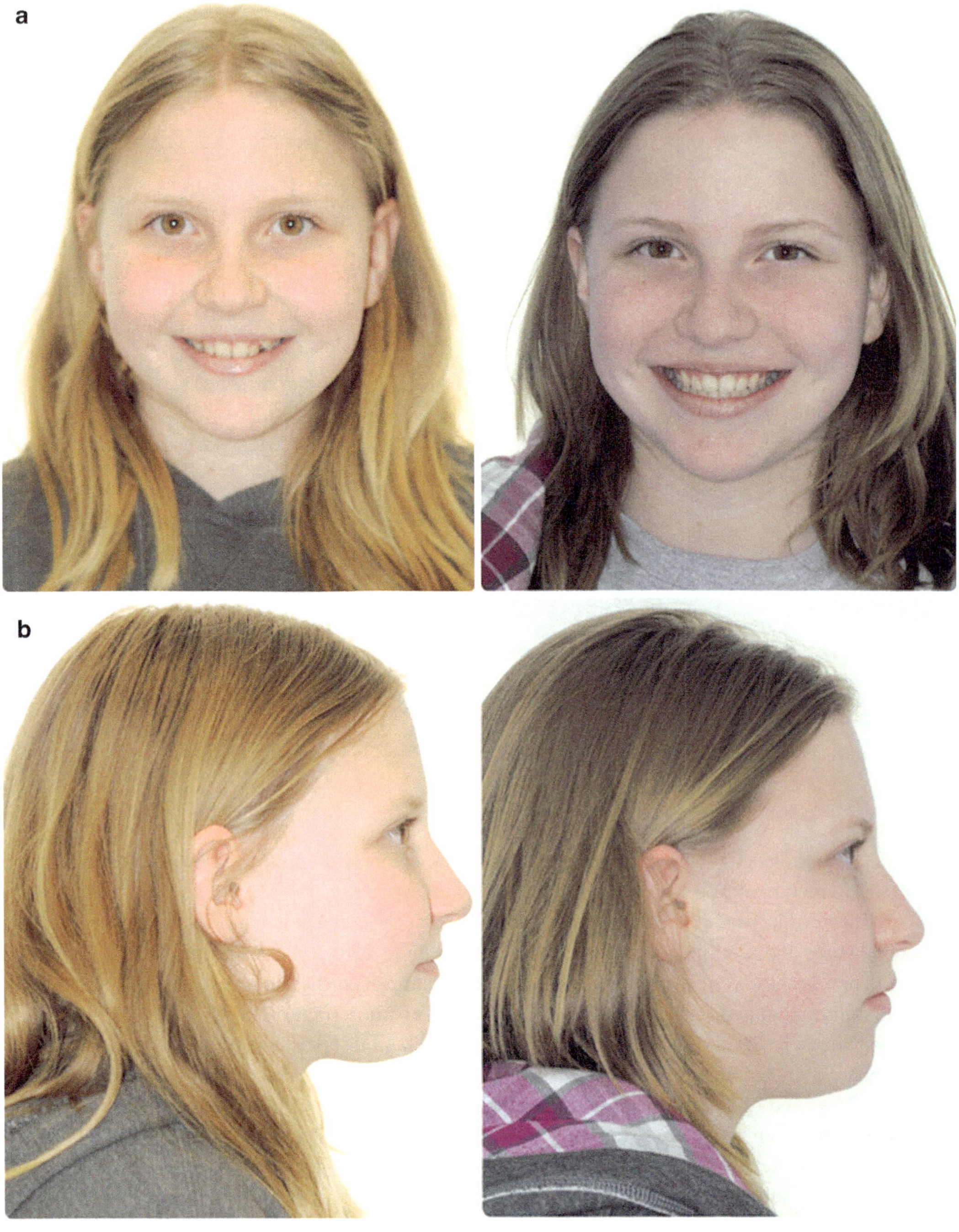

Fig. 6.8 (**a**) Case 1 pre- and posttreatment smiling photos. (**b**) Case 1 pre- and posttreatment profile photos

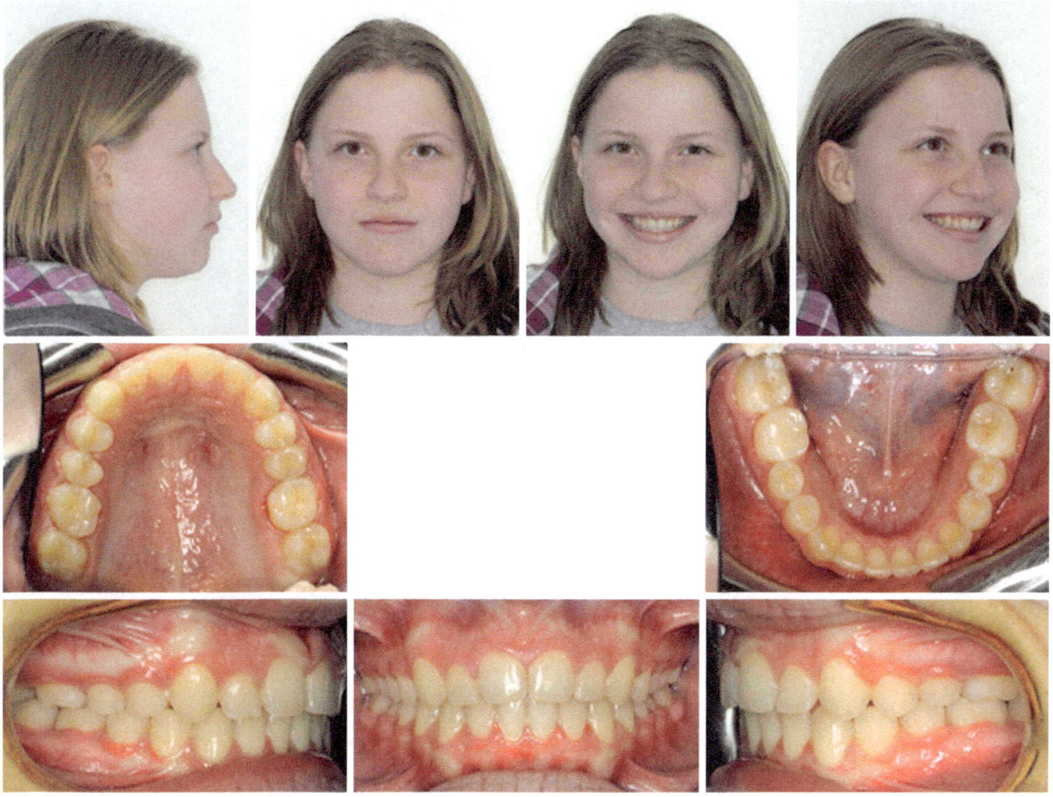

Fig. 6.9 Case 1 post-intraoral photos, right, left, and anterior

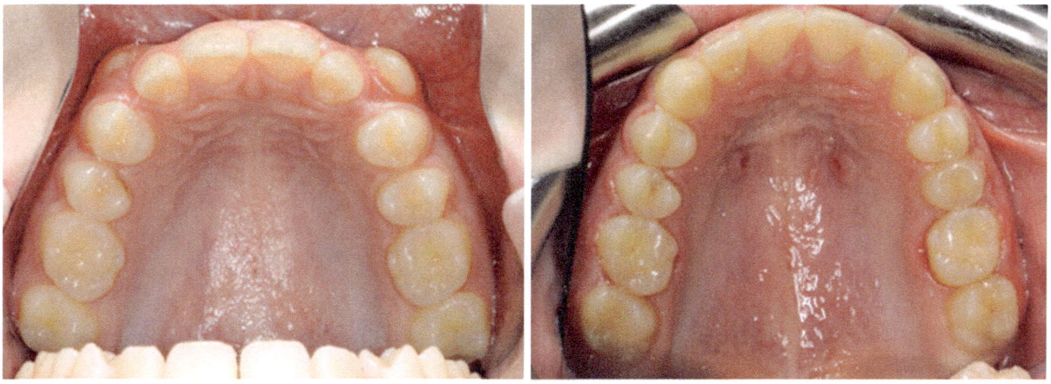

Fig. 6.10 Case 1 pre- and posttreatment maxillary occlusal photos

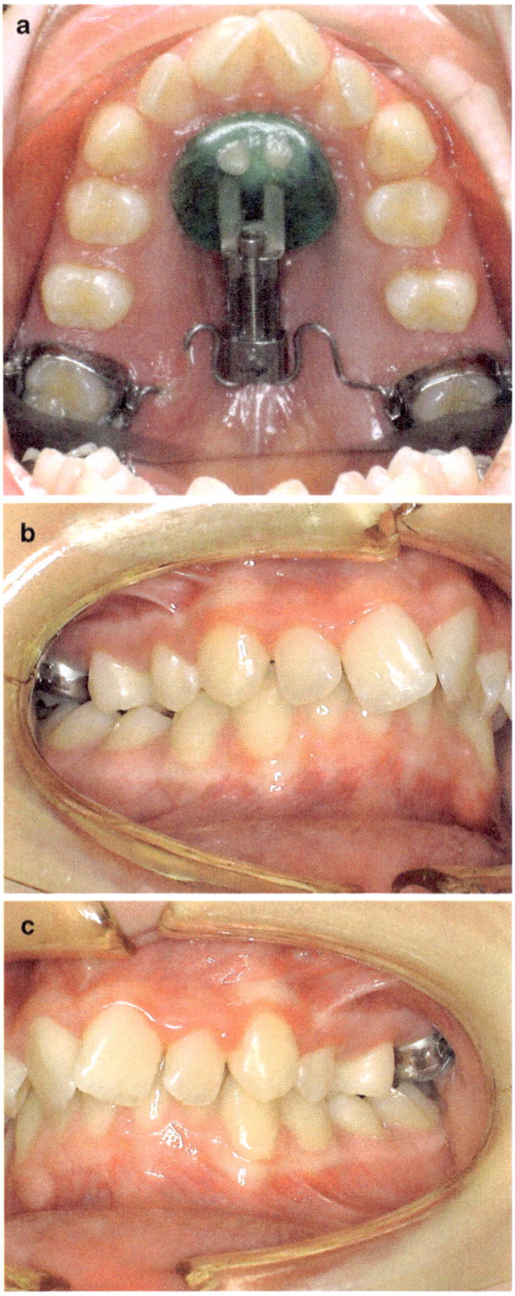

Fig. 6.11 (**a**) Case 2 maxillary occlusal photo after distalization. (**b**) Case 2 Frog removal right. (**c**) Frog removal left

a

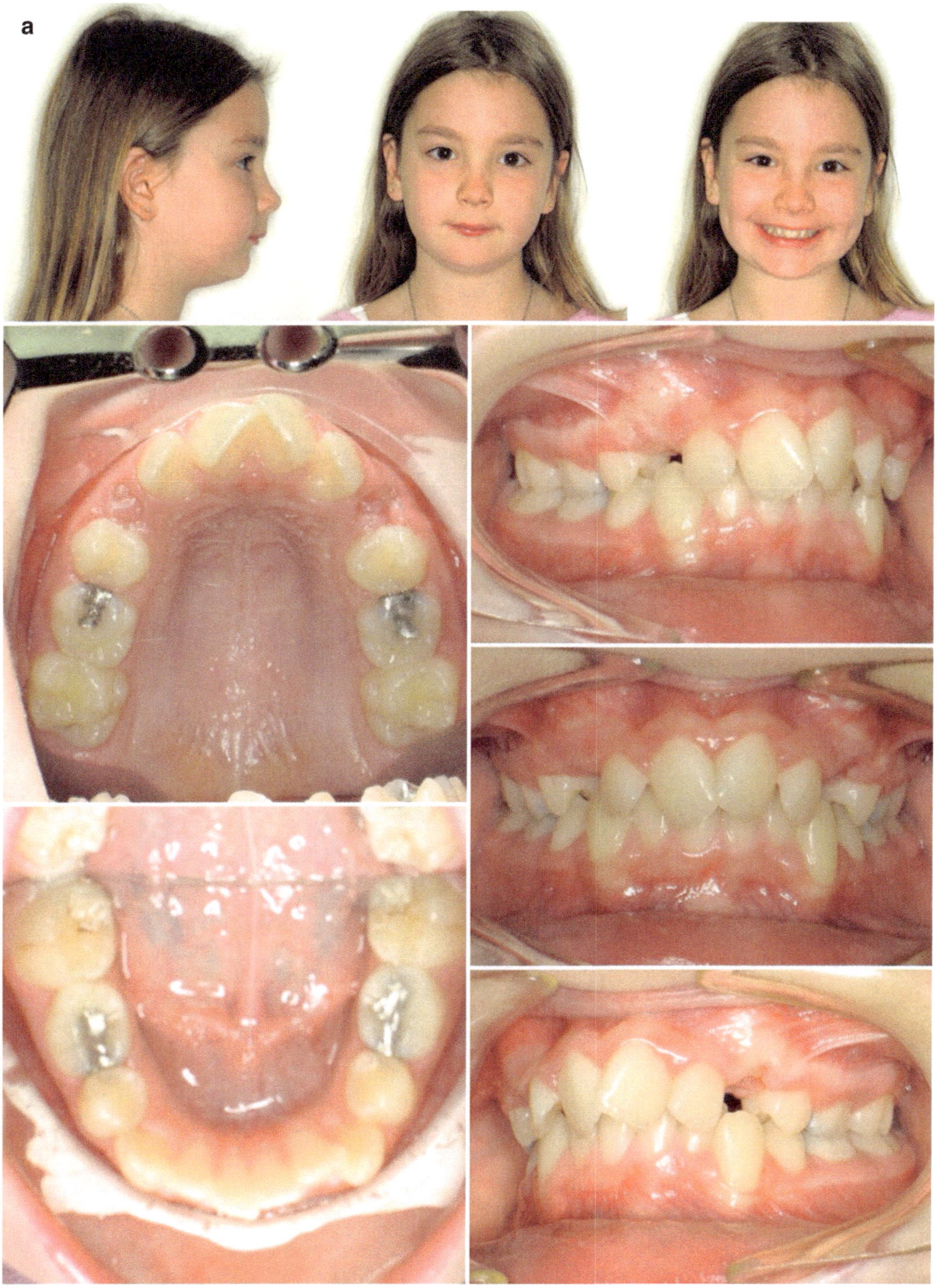

Fig. 6.12 (**a**) Initial composite of Case 2. (**b**) Case 2 composite at Frog removal. (**c**) Case 2 composite at appliance removal

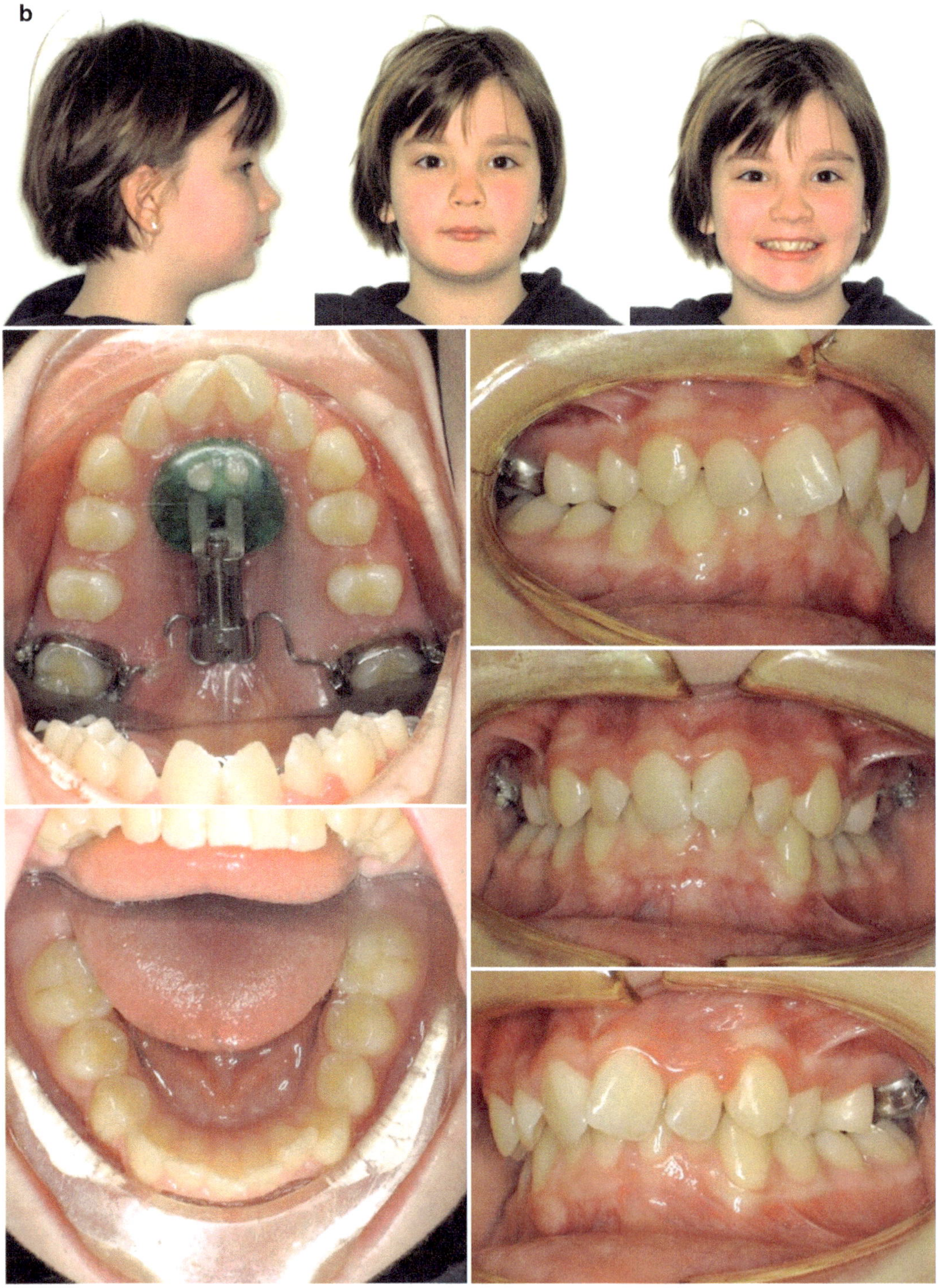

Fig. 6.12 (continued)

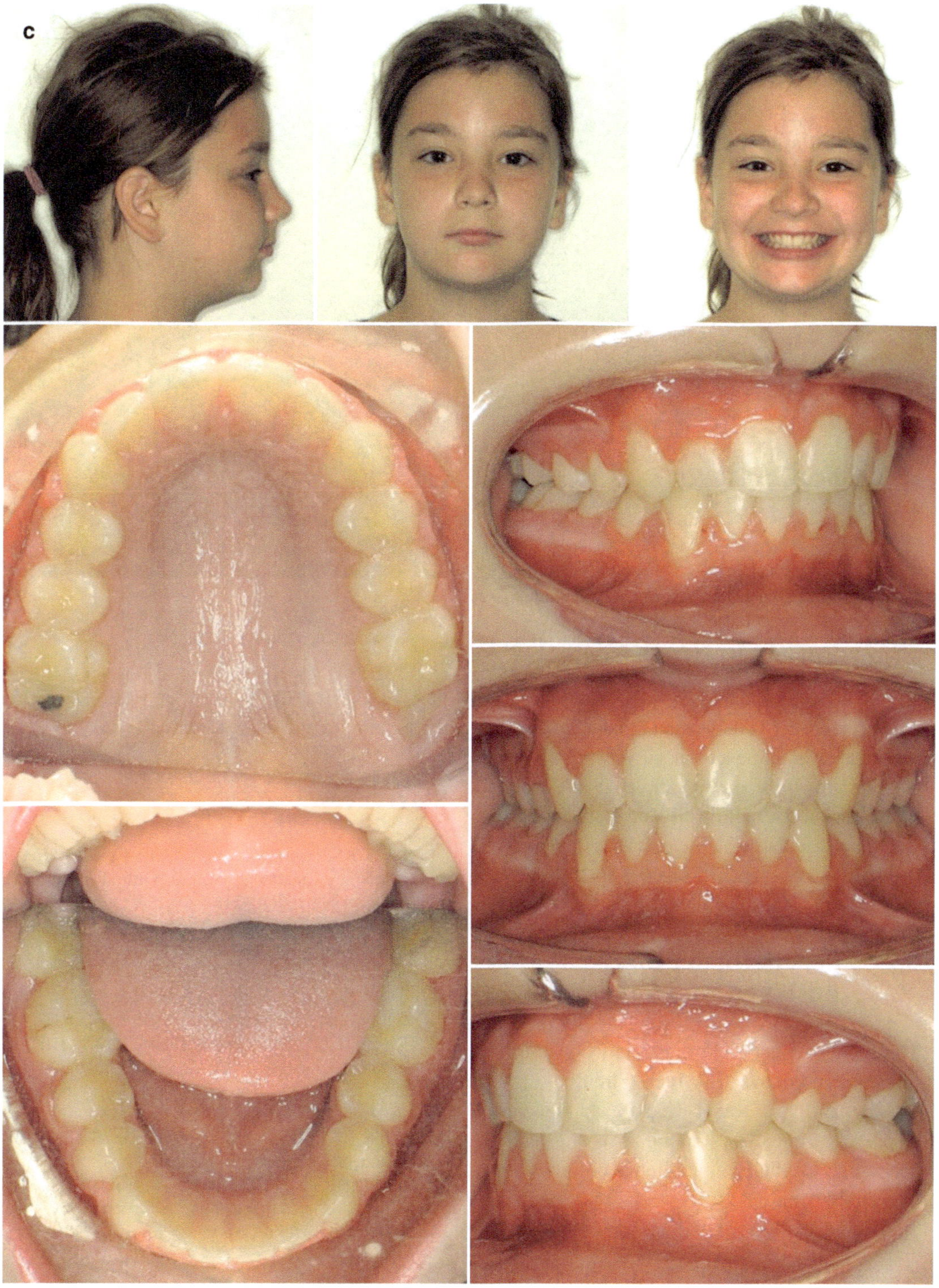

Fig. 6.12 (continued)

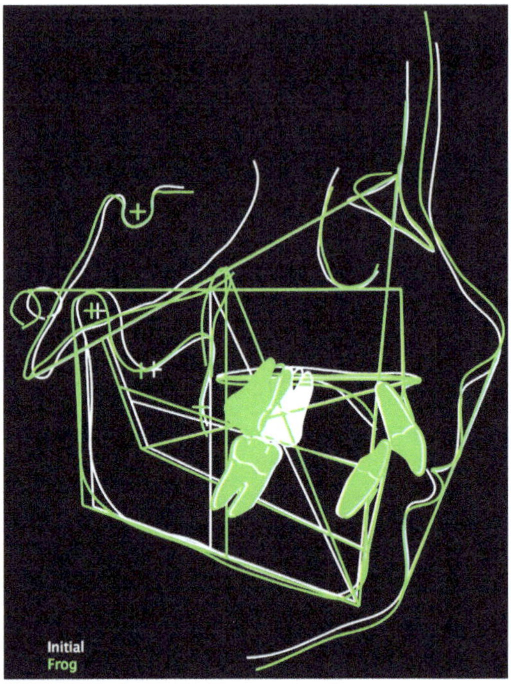

Fig. 6.13 Superimposition of pretreatment lateral cephalogram with Frog removal lateral cephalogram

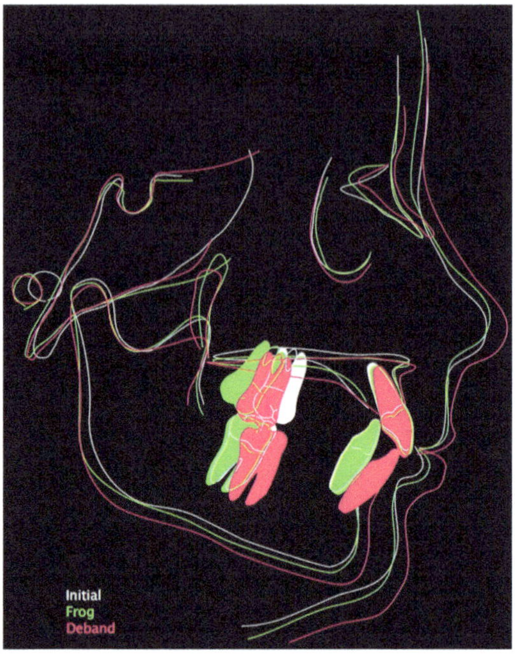

Fig. 6.14 Superimposition of pretreatment, Frog removal, and posttreatment lateral cephalograms

tracings (Fig. 6.14) shows that the outcome of this treatment was influenced positively by favorable anterior growth of the mandible. It also demonstrates that about half of the maxillary molar distalization was lost which emphasizes the need to overcorrect to a "super" Class I if possible.

6.7 Benefits of the TSAD-Anchored Frog Appliance

The TSAD-supported Frog is relatively simple to fabricate and deliver [6]. It is extremely easy to activate and is a very effective appliance for distalizing maxillary molars. Using TSAD anchorage for the Frog appliance eliminates any undesirable mesial forces on the teeth [7]. Additionally, the maxillary premolars can passively drift distally during activation reducing the amount of subsequent retraction required.

References

1. Nanda RS, Kierl MJ. Prediction of cooperation in orthodontic treatment. Am J Orthod Dentofacial Orthop. 1992;102:16–21.
2. Gianelly AA, Vaitas AS, Thomas WM, Berger DG. Distalization of molars with repelling magnets. J Clin Orthod. 1988;22:40–4.
3. Jones RD, White JM. Rapid Class II molar correction with an open-coil jig. J Clin Orthod. 1992;26:661–4.
4. Hilgers JJ. The Pendulum appliance for Class II non-compliance therapy. J Clin Orthod. 1992;26:706–14.
5. Carano A, Testa M. The Distal Jet for upper molar distalization. J Clin Orthod. 1996;30:374–80.
6. Walde KC. The simplified molar distalizer. J Clin Orthod. 2003;37(11):616–9.
7. Ludwig B, Glasl B, Kinzinger GS, Walde KC, Lisson JA. The skeletal frog appliance for maxillary molar distalization. J Clin Orthod. 2011;45(2):77–84.

Bone-Anchored Rapid Palatal Expansion

7

Ki Beom Kim

Abstract

Rapid palatal expansion (RPE) can cause significant periodontal consequences. Alternatives to traditional tooth-anchored RPE have been developed in an effort to offset these side effects. Bone-anchored RPE with support from miniscrew implants takes advantages over tooth-anchored RPE, as the expanders are directly attached to the posterior teeth. There are a few variations that can be used in different types of cases. Bone-anchored RPE without surgery can be an alternative to surgically assisted rapid palatal expansion in young adults.

It has been a common practice to use rapid palatal expansion (RPE) in correcting transverse maxillary deficiency and arch-length discrepancies. It is, however, known that RPE can cause significant periodontal problems such as excessive buccal crown tipping, root resorption, dehiscence, fenestration, and instability of results [1–5]. A few studies have reported that there is more dentoalveolar tipping than true skeletal expansion with RPE [6, 7]. Older patients have more dentoalveolar tipping after RPE becomes greater with its resultant gingival recessions.

There have been many attempts to minimize these side effects while maximizing the skeletal expansion [8–13]. One particular study, which compares a surgically assisted, bone-anchored RPE with a traditional tooth-anchored RPE, concludes that the bone-anchored expander produces more skeletal changes than dental changes [14]. However, another study has reported that both expanders show similar results [10]. It is still unclear whether bone-anchored RPE has less dentoalveolar tipping and more skeletal expansion. Therefore, there appears to be a need for a randomized clinical trial. It might seem logical that there would be advantages over tooth-borne RPE in regard to periodontal consequences, as the expanders are not directly attached to the posterior teeth. This chapter shows a few variations of bone-anchored RPE in different types of cases.

7.1 No Tooth Attachment Design

Four metal rings with a diameter of 1.6 mm were laser-welded with a jackscrew on the predetermined paramedial area. Four miniscrew

K.B. Kim, DDS, MSD, PhD
Department of Orthodontics, Center for Advanced Dental Education, Saint Louis University, 3320 Rutger Street, St. Louis, MO 6314, USA
e-mail: kkim8@slu.edu

K.B. Kim (ed.), *Temporary Skeletal Anchorage Devices*,
DOI 10.1007/978-3-642-55052-2_7, © Springer-Verlag Berlin Heidelberg 2014

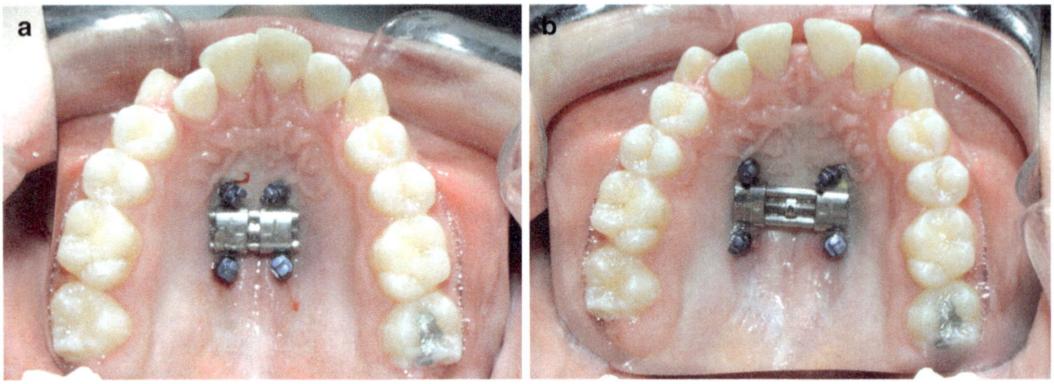

Fig. 7.1 Bone-anchored RPE. No tooth attachment design. (**a**) Pre-expansion. (**b**) Post-expansion

implants were placed through the metal rings that were fitted snuggly (Fig. 7.1). Four wire eyelets can be used for this design (Fig. 7.2). The amount of expansion at the maxillary first molar was only about 50 % of the expansion at the jackscrew (Fig. 7.3). The pressure from the cheek and palatal soft tissue may push the posterior teeth toward the median as a counterforce against the expansion that leads to the crown tipping palatally, quite opposite to the tooth-anchored RPE, which results in the buccal crown tipping (Fig. 7.4).

7.2 Supporting Wires Design

A Hyrax® expander was fabricated on a plaster cast marked with the locations for four or two miniscrew implants. Four metal rings were laser-welded to the expander screw. Stainless steel wires were extended to the lingual of the maxillary premolars and first molars to prevent palatal tipping. Four miniscrew implants were inserted in both palatal slopes using a template made with a vacuum-forming plastic (Fig. 7.5). If one side of the miniscrew implant is placed more gingivally than in the other side, then as the expansion progresses, the supporting wire on the same side can be embedded into the soft tissue, and this causes soft tissue irritation (Fig. 7.6).

7.3 Acrylic-Type Design

The average thickness of the palatal bone 2–4 mm from the midline was between 4 and 7 mm [15]. A careful evaluation of the bone thickness is essential for locating and directing the miniscrew implant placement to prevent unwanted tissue injury. First, four miniscrew implants were placed paramedially in the palate. An impression was taken for fabrication of an RPE with palatal acrylic, which was secured to the miniscrews with flowable composite. A small amount of relief underneath the acrylic is required to prevent soft tissue irritation. The cross-slot head design or higher-profile miniscrew implants are preferable to increase the mechanical retention. Small occlusal rests on the premolars are needed to keep the acrylic away from the palatal tissue. Once the flowable composite is cured, then the wires for the occlusal rest can be removed (Fig.7.7).

7.4 Hybrid Design

It is quite possible to use both bone anchorage and tooth anchorage for RPE at the same time. There have been only a few articles to show two anterior miniscrew implants and two posterior bands [16–17]. When teeth normally used for anchorage are missing, hybrid RPE can be used (Fig. 7.8). The finite element simulations suggest

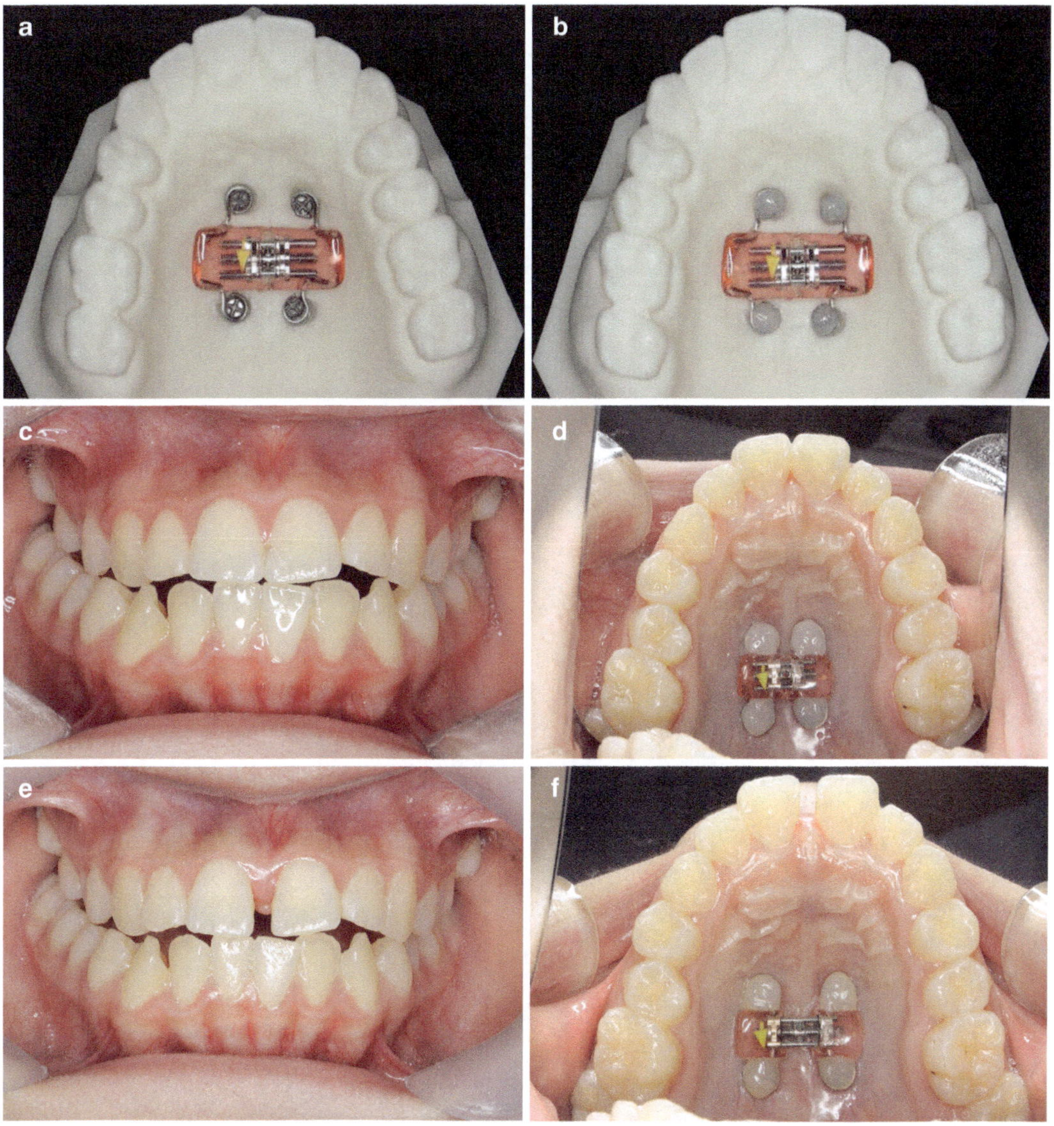

Fig. 7.2 No tooth attachment design (Courtesy of Dr. Yoon-Ah Kook, Dr. Seong-Hun Kim). (**a**) Bone-anchored RPE. (**b**) Bone-anchored RPE was secured with the flowable composite. (**c**) Frontal view of pre-expansion. (**d**) Occlusal view of pre-expansion. (**e**) Frontal view of post-expansion. (**f**) Occlusal view of post-expansion

that the hybrid RPE appliance is capable of minimizing many of the periodontal side effects associated with the tooth-anchored RPE [16–19].

7.4.1 Considerations

With no direct attachment of the posterior teeth, banding and bonding are carried out with the expander in place; as a result, leveling and alignment can be started while keeping the expander for the purpose of consolidating the expansion. It may be that the overall treatment time is shortened. One of the common problems of a tooth-anchored RPE is bite-opening effect due to the extrusion of the palatal cusps of the maxillary posterior teeth along with the buccal crown tipping. However, bone-anchored RPEs for open

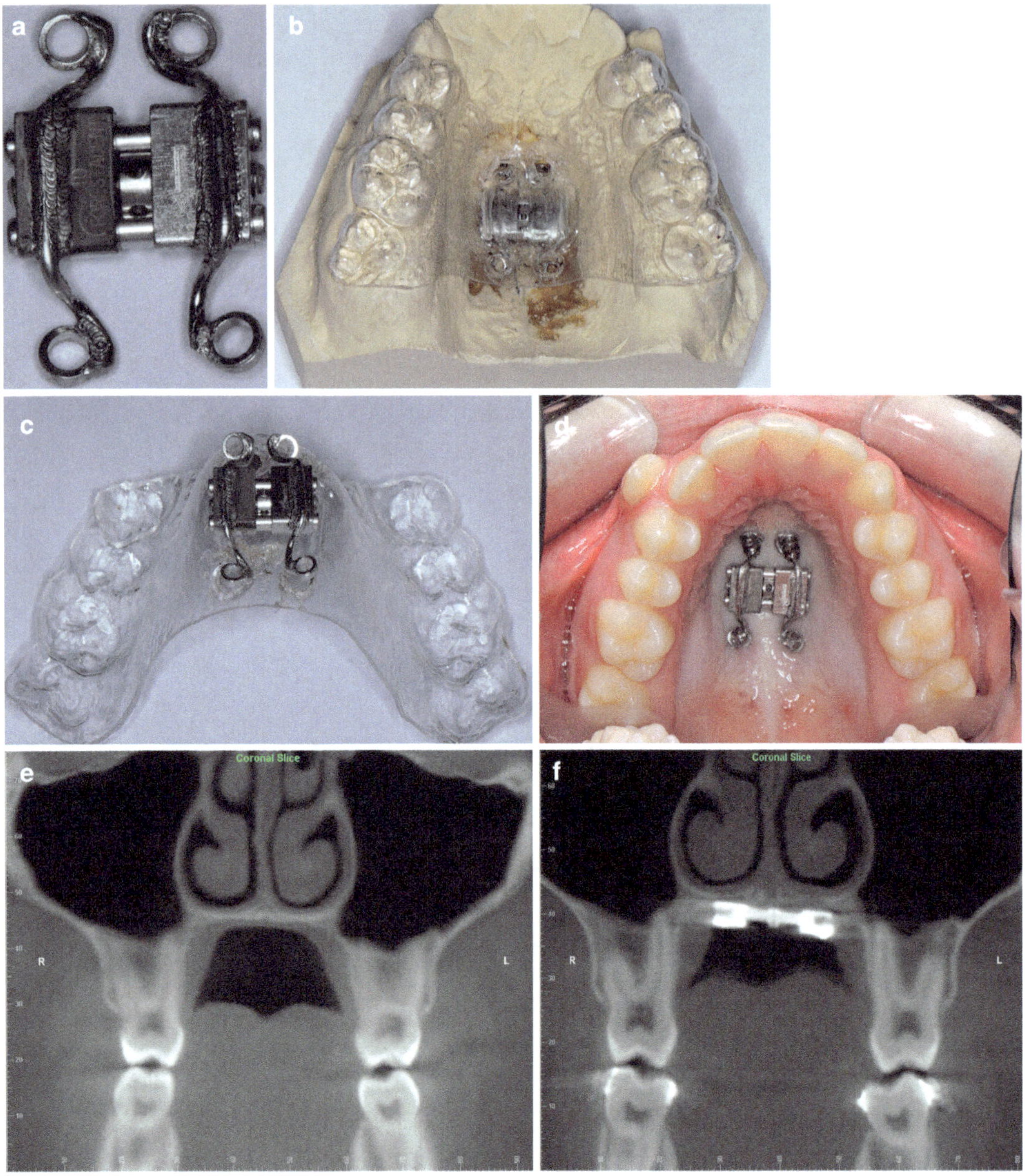

Fig. 7.3 No tooth attachment design. (**a**) Expansion screw. (**b**) Expansion screw with vacuum-formed template on the model. (**c**) Expansion screw with vacuum-formed template. (**d**) Expansion screw applied to a patient. (**e**) Coronal view of CBCT, pre-expansion. (**f**) Coronal view of CBCT, post-expansion. RPE screw was expanded by 6 mm, but intermolar distance was increased by 2.8 mm

bite patients seem not to show much vertical change after the expansion because dentoalveolar tipping happens much less than tooth-borne RPE. For patients who have periodontal disease or very thin alveolar bones around the posterior teeth, bone-anchored RPE may be a good option for expanding the maxilla without compromising the periodontal health.

7.4.2 Surgically Assisted RPE (SARPE) with Bone-Anchored Expander

Recently there have been reports of successful nonsurgical maxillary expansion in adult patients [20–21]. However, SARPE is considered as the standard procedure to correct the narrow maxilla

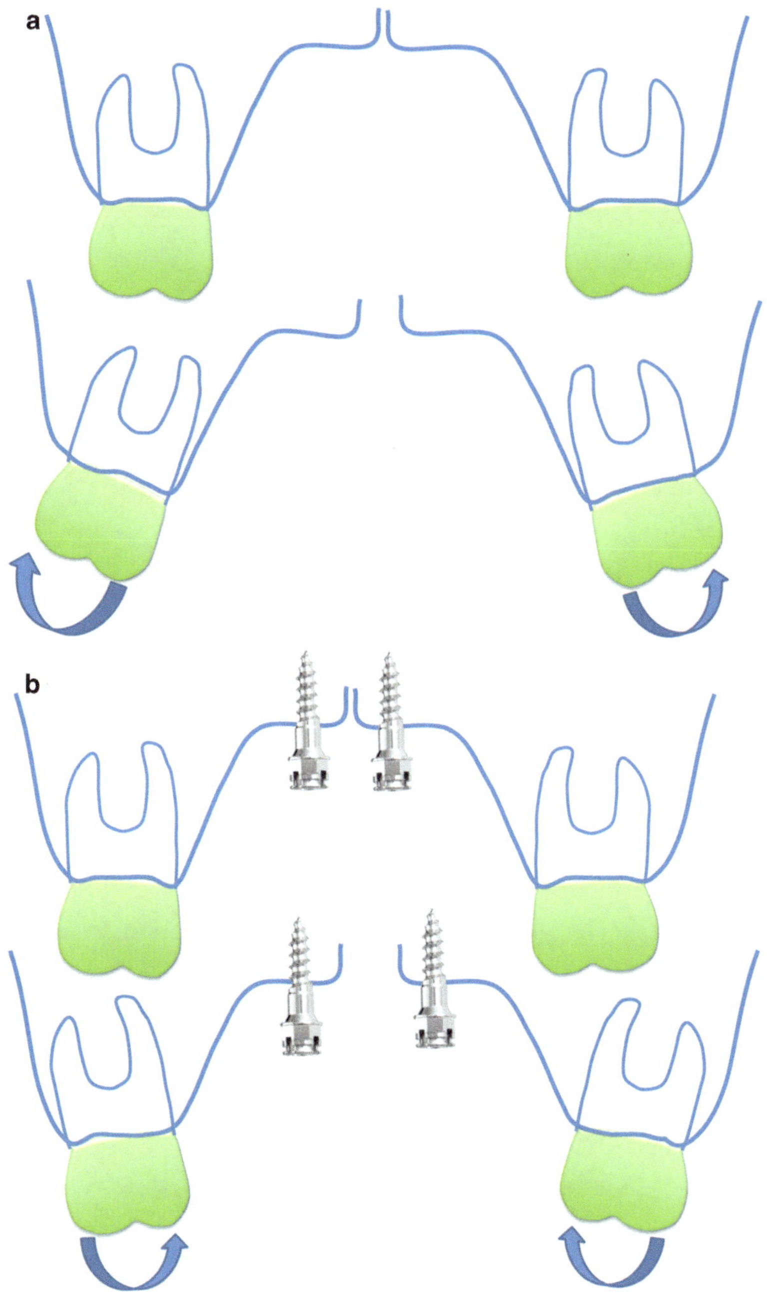

Fig. 7.4 Dentoalveolar response after RPE. (**a**) Buccal crown tipping with tooth-anchored RPE. (**b**) Palatal crown tipping with bone-anchored RPE

width in adult patients [22–23]. Typically a tooth-anchored expander is used in SARPE, but it has been shown that there may be periodontal complications as a result of stress on the anchoring teeth [24–28]. Bone-anchored expanders followed by Le Fort I surgery have been used, and they have produced successful results [24, 25, 29, 30–32]. Reportedly, the benefits of bone-anchored expanders for SARPE [11, 12, 27, 33–35] have proven to be a reliable and suitable technique for maxillary expansion without causing significant dental and periodontal damage [13, 36].

7.4.3 Possible Alternative for SARPE

One study showed that nonsurgical maxillary expansion was achieved with hybrid expander in

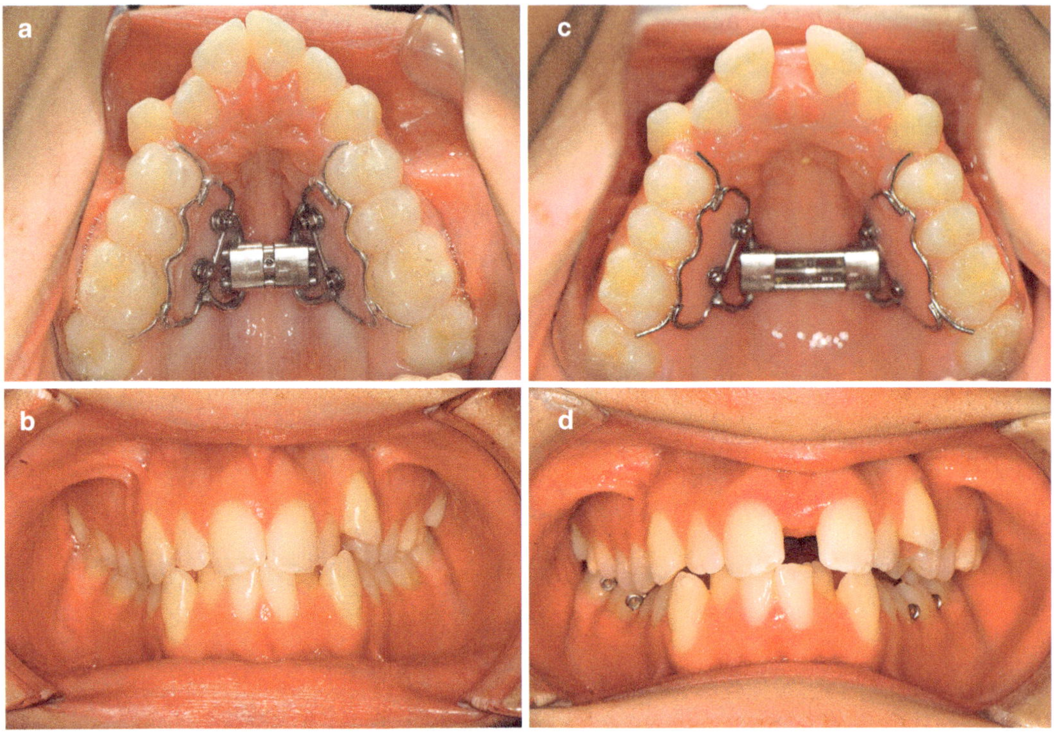

Fig. 7.5 Supporting wire design. (**a**) Occlusal view of pre-expansion. (**b**) Frontal view of pre-expansion. (**c**) Occlusal view of post-expansion. (**d**) Frontal view of post-expansion

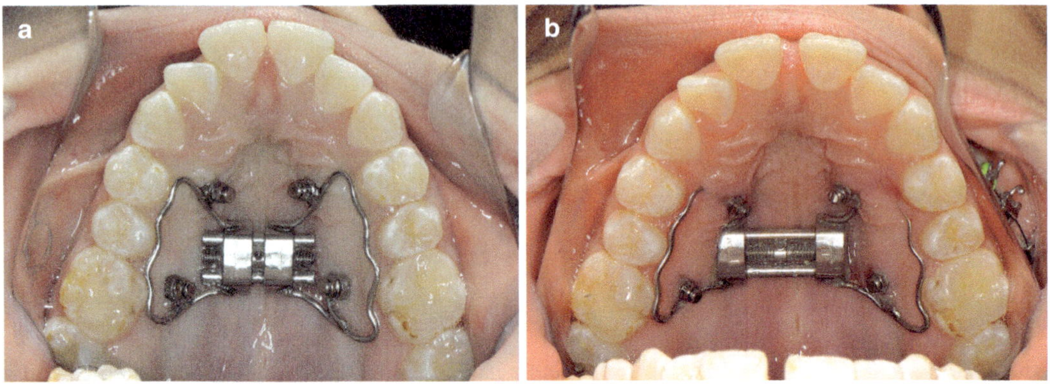

Fig. 7.6 Supporting wire design problem. (**a**) Occlusal view of pre-expansion. (**b**) Occlusal view of post-expansion. Note two anterior miniscrews and supporting wires are impinging the palatal soft tissue

a young adult male patient [37]. According to the adult cadaver simulation with a tooth-anchored RPE, there was no sutural opening, but rather an unwanted rupture of the alveolar process or a tooth rupture through the alveolar bone [38]. In contrast, there was a successful separation of the intermaxillary suture, which was achieved in a bone-anchored RPE. A finite element model simulation shows that it needs a relatively low transverse force to open the intermaxillary suture with a bone-anchored RPE. A high tensile stress was concentrated only on the palatine suture, and the

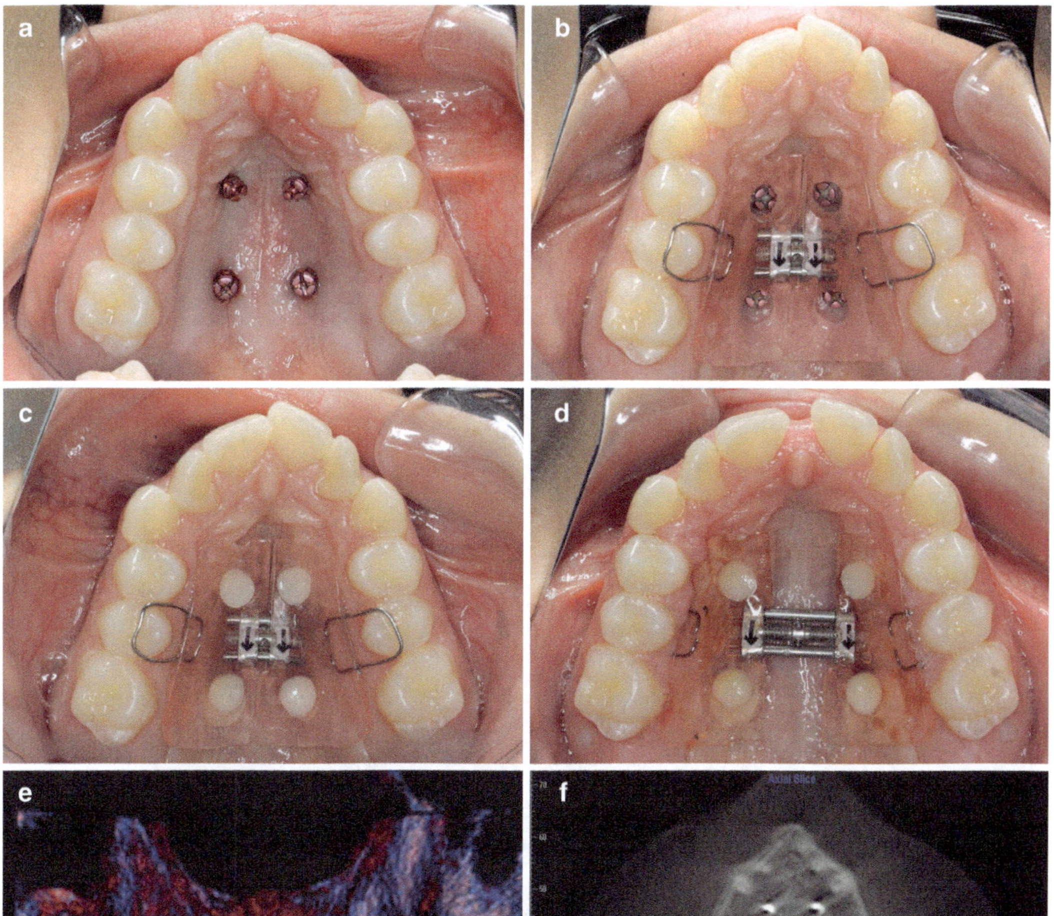

Fig. 7.7 Acrylic-type design. (**a**) Four miniscrew implants were placed in midpalatal region. (**b**) Acrylic-type RPE was tried in. There was a relief under the acrylic and occlusal rests were preventing the acrylic touching the palatal tissue. (**c**) RPE was secured with the flowable composite. (**d**) Occlusal view of post-expansion. (**e**) 3D surface rendering from CBCT, pre-expansion. (**f**) Transverse view of CBCT, pre-expansion. (**g**) Coronal view of CBCT, pre-expansion. (**h**) 3D surface rendering from CBCT, post-expansion. (**i**) Transverse view of CBCT, post-expansion. (**j**) Coronal view of CBCT, post-expansion

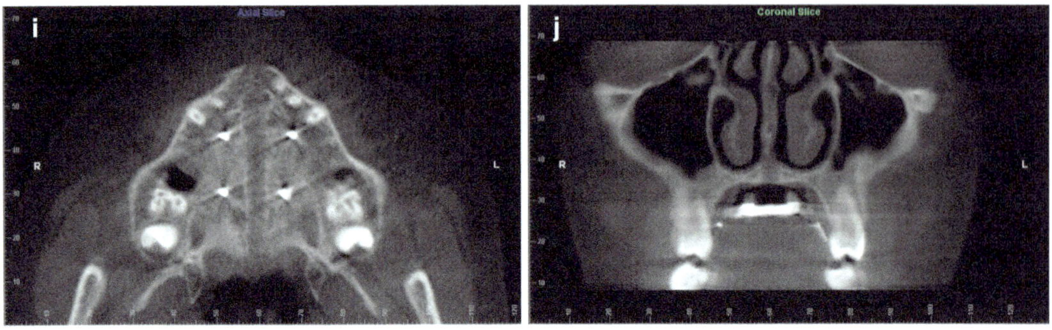

Fig. 7.7 (continued)

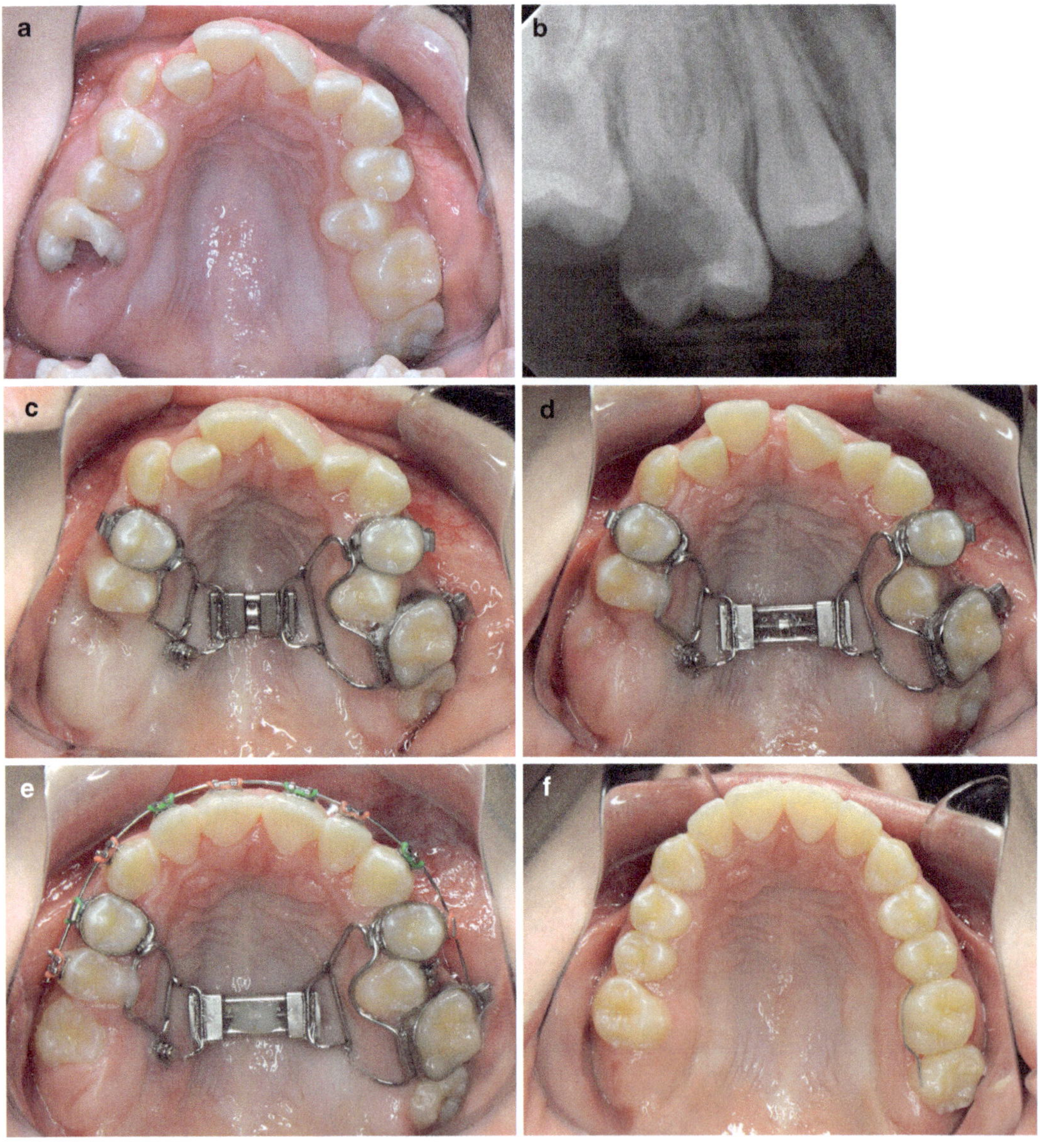

Fig. 7.8 Hybrid design. (**a**) Note severe caries on the maxillary right first molar. (**b**) Periapical radiograph of the maxillary right first molar. (**c**) Occlusal view of pre-expansion. (**d**) Occlusal view of post-expansion. (**e**) Bond the upper arch. (**f**) Occlusal view of posttreatment

overall stress distribution on the remaining skull is almost negligible [39]. The bone-anchored RPE does not affect the position of the teeth, and the effect on the alveolar process is insignificant (Fig. 7.9). Lee et al. studied the stress distribution and the displacement of the maxilla and teeth according to the different designs of bone-anchored RPE [19]. According to their results, the acrylic-type design expanders with miniscrew implants placed at the palatal slope showed the palatal expansion without buccal inclination of the dentition (Fig. 7.10). Although there needs to be more studies done to prove this, a bone-anchored RPE without surgery may be a possible alternative to SARPE in certain cases, especially for young adults (Fig.7.11).

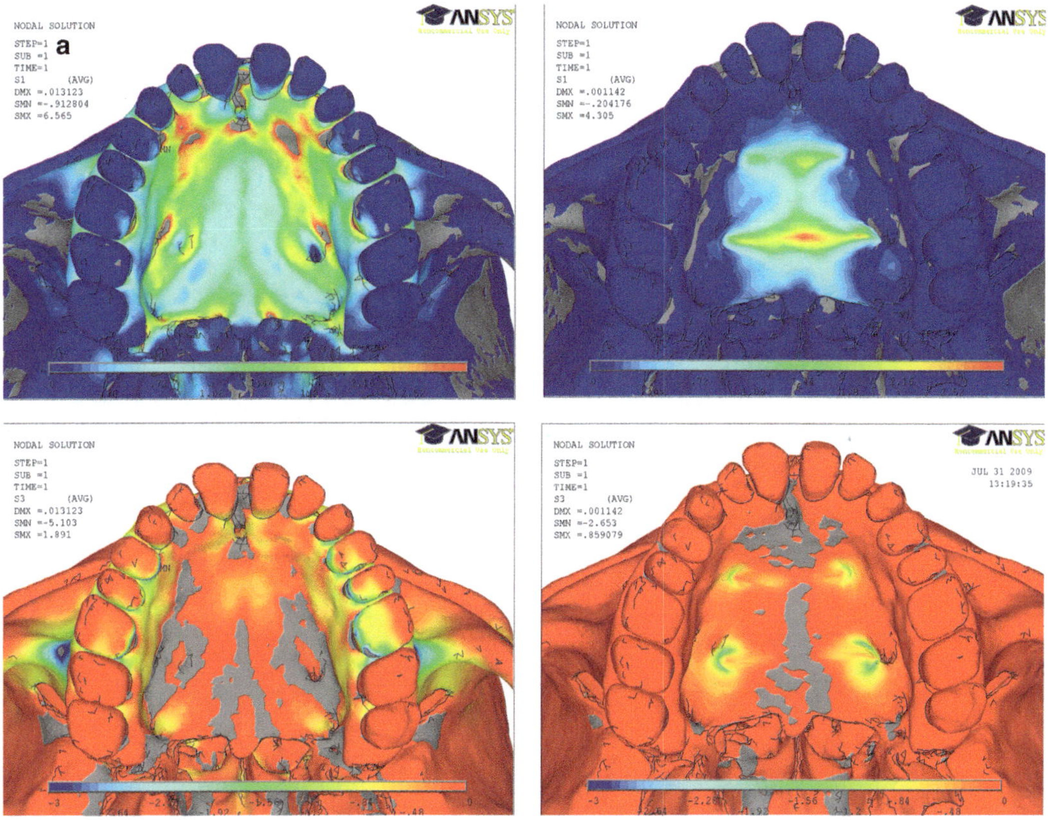

Fig. 7.9 Finite element simulation with the tooth-anchored RPE and bone-anchored RPE. (**a**) Finite element simulation of a transverse force application with the tooth-anchored RPE and bone-anchored RPE (From Boryor et al. [39]). *Upper left*: Tensile stress distribution with the tooth-anchored RPE. *Lower left*: Compressive stress distribution with the tooth-anchored RPE. *Upper right*: Tensile stress distribution with the bone-anchored RPE. *Lower right*: Compressive stress distribution with the bone-anchored RPE. (**b**) Finite element simulation results of the stress distribution on the inner cranial base with the tooth-anchored RPE and bone-anchored RPE. *Upper left*: Compressive stress distribution on the inner cranial base is mainly concentrated in the regions where blood vessels and nerves are located with the tooth-anchored RPE. *Lower left*: High tensile stress distribution in the inner cranial base is exerted with the tooth-anchored RPE. *Upper right*: Very low compressive stress distribution is seen in the inner cranial base with the bone-anchored RPE. *Lower right*: Very low tensile stress distribution in the inner cranial base is applied with the bone-anchored RPE

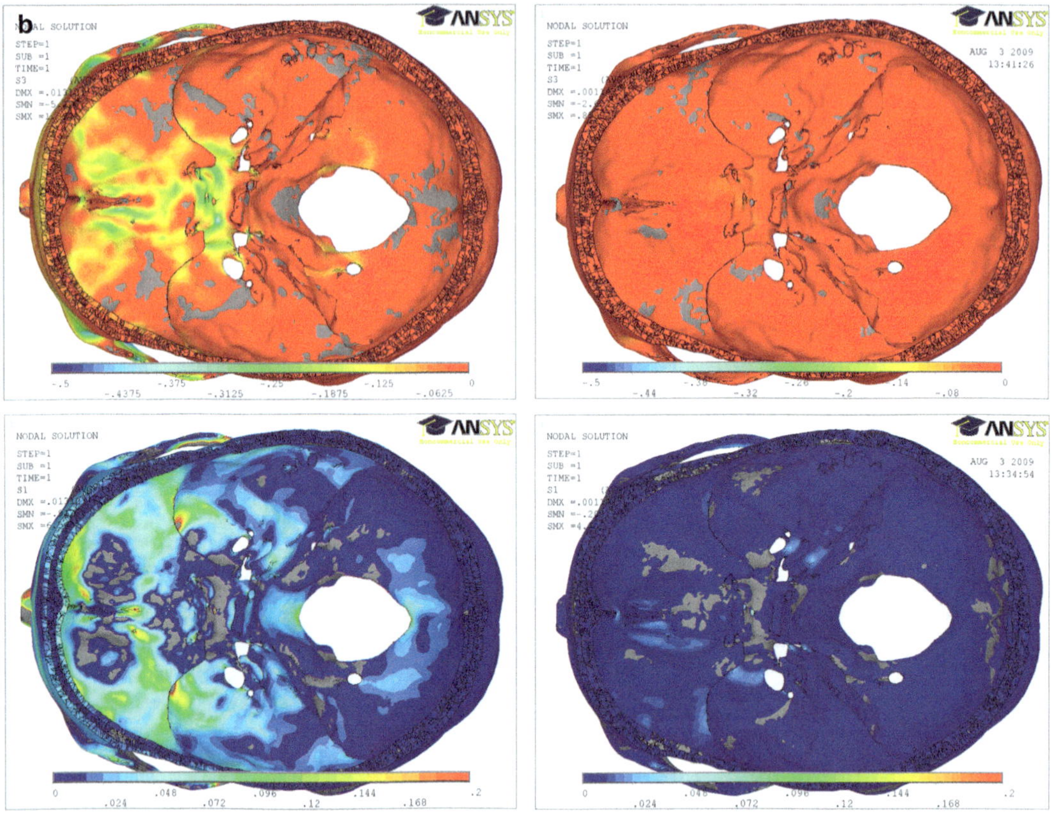

Fig. 7.9 (continued)

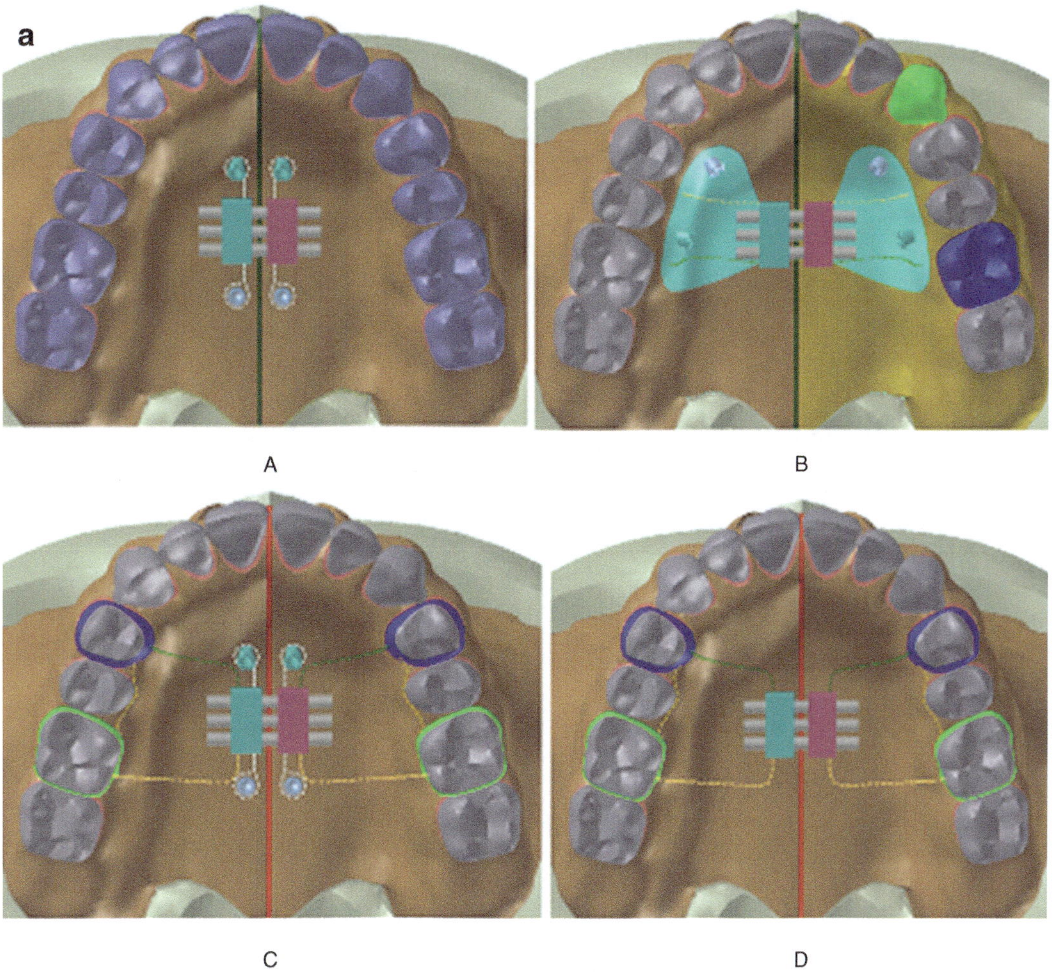

Fig. 7.10 Stress distribution and displacement by tooth-anchored RPE and bone-anchored RPE. (From Lee et al. [19]). (**a**) Designs of the RPE types (*A*) Bone-anchored RPE with miniscrews placed 3 mm lateral to midpalatal suture (type 1). (*B*) Bone-anchored RPE with miniscrews placed at the palatal slope (type 2). (*C*) Combined tooth-anchored RPE with four bands and bone-anchored RPE with miniscrews placed 3 mm lateral to midpalatal suture (type 3). (*D*) Surgically assisted tooth-anchored RPE with four bands (type 4). (**b**) Von Mises stress distribution in occlusal view. (*A*) Type 1, (*B*) Type 2, (*C*) Type 3, (*D*) Type 4. (**c**) Von Mises stress distribution in cross section at the first premolar area (*A*) Type 1, (*B*) Type 2, (*C*) Type 3, (*D*) Type 4

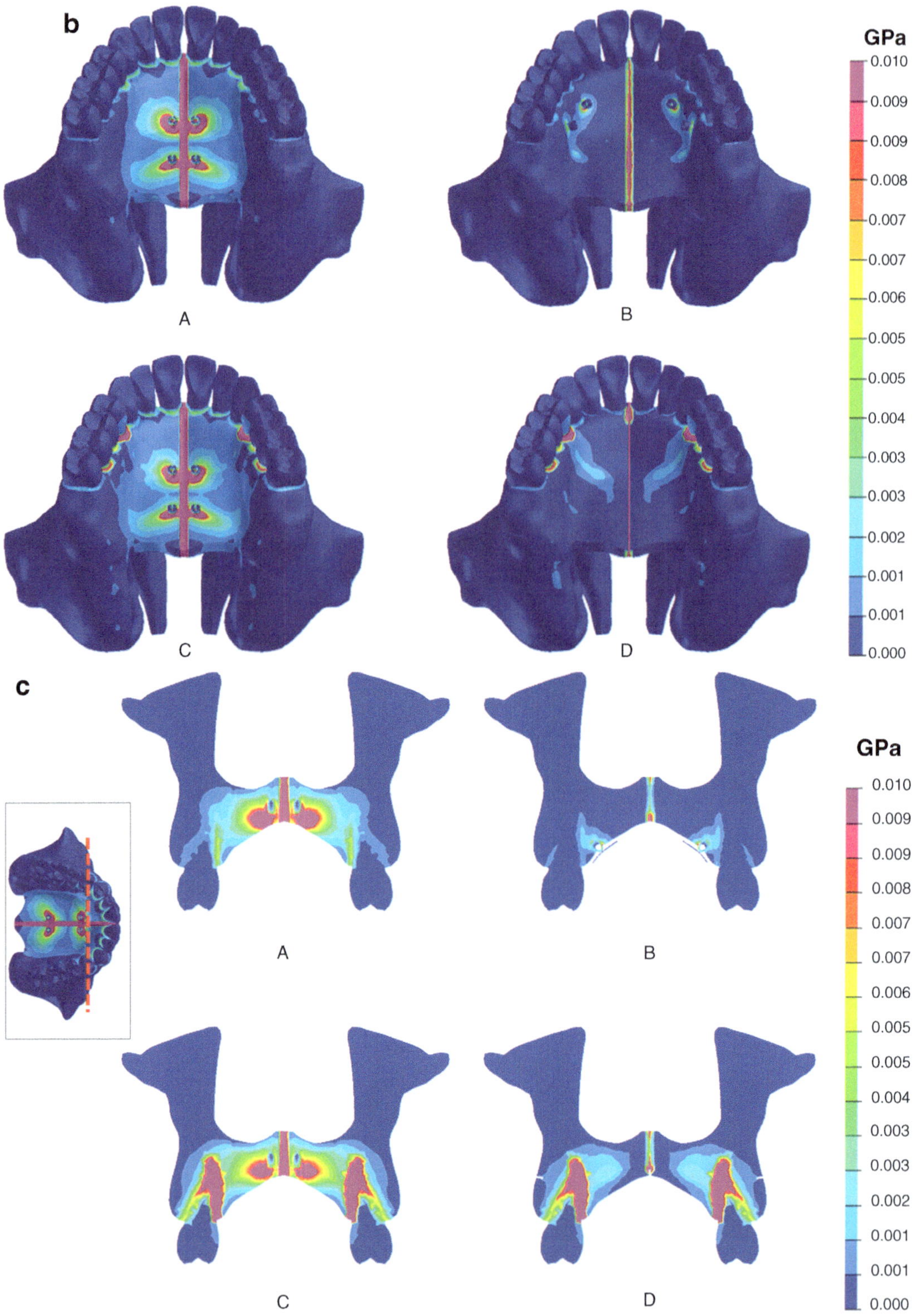

Fig. 7.10 (continued)

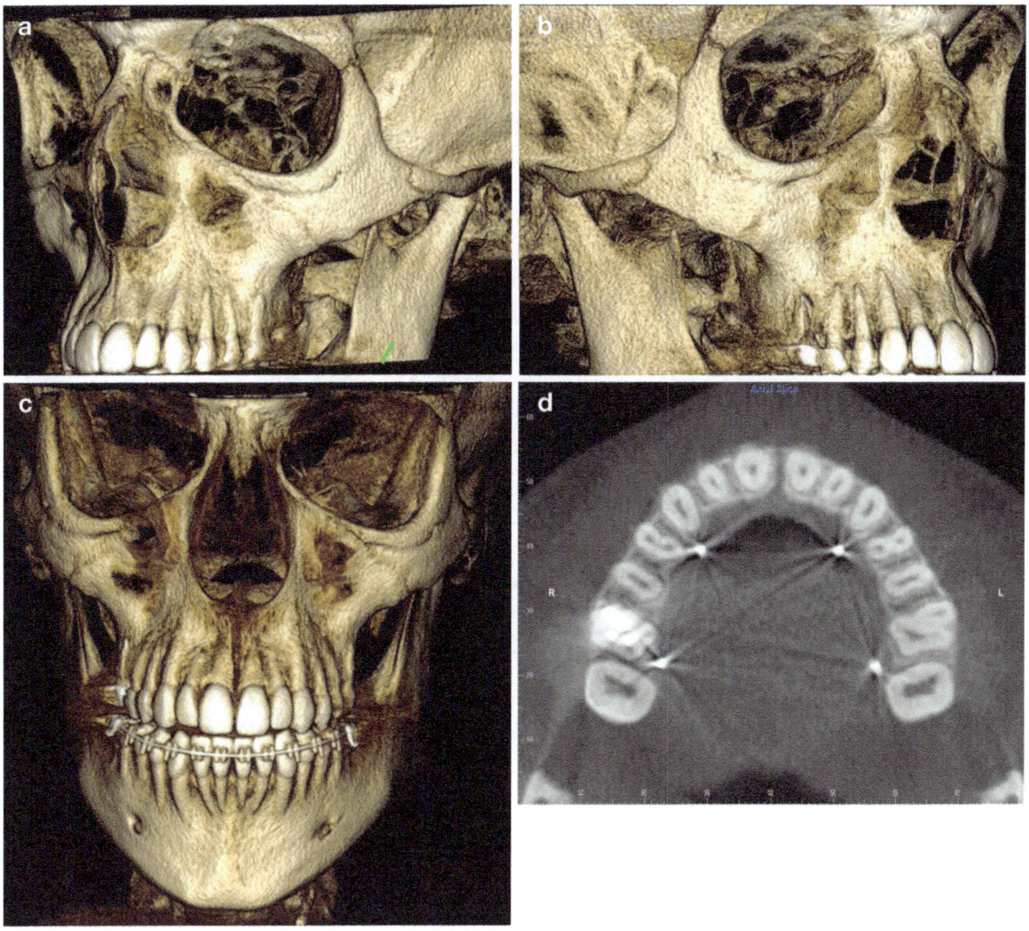

Fig. 7.11 A 20-year-and-7-month-old female patient. (**a**) 3D surface rendering from CBCT, pre-expansion. Note very thin buccal alveolar bones around her posterior teeth. (**b**) 3D surface rendering from CBCT, pre-expansion. (**c**) 3D surface rendering from CBCT, post-expansion. Note the midpalatal suture opening. (**d**) Transverse view of CBCT, post-expansion. Note the diastema. (**e**) Cross-sectional images at premolar region, pre-expansion. (**f**) Cross-sectional images at premolar region, post-expansion. There was no angular change in the premolars. (**g**) Cross-sectional images at the first molar, pre-expansion. (**h**) Cross-sectional images at the first molar, post-expansion. There was no tipping of the first molar

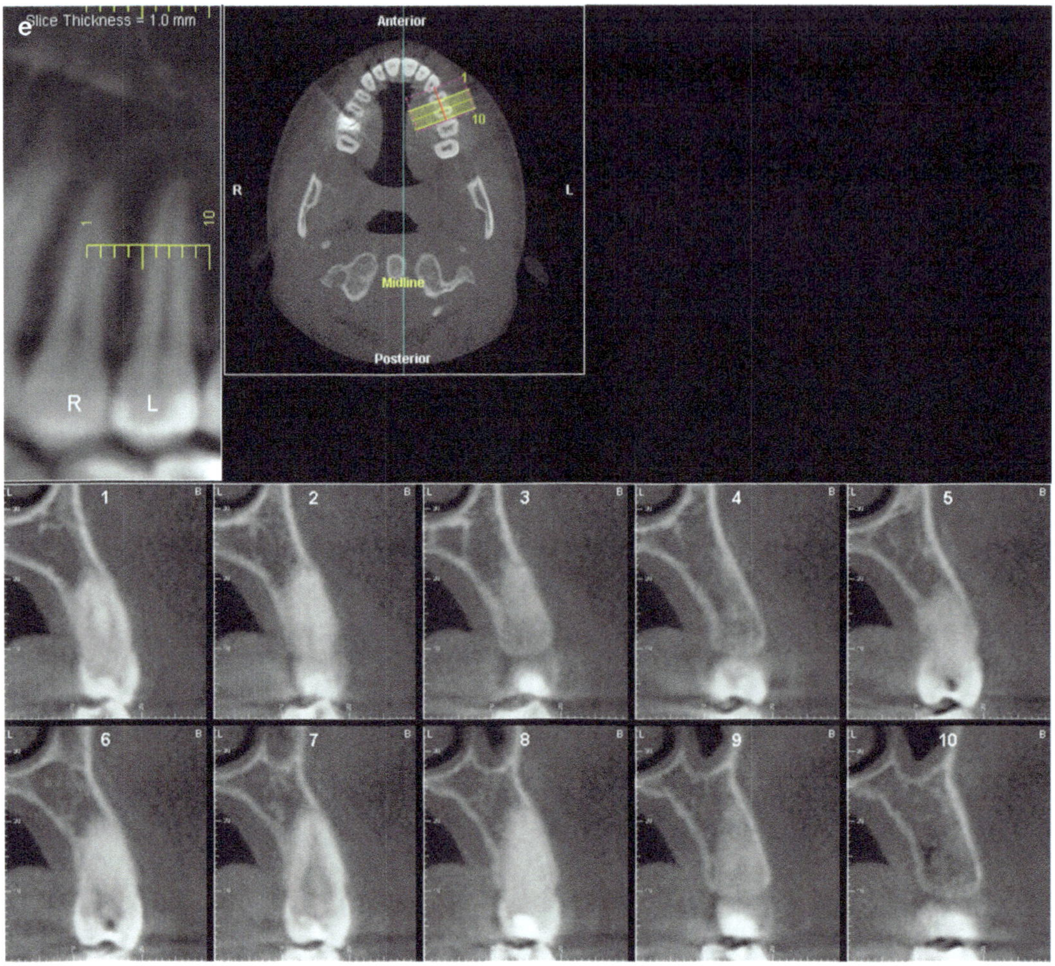

Fig. 7.11 (continued)

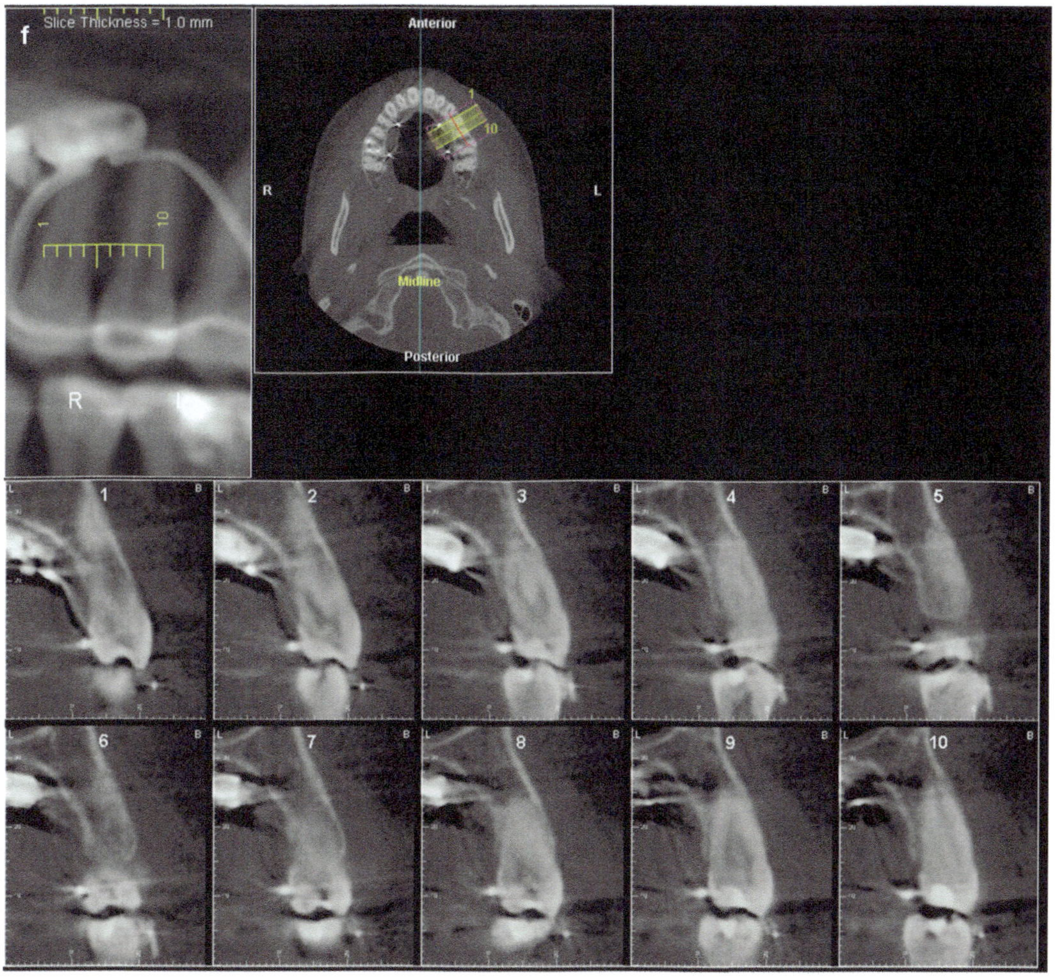

Fig. 7.11 (continued)

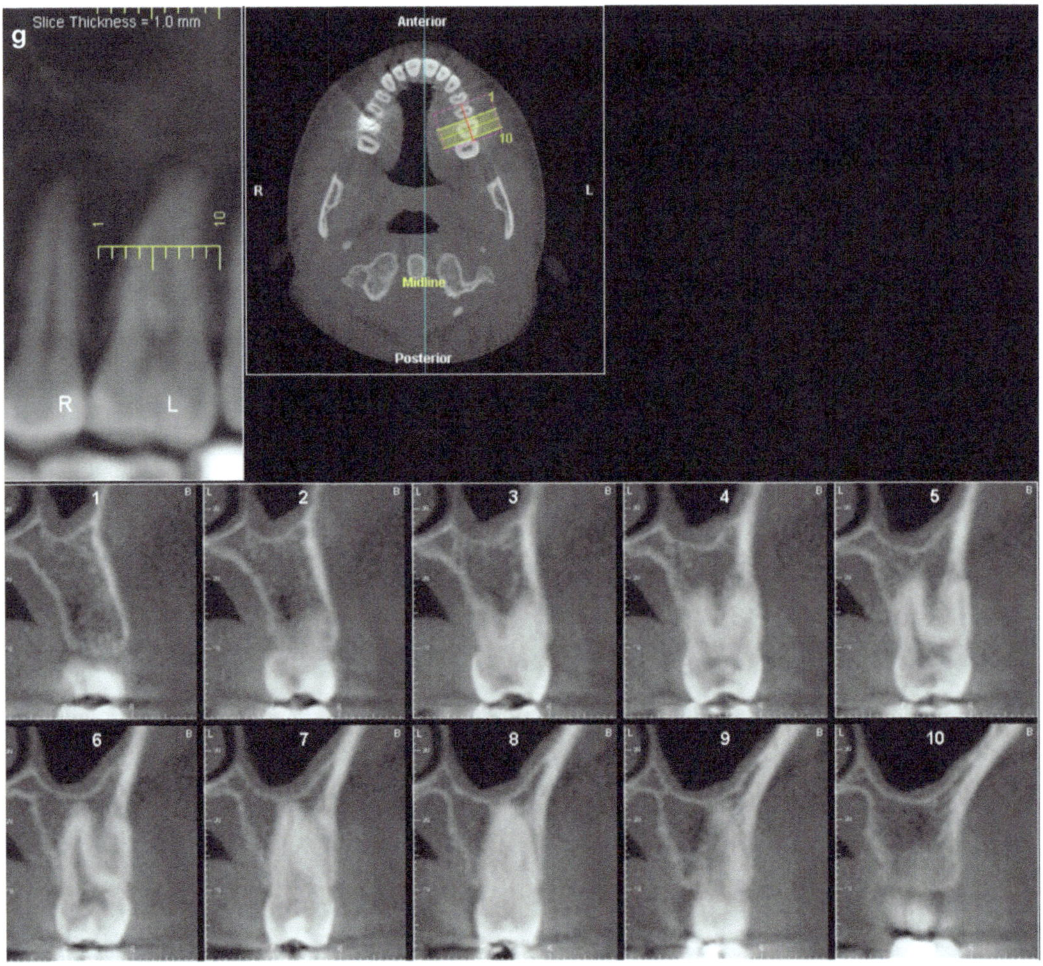

Fig. 7.11 (continued)

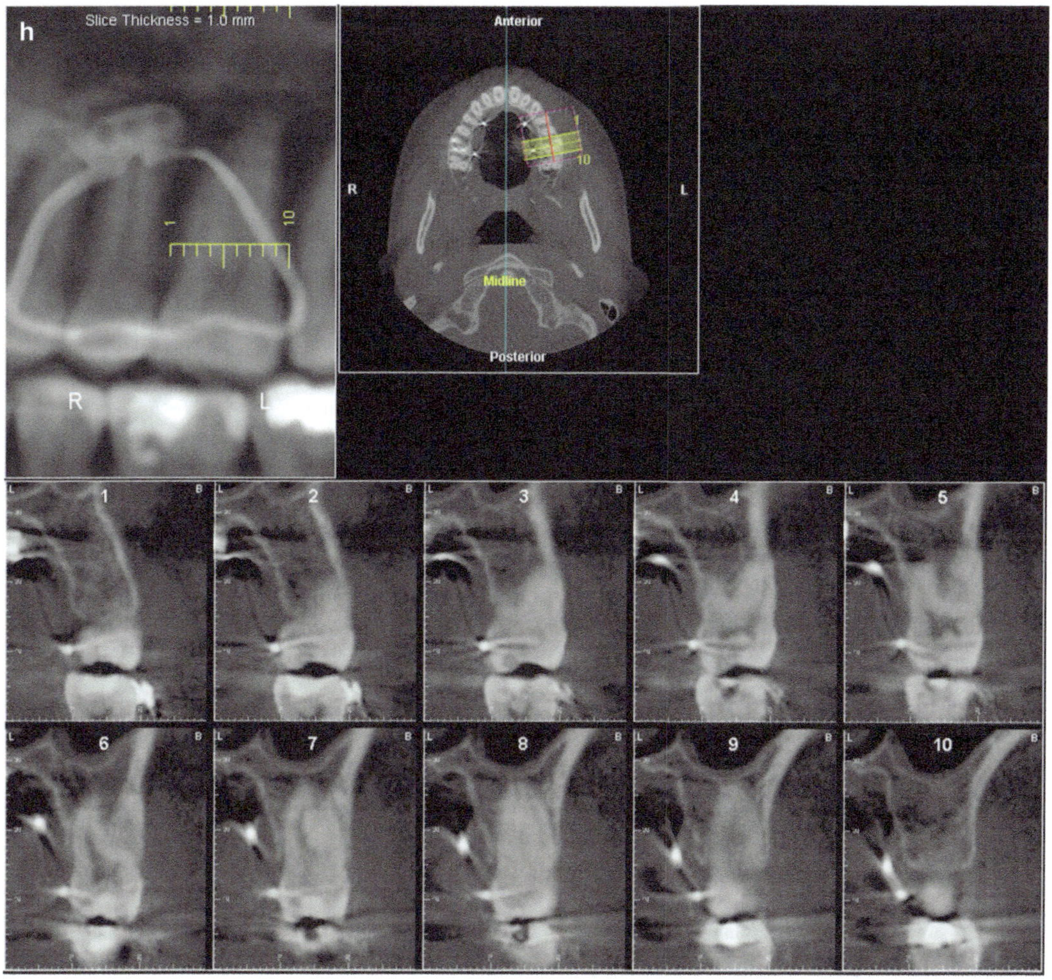

Fig. 7.11 (continued)

References

1. Thilander B, Nyman S, Karring T, Magnusson I. Bone regeneration in alveolar bone dehiscences related to orthodontic tooth movements. Eur J Orthod. 1983;5(2):105–14.
2. Erverdi N, Okar I, Kücükkeles N, Arbak S. A comparison of two different rapid palatal expansion techniques from the point of root resorption. Am J Orthod Dentofacial Orthop. 1994;106(1):47–51.
3. Garib DG, Henriques JFC, Janson G, de Freitas MR, Fernandes AY. Periodontal effects of rapid maxillary expansion with tooth-tissue-borne and tooth-borne expanders: a computed tomography evaluation. Am J Orthod Dentofacial Orthop. 2006;129(6):749–58.
4. Bassarelli T, Dalstra M, Melsen B. Changes in clinical crown height as a result of transverse expansion of the maxilla in adults. Eur J Orthod. 2005;27(2):121–8.
5. Lagravere MO, Major PW, Flores-Mir C. Long-term dental arch changes after rapid maxillary expansion treatment: a systematic review. Angle Orthod. 2005;75(2): 155–61.
6. Garrett BJ, Caruso JM, Rungcharassaeng K, Farrage JR, Kim JS, Taylor GD. Skeletal effects to the maxilla after rapid maxillary expansion assessed with cone-beam computed tomography. Am J Orthod Dentofacial Orthop. 2008;134(1):8–9.
7. Lagravère MO, Heo G, Major PW, Flores-Mir C. Meta-analysis of immediate changes with rapid maxillary expansion treatment. J Am Dent Assoc. 2006;137(1): 44–53.
8. Parr JA, Garetto LP, Wohlford ME, Arbuckle GR, Roberts WE. Sutural expansion using rigidly integrated endosseous implants: an experimental study in rabbits. Angle Orthod. 1997;67(4):283–90.
9. Sarı E, Uçar C, Ceylanoglu C. Transpalatal distraction in a patient with a narrow maxilla. Angle Orthod. 2007;77(6):1126–31.
10. Lagravère MO, Carey J, Heo G, Toogood RW, Major PW. Transverse, vertical, and anteroposterior changes from bone-anchored maxillary expansion vs traditional rapid maxillary expansion: a randomized clinical trial. Am J Orthod Dentofacial Orthop. 2010;137(3):304.e1–12.
11. Harzer W, Schneider M, Gedrange T, Tausche E. Direct bone placement of the hyrax fixation screw for Surgically Assisted Rapid Palatal Expansion (SARPE). J Oral Maxillofac Surg. 2006;64(8):1313–7.
12. Pinto PX, Mommaerts MY, Wreakes G, Jacobs WV. Immediate postexpansion changes following the use of the transpalatal distractor. J Oral Maxillofac Surg. 2001;59(9):994–1000; discussion 1001.
13. Verlinden CRA, Gooris PG, Becking AG. Complications in transpalatal distraction osteogenesis: a retrospective clinical study. J Oral Maxillofac Surg. 2011;69(3):899–905.
14. Tausche E, Hansen L, Hietschold V, Lagravère MO, Harzer W. Three-dimensional evaluation of surgically assisted implant bone-borne rapid maxillary expansion: a pilot study. Am J Orthod Dentofacial Orthop. 2007;131(4 Suppl):S92–9.
15. Ryu J-H, Park JH, Vu Thi Thu T, Bayome M, Kim Y, Kook Y-A. Palatal bone thickness compared with cone-beam computed tomography in adolescents and adults for mini-implant placement. Am J Orthod Dentofacial Orthop. 2012;142(2):207–12.
16. Wilmes B, Nienkemper M, Drescher D. Application and effectiveness of a mini-implant- and tooth-borne rapid palatal expansion device: the hybrid hyrax. World J Orthod. 2010;11(4):323–30.
17. Ludwig B, Glas B, Bowman SJ, Drescher D, Wilmes B. Miniscrew-supported Class III treatment with the hybrid RPE advancer. J Clin Orthod. 2010;44(9):533–9, quiz 561.
18. Ludwig B, Baumgaertel S, Zorkun B, Bonitz L, Glasl B, Wilmes B, et al. Application of a new viscoelastic finite element method model and analysis of miniscrew-supported hybrid hyrax treatment. Am J Orthod Dentofacial Orthop. 2013;143(3):426–35.
19. Lee HK, Bayome M, Ahn CS, Kim S-H, Kim KB, Mo S-S, et al. Stress distribution and displacement by different bone-borne palatal expanders with micro-implants: a three-dimensional finite-element analysis. Eur J Orthod. 2012. [Epub ahead of print]
20. Stuart DA, Wiltshire WA. Rapid palatal expansion in the young adult: time for a paradigm shift? J Can Dent Assoc. 2003;69(6):374–7.
21. Handelman CS, Wang L, BeGole EA, Haas AJ. Nonsurgical rapid maxillary expansion in adults: report on 47 cases using the Haas expander. Angle Orthod. 2000;70(2):129–44.
22. Shetty V, Caridad JM, Caputo AA, Chaconas SJ. Biomechanical rationale for surgical-orthodontic expansion of the adult maxilla. J Oral Maxillofac Surg. 1994;52(7):742–9; discussion 750–1.
23. Koudstaal MJ, Poort LJ, van der Wal KGH, Wolvius EB, Prahl-Andersen B, Schulten AJM. Surgically assisted rapid maxillary expansion (SARME): a review of the literature. Int J Oral Maxillofac Surg. 2005;34(7):709–14.
24. Mommaerts MY. Transpalatal distraction as a method of maxillary expansion. Br J Oral Maxillofac Surg. 1999;37(4):268–72.
25. Neyt NMF, Mommaerts MY, Abeloos JVS, De Clercq CAS, Neyt LF. Problems, obstacles and complications with transpalatal distraction in non-congenital deformities. J Craniomaxillofac Surg. 2002;30(3):139–43.
26. Koudstaal MJ, Wolvius EB, Schulten AJM, Hop WCJ, van der Wal KGH. Stability, tipping and relapse of bone-borne versus tooth-borne surgically assisted rapid maxillary expansion; a prospective randomized patient trial. Int J Oral Maxillofac Surg. 2009;38(4):308–15.
27. Landes CA, Laudemann K, Schübel F, Petruchin O, Mack M, Kopp S, et al. Comparison of tooth- and bone-borne devices in surgically assisted rapid maxillary expansion by three-dimensional computed tomography monitoring: transverse dental and skeletal maxillary expansion, segmental inclination, dental

tipping, and vestibular bone resorption. J Craniofac Surg. 2009;20(4):1132–41.
28. Seeberger R, Kater W, Schulte-Geers M, Davids R, Freier K, Thiele O. Changes after surgically-assisted maxillary expansion (SARME) to the dentoalveolar, palatal and nasal structures by using tooth-borne distraction devices. Br J Oral Maxillofac Surg. 2011;49(5):381–5.
29. Ramieri GA, Spada MC, Austa M, Bianchi SD, Berrone S. Transverse maxillary distraction with a bone-anchored appliance: dento-periodontal effects and clinical and radiological results. Int J Oral Maxillofac Surg. 2005;34(4):357–63.
30. Iida S, Haraguchi S, Aikawa T, Yashiro K, Okura M, Kogo M. Conventional bone-anchored palatal distractor using an orthodontic palatal expander for the transverse maxillary distraction osteogenesis: technical note. Oral Surg Oral Med Oral Pathol Oral Radiol Endod. 2008;105(2):e8–11.
31. Gerlach KL, Zahl C. Transversal palatal expansion using a palatal distractor. J Orofac Orthop. 2003;64(6): 443–9.
32. Gerlach KL, Zahl C. Surgically assisted rapid palatal expansion using a new distraction device: report of a case with an epimucosal fixation. J Oral Maxillofac Surg. 2005;63(5):711–3.
33. Koudstaal MJ, van der Wal KGH, Wolvius EB, Schulten AJM. The Rotterdam Palatal Distractor: introduction of the new bone-borne device and report of the pilot study. Int J Oral Maxillofac Surg. 2006;35(1):31–5.
34. Günbay T, Akay MC, Günbay S, Aras A, Koyuncu BO, Sezer B. Transpalatal distraction using bone-borne distractor: clinical observations and dental and skeletal changes. J Oral Maxillofac Surg. 2008;66(12):2503–14.
35. Hansen L, Tausche E, Hietschold V, Hotan T, Lagravère M, Harzer W. Skeletally-anchored rapid maxillary expansion using the Dresden Distractor. J Orofac Orthop/Fortschr Kieferorthop. 2007;68(2):148–58.
36. Swennen GRJ, Treutlein C, Brachvogel P, Berten J-L, Schwestka-Polly R, Hausamen J-E. Segmental unilateral transpalatal distraction in cleft patients. J Craniofac Surg. 2003;14(5):786–90.
37. Lee K-J, Park Y-C, Park J-Y, Hwang W-S. Miniscrew-assisted nonsurgical palatal expansion before orthognathic surgery for a patient with severe mandibular prognathism. Am J Orthod Dentofacial Orthop. 2010;137(6):830–9.
38. Boryor A, Hohmann A, Wunderlich A, Geiger M, Kilic F, Sander M, et al. In-vitro results of rapid maxillary expansion on adults compared with finite element simulations. J Biomech. 2010;43(7):1237–42.
39. Boryor A, Hohmann A, Wunderlich A, Geiger M, Kilic F, Kim KB, et al. Use of a modified expander during rapid maxillary expansion in adults: an in vitro and finite element study. Int J Oral Maxillofac Implants. 2013;28(1):e11–6.

8 Molar Protraction: Orthodontic Substitution of Missing Posterior Teeth

Unbong B. Baik

Abstract

The main focus of this chapter is on the closure of missing posterior spaces by protraction of the second and third molars using TSAD (Temporary Skeletal Anchorage Device). The missing spaces are from upper first molar (U-6), lower first molar (L-6), and missing lower second bicuspid with extraction of deciduous second molar (L-E). In this chapter, cases of second molar extraction or missing will not be discussed.

Total 110 cases of missing teeth were treated (U-6: 27, L-6: 63, L-E: 20) and three cases have failed; therefore, the success rate was 97.3 %. In many cases, the impacted third molar erupted well and it became usable. This treatment can replace traditional treatment method, such as bridges or implants. If we can use the third molar, which was to be discarded, the significance of this treatment will become great.

When patient has missing tooth, orthodontic evaluation should be done prior to other treatment options, because orthodontic treatment course becomes much more complex and difficult for the cases when implants or bridges are already applied.

As one of most up-to-date revolutions in orthodontics, TSAD (Temporary Skeletal Anchorage Device) has enabled mesial and distal movement of the molars [1–5]. Between the two types of molar movement, distal movement has been discussed more than mesial movement [6–12]. Prior to TSAD, small amount of mesial movement was enabled into the extraction space by controlling anchorage, such as anchorage reinforcement and elastics. On the other hand, distal movement of molars had much difficulty not only because posterior anchorage was almost impossible but also because posterior anchorage, if possible, needed uncomfortable and inconvenient appliances, for instance, headgear [13–16].

However, we will have a far better and more efficient prospect, if we expand our concern about mesial movement from a small to a large amount, so that such a movement closes the missing posterior teeth space that occurred by other reasons, such as caries or congenital missing. If we can easily use molar protraction for closing missing posterior teeth spaces, this treatment will

U.B. Baik, DDS, MS, PhD
Private Practice, 35-5 Songjung-dong, Gangbuk-ku, Ecopia 7F, Seoul 142-100, South Korea
e-mail: baikub222@naver.com

K.B. Kim (ed.), *Temporary Skeletal Anchorage Devices*,
DOI 10.1007/978-3-642-55052-2_8,

provide a particularly useful treatment modality to replace dental implants and bridges as well as orthodontic treatment [17]. If we can use the third molar, which was to be discarded, the significance of this treatment will become exponentially greater [18–20].

However, this treatment has some difficulties. The mesiodistal length of the mandibular first molar (10–11.5 mm) is longer than that of the bicuspid (7–7.5 mm). The longer the distance to be moved, the greater the side effects will become. It is almost inconceivable without TSAD, and, even with TSAD, it is not so simple to control horizontal, vertical, and transverse problems [21]. Periodontal and alveolar bone problems must also be considered simultaneously. To what extent is this treatment possible? How much clinical and scientific evidence is there?

In this chapter, a total of 110 missing first molar and lower E spaces (87 patients) have been closed by second molar protraction. The aim of this chapter is to introduce these cases for further analysis and to discuss the validity of this treatment.

The main focus of this chapter is on the closure of first molar missing spaces by protraction of the second and third molars. Third molar eruption when the second molar is missing or extracted will not be discussed in this chapter. When the second molar is missing, protraction of only the third molar is necessary. On the other hand, when the first molar is missing, the protraction of both the second and third molars is necessary. Accordingly, the case of a missing first molar is more difficult to treat than the case of a missing second molar. For a quite long period of time, the second molar has been extracted to solve anterior crowding and protrusion, and that space would be closed by distal movement of the first molar and the eruption of the impacted third molar. The traditional second molar extraction treatment can be characterized by molar distalization rather than molar protraction.

8.1 Classifications of Molar Protraction

Molar protraction with TSAD can be classified by the missing area and amount of the movement of the posterior teeth.

1. By the missing area
   (i) Missing maxillary first molar (Fig. 8.1a)
   (ii) Missing mandibular first molar (Fig. 8.1b)
   (iii) Closure of E (deciduous second molar) space (mandible) (Fig. 8.1c) when the permanent second bicuspid is missing
2. By the amount of mesial movement of the posterior teeth
   (i) Pure retraction of anterior teeth: In practice, there are very few cases of pure retraction of anterior teeth because the mesiodistal length of the first molar is very long.

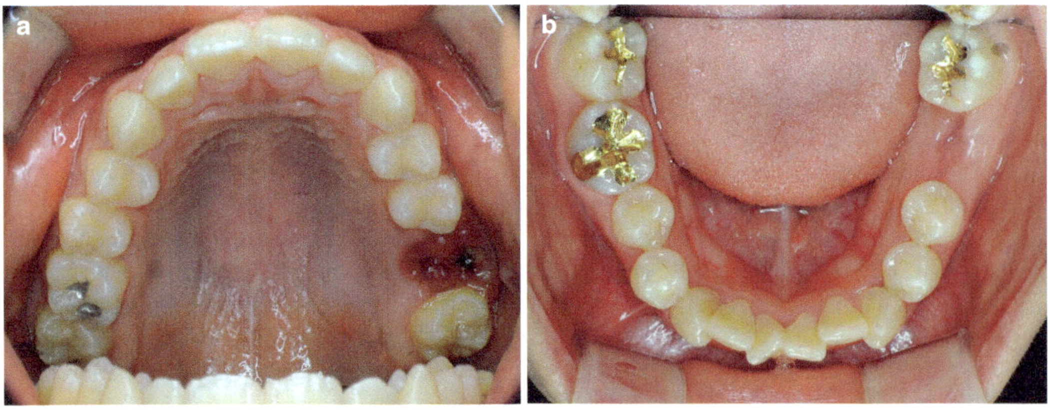

Fig. 8.1 Three areas of missing posterior teeth. (**a**) Missing maxillary first molar. (**b**) Missing mandibular first molar. (**c**) Closure of E (deciduous second molar) space (mandible) when the permanent second bicuspid is missing

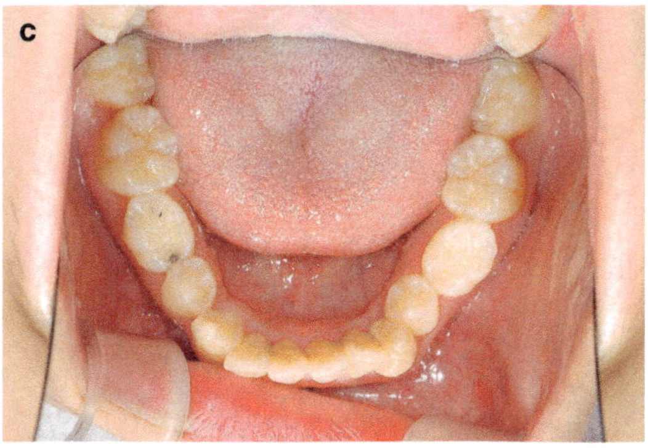

Fig. 8.1 (continued)

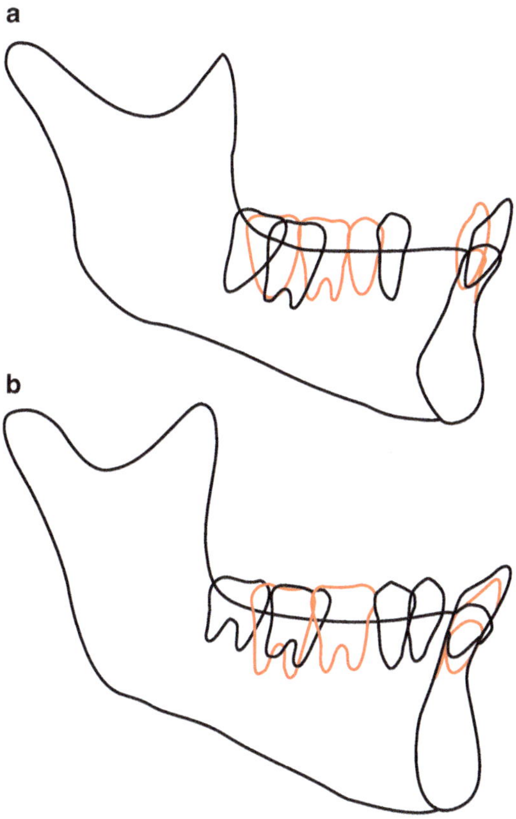

Fig. 8.2 (**a**) Reciprocal traction. (**b**) Pure protraction of the posterior teeth

(ii) Reciprocal traction (Fig. 8.2a): Many cases fall under this category.

(iii) Pure protraction of posterior teeth (Fig. 8.2b): The missing first molar space is closed by pure protraction of the posterior teeth. If the first molar were intact, these cases could be treated by non-extraction. This is the most difficult type of teeth movement because the distance to be moved is the longest.

8.2 Cases of Molar Protraction

1. Missing maxillary first molar (Fig. 8.3)
2. Missing mandibular first molar (Fig. 8.4)
3. Closure of E (deciduous second molar) space (mandible) when permanent second bicuspid is missing (Figs. 8.5, 8.6 and 8.7)

8.3 Formation of Molar and Canine Relation

In this chapter, the term "Class I molar relationship" is used to specify the position of the second molars moved into the first molar location.

1. Class I molar and Class I canine relation
   (i) Missing maxillary first molar and mandibular non-extraction (Fig. 8.8a)
   (ii) Missing maxillary and mandibular first molar (Fig. 8.8b)
   (iii) Maxillary non-extraction and missing mandibular first molar (Fig. 8.8c)
2. Class II molar and Class I canine relation
   (i) Maxillary bicuspid extraction and missing mandibular first molar (Fig. 8.9)
3. Class III molar and Class I canine relation
   (i) Missing maxillary first molar and mandibular bicuspid extraction (Fig. 8.10)

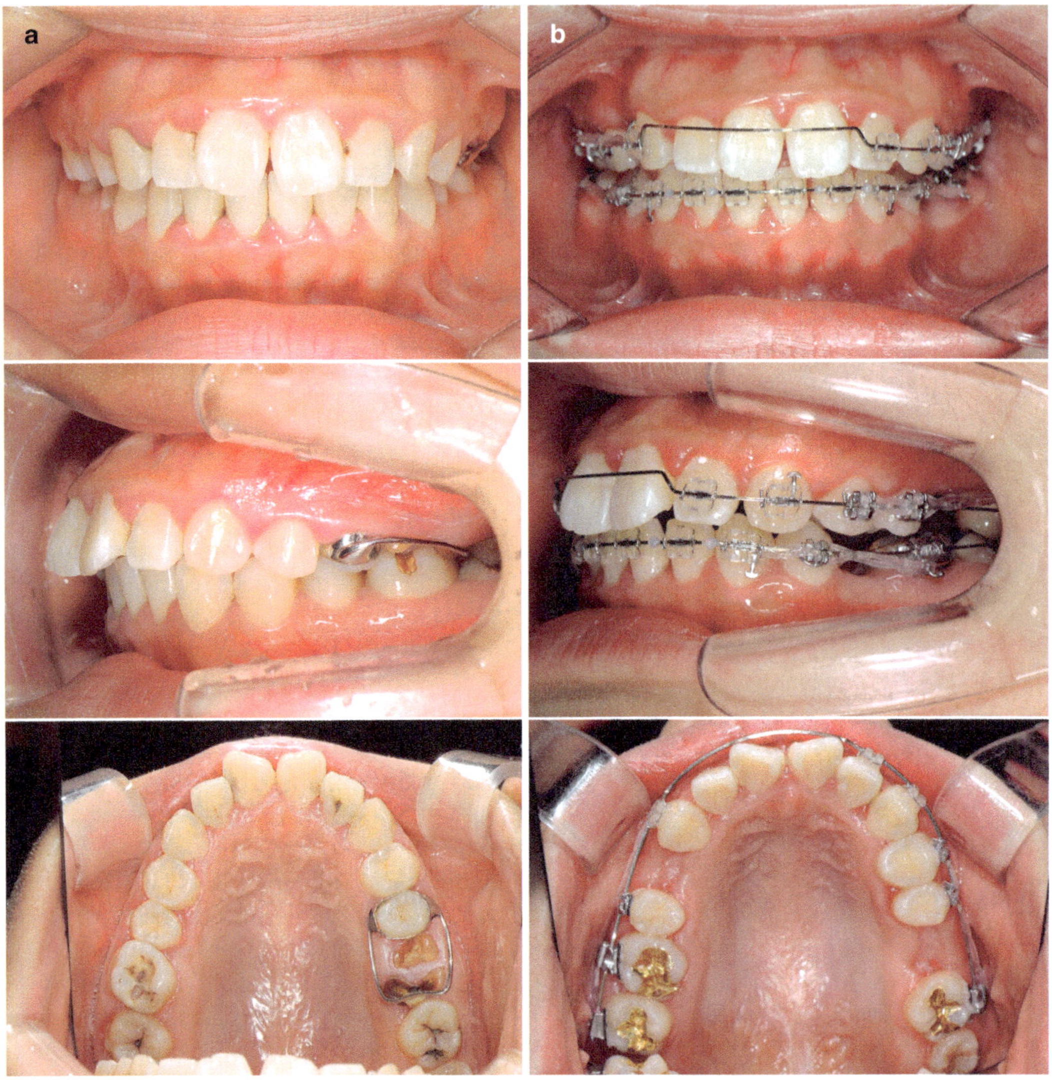

Fig. 8.3 (**a**) Initial, (**b**) during treatment, (**c**) debonding, (**d**) 1 year 8 months after debonding, (**e**) X-ray. A 20-year, 7-month-old female patient came for the correction of lip protrusion and crowding. Her maxillary left first molar was in a root rest state due to severe caries; therefore, the first molar was extracted instead of the bicuspid of the maxillary left side. At debonding, the missing first molar space closed completely. The lip protrusion and crowding improved. At 1 year and 8 months after debonding, there was no space relapse. The second and third molars looked like the first and second molars

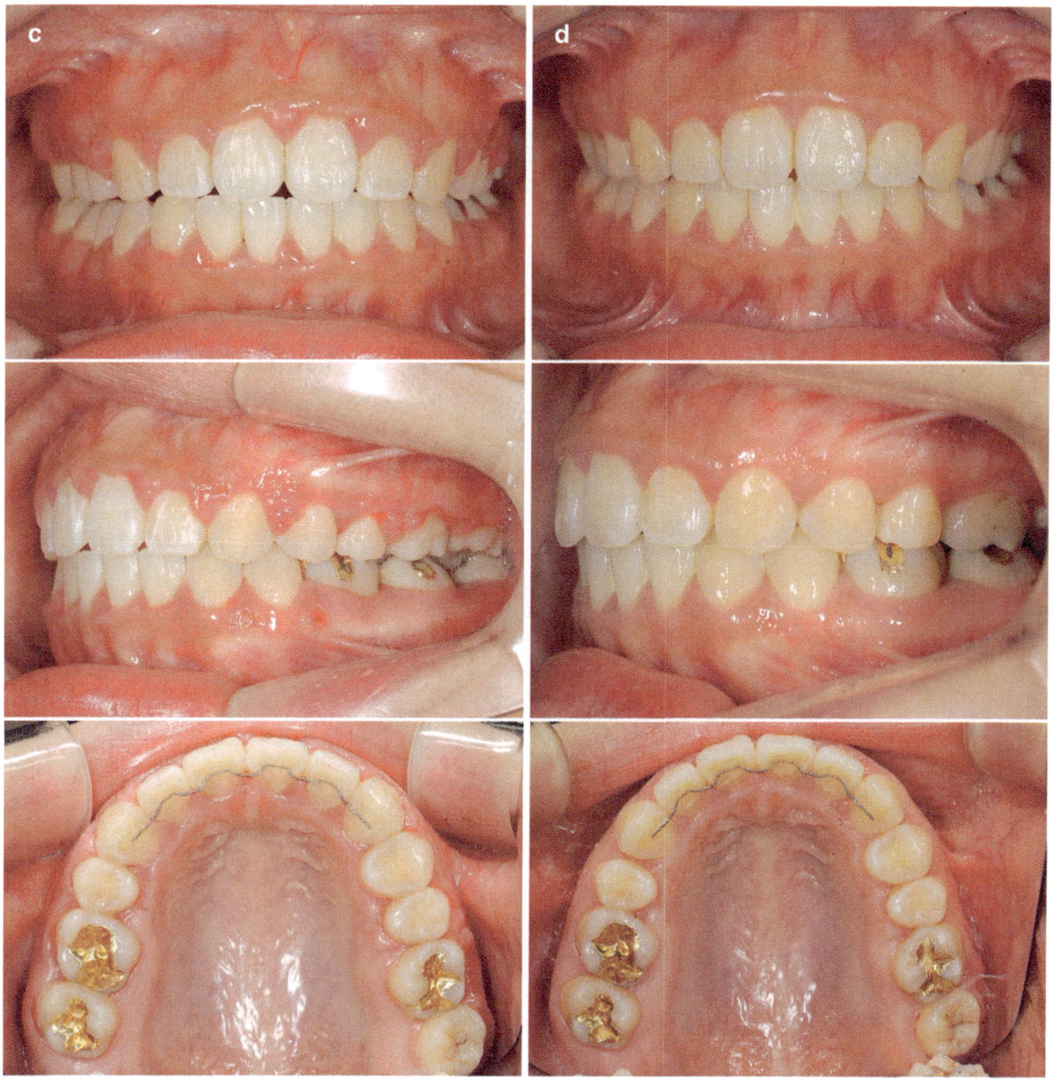

Fig. 8.3 (continued)

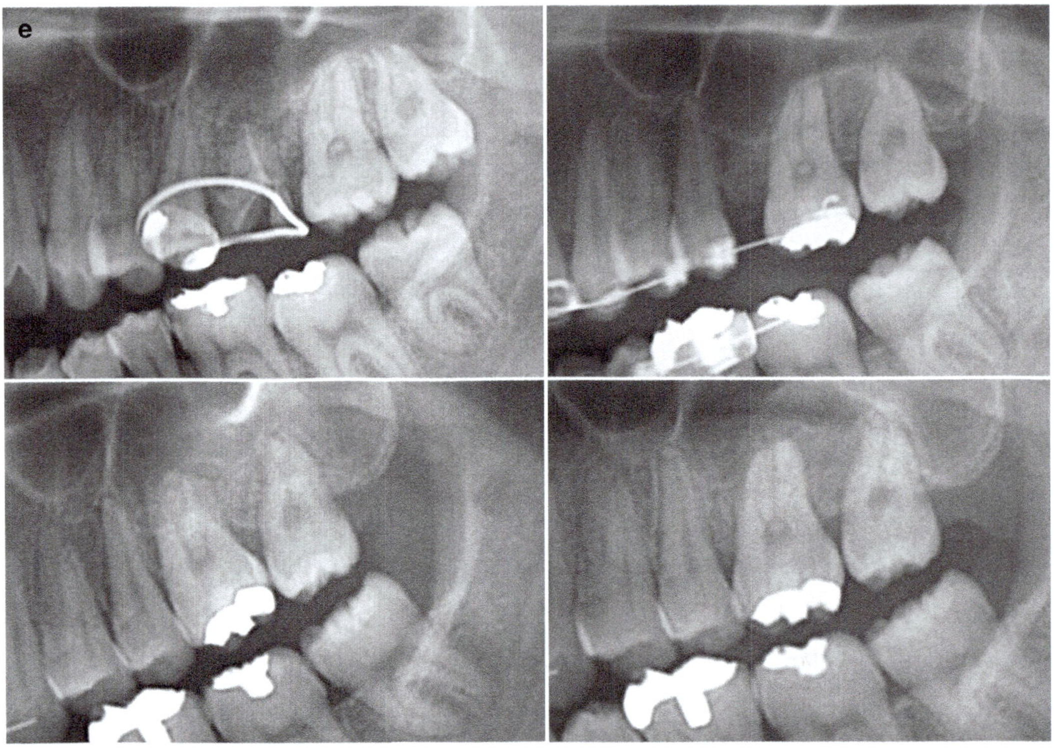

Fig. 8.3 (continued)

8.4 Possible Problems and Biomechanics

8.4.1 Tipping of Adjacent Teeth

This 33-year-old female had been referred by other clinic (Fig. 8.11a, b). Her chief complaint was protrusion and she had a bad mandibular left first molar. Three bicuspids and the mandibular first molar had been extracted with the space closed at the previous clinic. At this stage (Fig. 8.11c), when she came to my clinic, the second molar showed severe tilting. Within 4 years and 6 months after the start of treatment, the periodontium had been severely damaged. The root barely moved. This is the most common complication of this treatment.

8.4.2 Mesial Rotation and Buccal Sweeping

When protracting the second molars, mesial rotation and swinging into the buccal side of the protracted second molars may occur, which can create a posterior crossbite (Fig. 8.12). To prevent this, a rigid lingual arch and a lingually placed TSAD can be used. However, the lingual

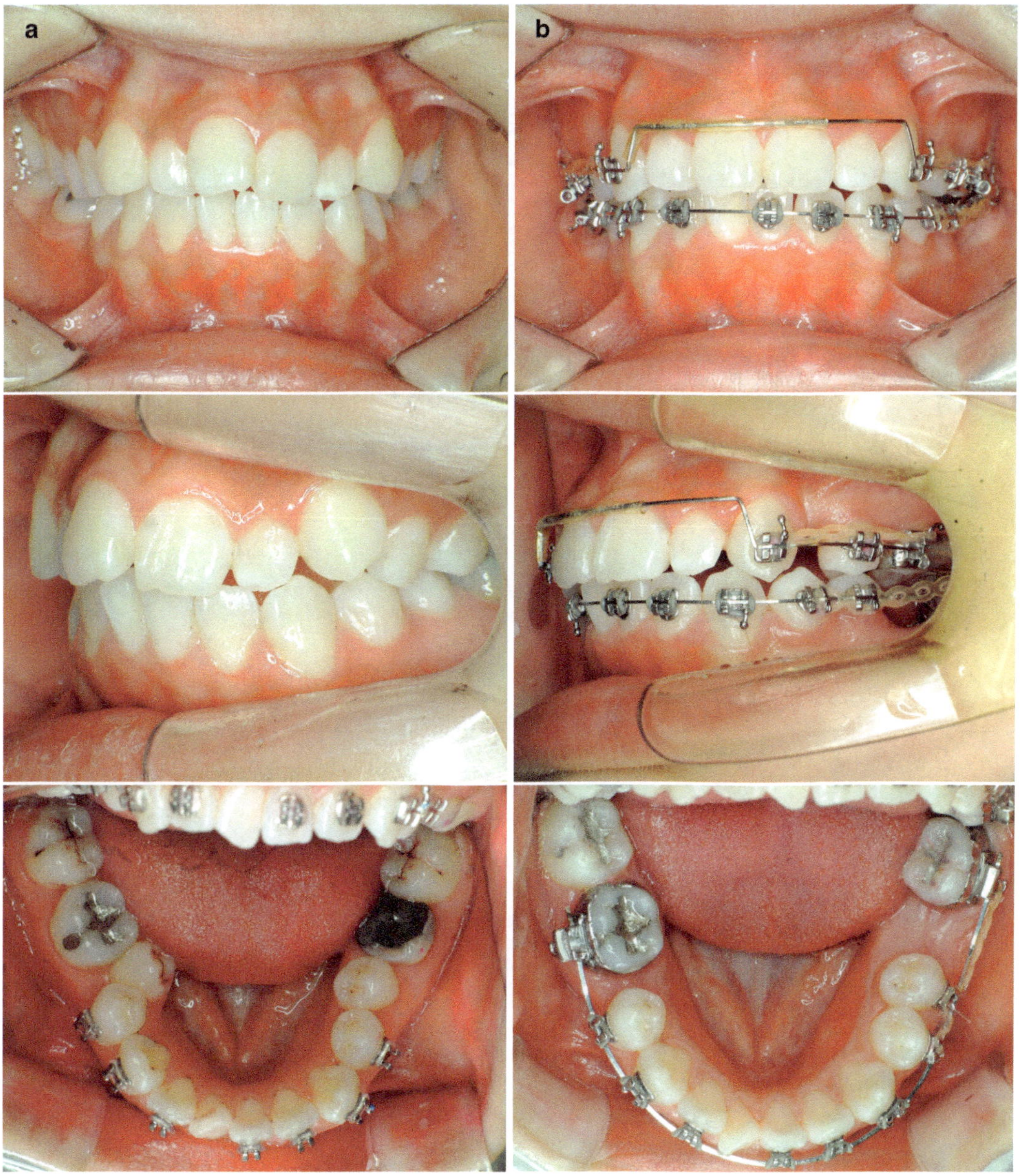

Fig. 8.4 (**a**) Initial, (**b**) during treatment, (**c**) debonding, (**d**) 5 years and 8 months after treatment, (**e**) X-ray. A 16-year, 11-month-old female patient came for the correction of anterior crowding and protrusion. Her mandibular left first molar was severely damaged by caries. The first molar was extracted at that site, and on the other side, three bicuspids were extracted. The long distance of the mandibular left first molar extraction space was closed successfully. There was no space relapse 5 years and 8 months after debonding, despite no usage of a fixed wire retainer. The impacted third molar erupted well even though the configuration was not good. It will be usable for a considerable amount of time without major problems

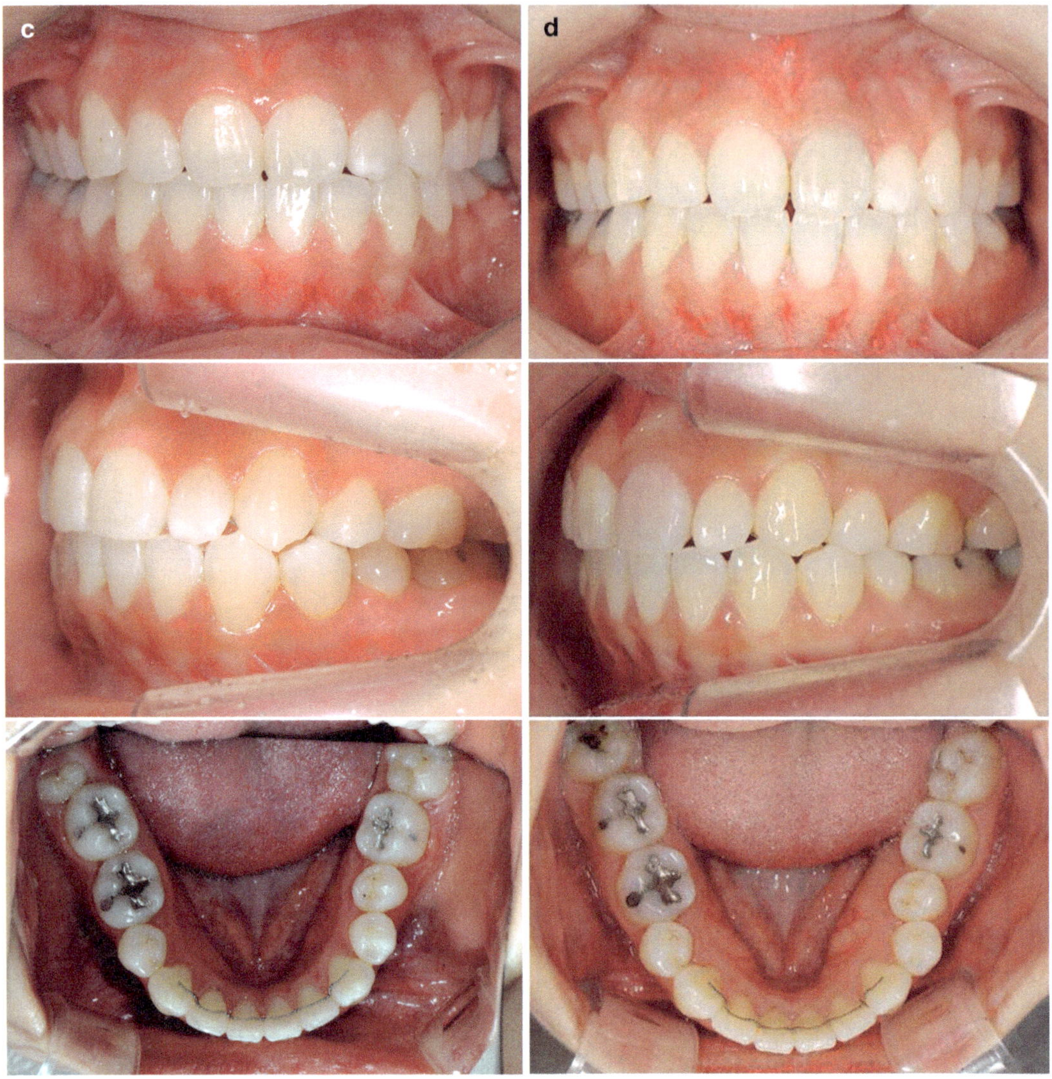

Fig. 8.4 (continued)

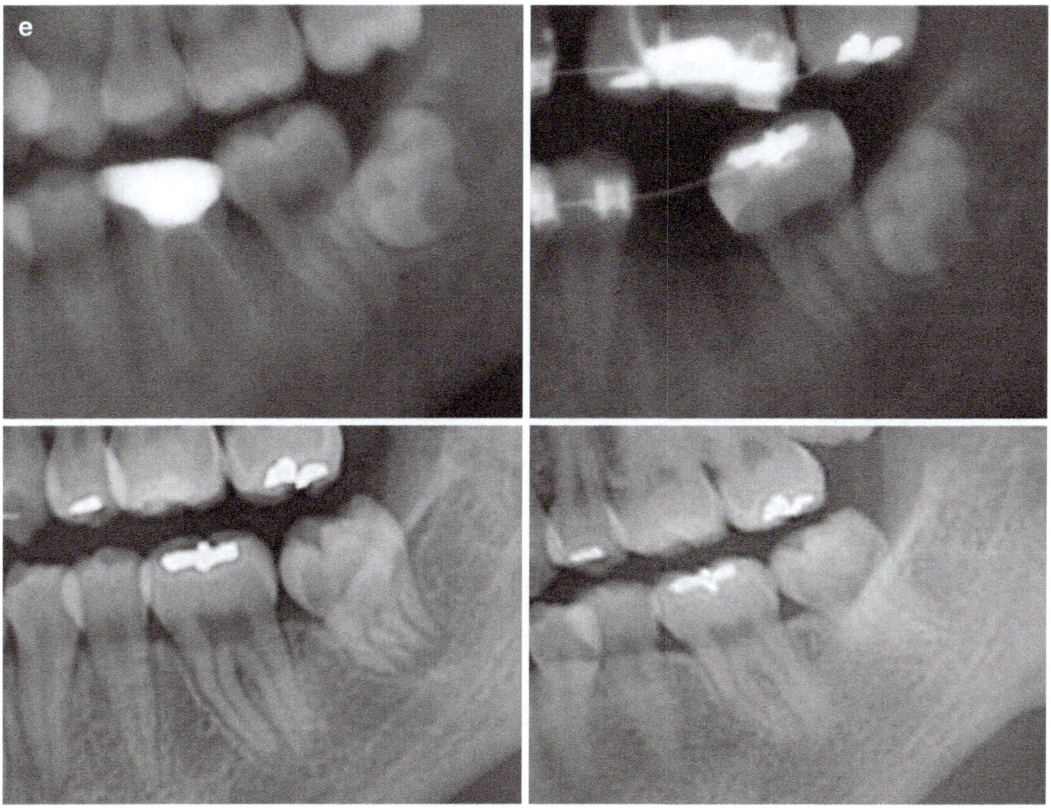

Fig. 8.4 (continued)

arch may not only cause discomfort to the patient but also interfere with further mesial movement. In addition, the lingual arch needs to be remade when it touches the lingual side of the anterior teeth. Lingual placement of the TSAD is very difficult because of poor vision and accessibility. Other methods are placing an elastic chain from the lingual side of the molars to a button on the canine or a sliding band with a lingual arch. In the cases in this book, this problem was minimized by inserting an anti-rotation bend in the posterior portion of the arch wire.

8.4.3 Extrusion of the Posterior Teeth

During the protraction, the extrusion of the posterior teeth caused an anterior open bite (Fig. 8.13). The entire arch rotates around the center of rotation of the whole dentition in the TSAD retraction system (Fig. 8.14). As a result, when the posterior teeth were protracted, the molars are extruded, causing an anterior open bite.

To solve these problems, the following methods are suggested: (1) A long hook can be attached to the second molar brackets to relocate the protracting force near the center of rotation. (2) The maxillary and mandibular molar intrusion can be done by TSAD.

8.5 Other Cases

1. Case of three missing first molars (Figs. 8.15 and 8.16)
2. Difficult case (Figs. 8.17 and 8.18)
3. Failed case (Fig. 8.19)

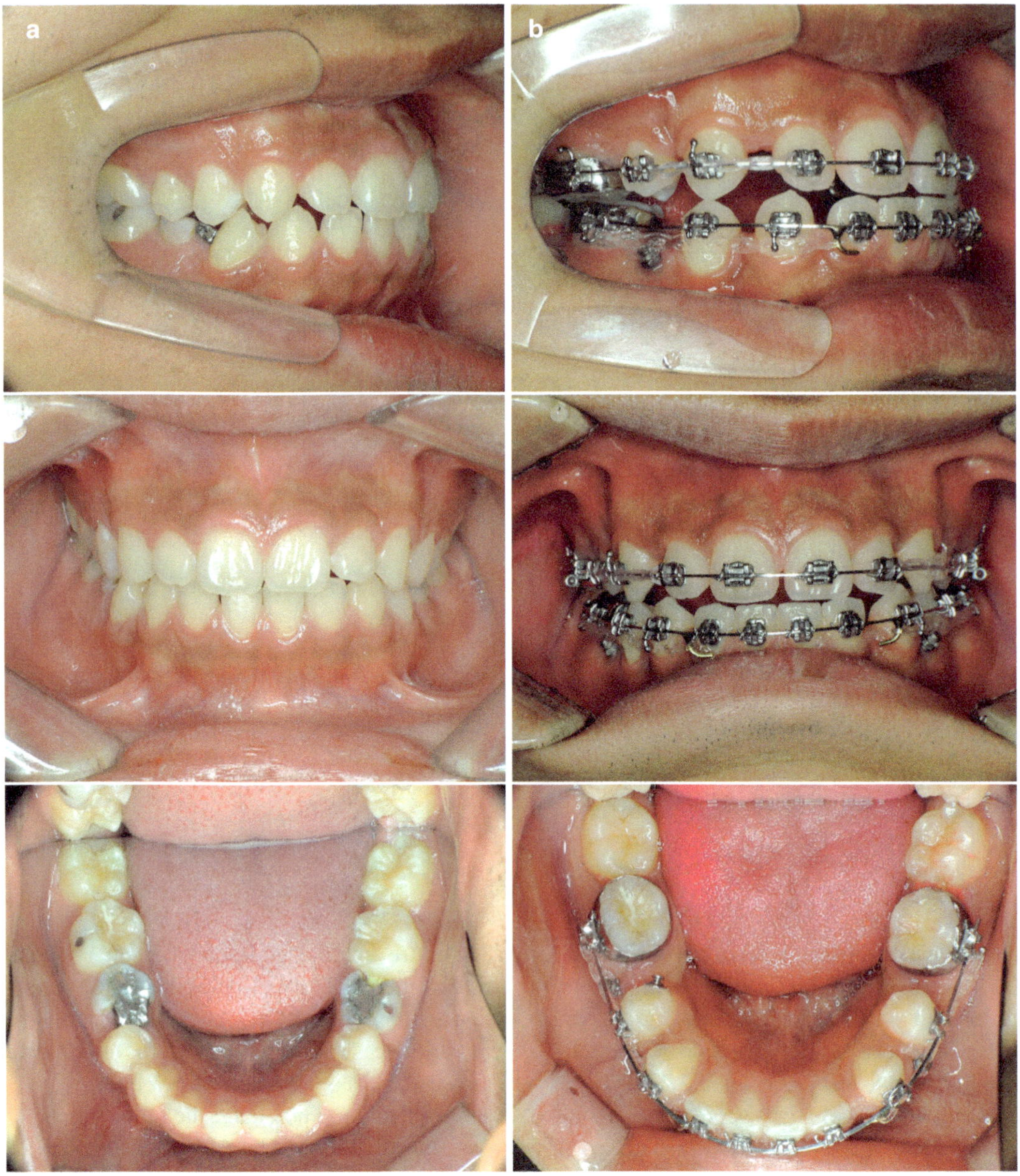

Fig. 8.5 (**a**) Initial, (**b**, **c**) during treatment, (**d**) debonding, (**e**) 4 years and 9 months after treatment. A 15-year, 11-month-old male patient came for the correction of anterior protrusion. The mandibular left and right second deciduous molars were retained and their successors (second bicuspids) were missing. Those teeth and the maxillary right and left first bicuspids were extracted. At debonding, bilateral Class I molar and canine relation had been achieved. The retraction of the anterior teeth reduced the protrusion of the lips. At 4 years and 9 months after treatment, stable occlusion and good function could be seen and there was no space relapse

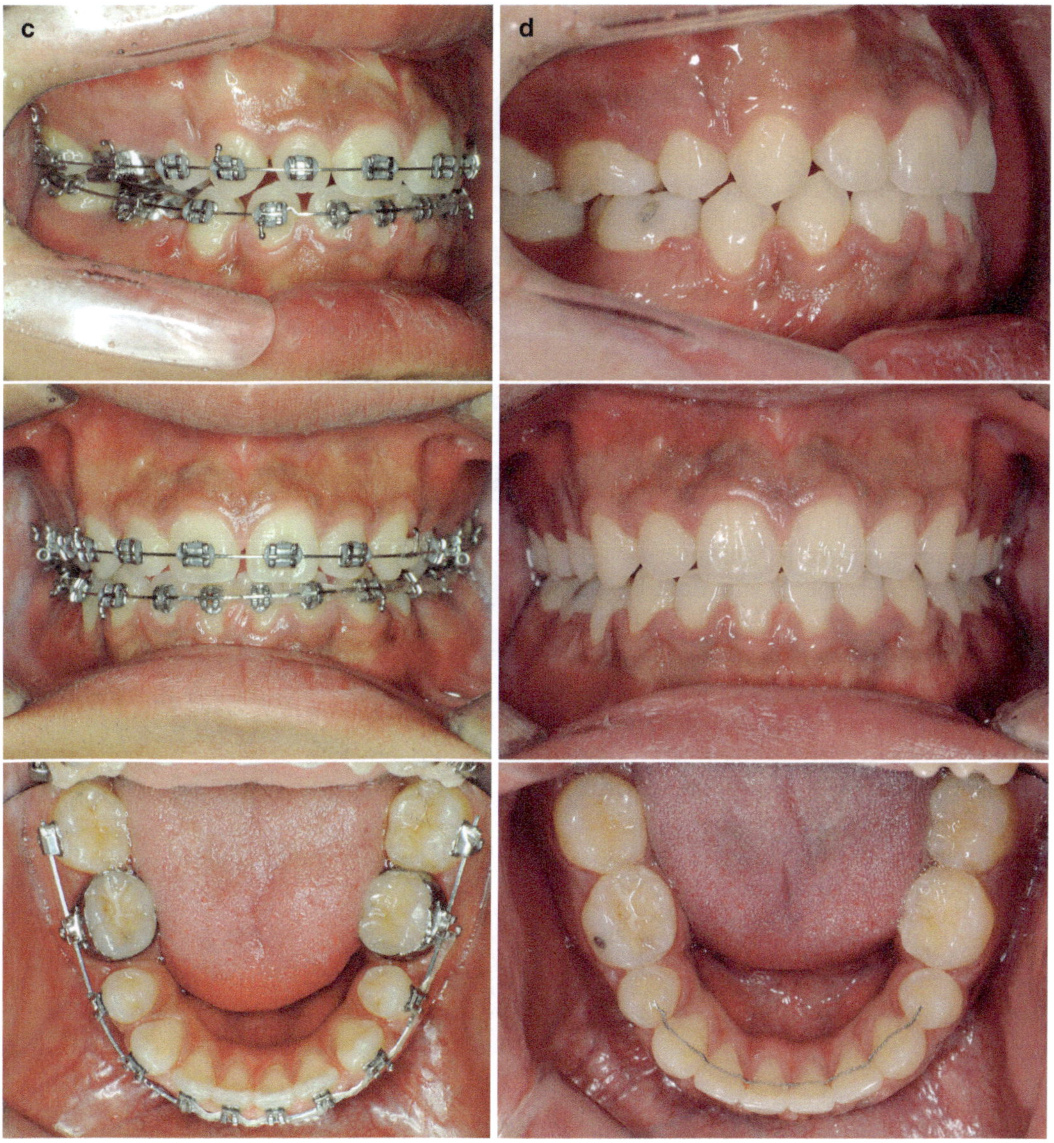

Fig. 8.5 (continued)

8.6 Summary of Finished Cases

8.6.1 Patients and Teeth

Only patients who had permanent dentition at the initial stage were collected and analyzed. In this study, the total number of teeth treated was 110 and the number of the patients was 87. The subjects were divided into three groups.

(i) Closure of maxillary (upper) first molar missing space (U-6)
(ii) Closure of mandibular (lower) first molar missing space (L-6)
(iii) Closure of mandibular (lower) deciduous second molar extraction space with second bicuspid missing (L-E)

The number of U-6 was 27; L-6, 63; and L-E, 20 (Table 8.1). The number of teeth treated in female patients was two times higher than that of teeth treated in male patients. Of the three groups, the number of female patients was the highest in the L-6 group. There were three cases of a patient with three missing posterior teeth and the case of one patient with four missing first molars (Table 8.2).

8.6.2 Age Distribution

This data shows only the patients with permanent dentition. The average age of all patients was 20.8 years old (Table 8.3). The age distribution of the U-6 and L-6 group had no significant

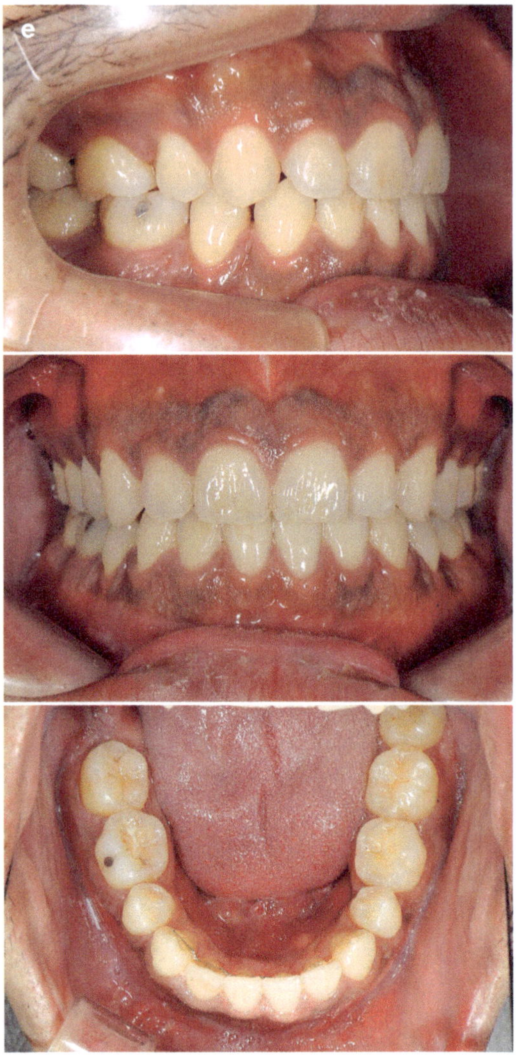

Fig. 8.5 (continued)

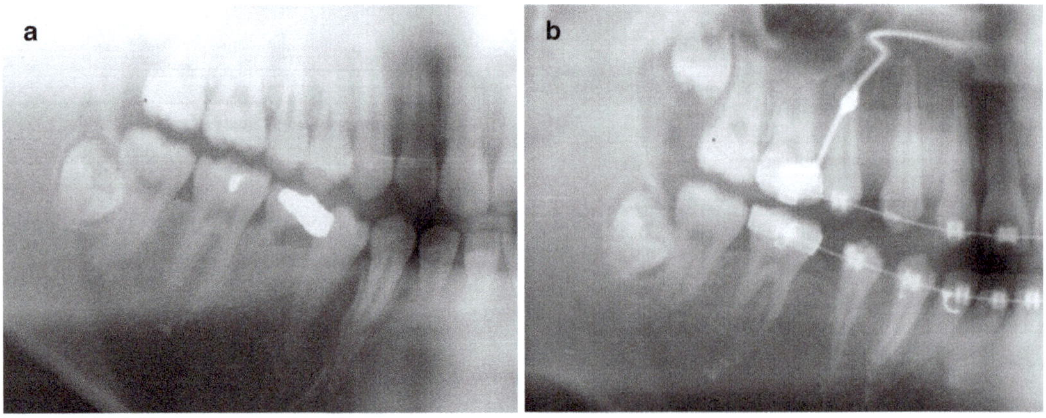

Fig. 8.6 (Continued) *Right side*. (**a**) Initial, (**b–d**) during treatment, (**e**) debonding, (**f**) 4 years and 9 months after treatment

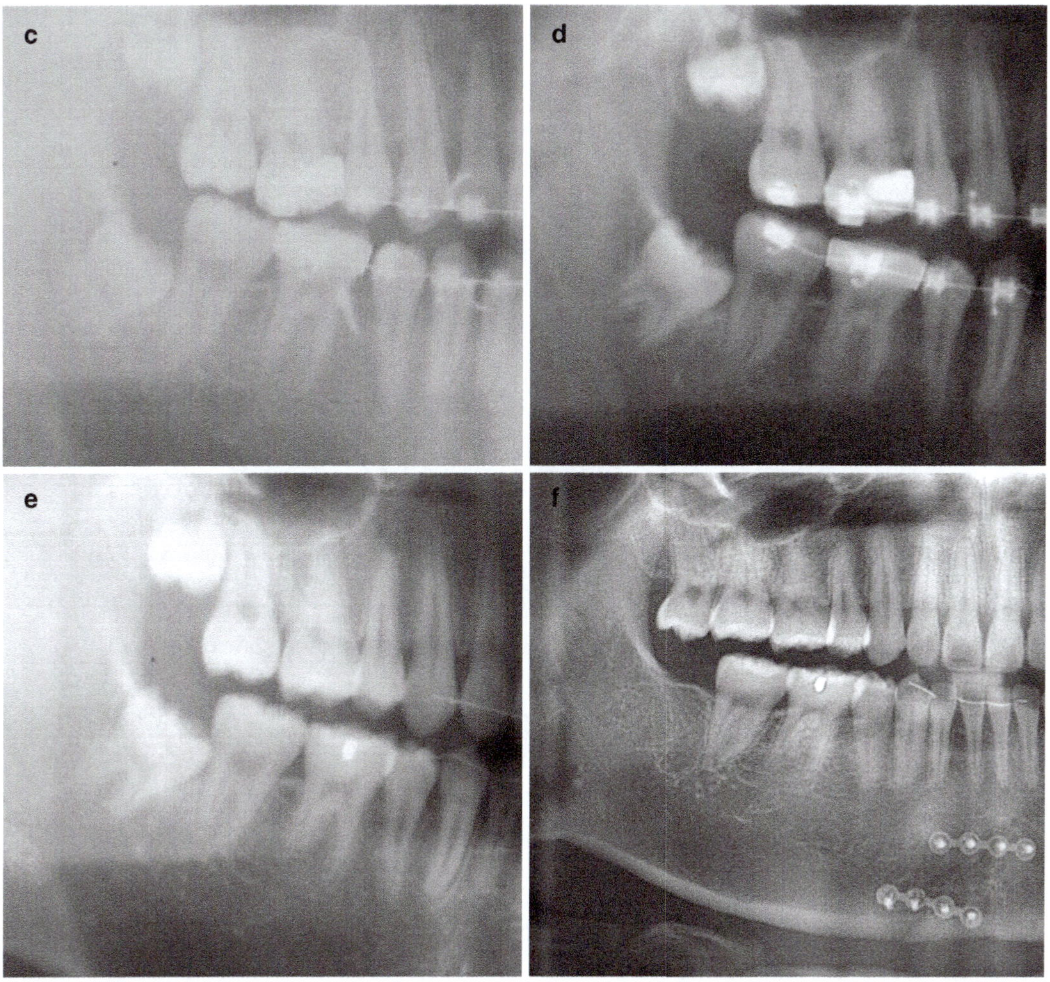

Fig. 8.6 (continued)

difference, whereas the age of the L-E group was younger than the others.

The youngest patient was 13.8 years old (L-E), and the oldest patient was 39.8 years old (U-6, L-6). In the L-6 group, there were quite a number of patients above 30 years old (Figs. 8.20, 8.21 and 8.22).

8.6.3 Treatment Time

The treatments required the period of an average of 2 years and 10 months (Table 8.4). In the same clinic, it took approximately 2 years and 3 months to treat the typical bicuspid extraction. As a result, the first molar substitution treatment took 7 more months, but the treatment time will be expected to decrease in a near future because of accumulated skills.

Among the three groups (U-6, L-6, L-E), there was no significant difference in the treatment time (Figs. 8.23, 8.24 and 8.25).

8.6.4 Success Rate

Prior to analyzing failed or successful cases, the standards of failure and success must be established, difficult as it may be. If the parameter of failure is set as second molar becoming bad that

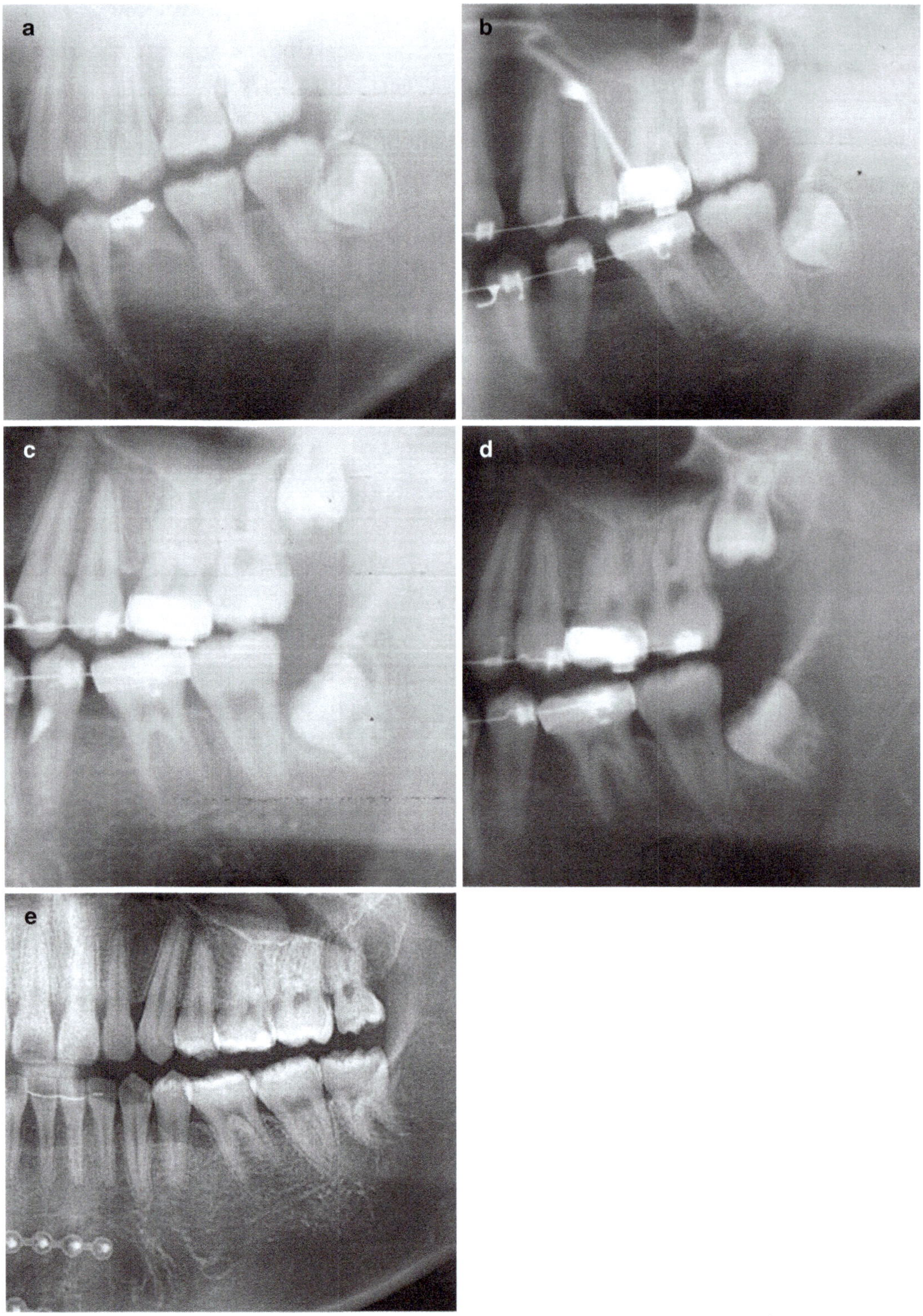

Fig. 8.7 (Continued) *Left side*. (**a**) Initial, (**b**, **c**) during treatment, (**d**) right before debonding, (**e**) 4 years and 9 months after treatment. Because of Leeway space, the mesiodistal length of the mandibular second deciduous molar was longer than that of its successors (second bicuspid). At debonding, the root arranged parallelly. The impacted mandibular third molar erupted successfully. His mandible was fractured 2 months before the follow-up and was operated on

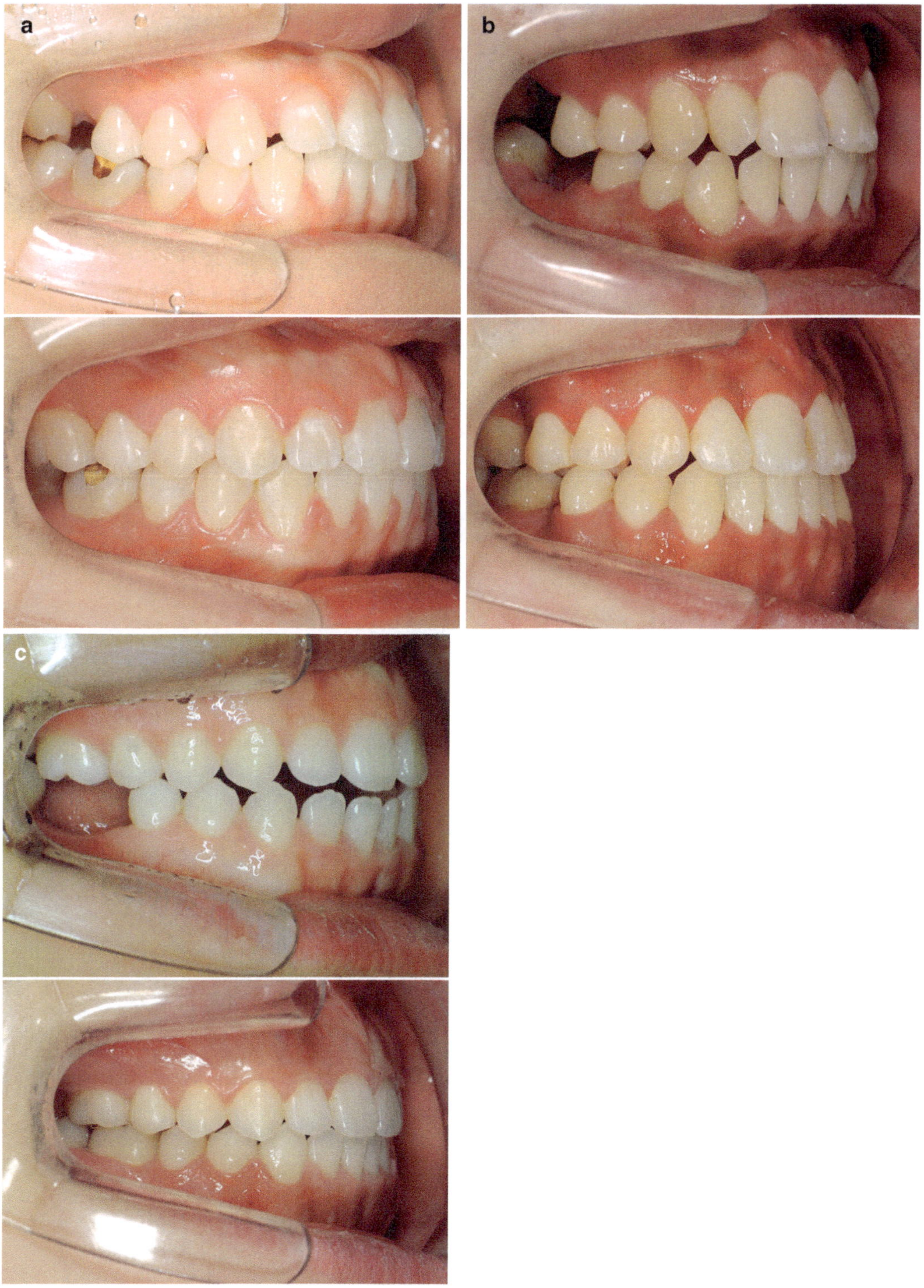

Fig. 8.8 Class I molar and Class I canine relation. (**a**) Missing maxillary first molar and mandibular non-extraction. (**a-1**) Before treatment. (**a-2**) After treatment. (**b**) Missing maxillary and mandibular first molar. (**b-1**) Before treatment. (**b-2**) After treatment. (**c**) Maxillary non-extraction and missing mandibular first molar. (**c-1**) Before treatment. (**c-2**) After treatment

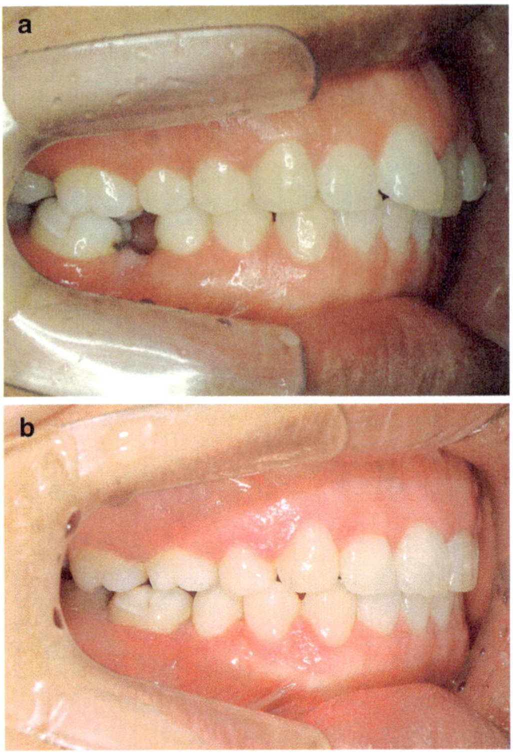

Fig. 8.9 Class II molar and Class I canine relation: maxillary bicuspid extraction and missing mandibular first molar. (**a**) Before treatment. (**b**) After treatment

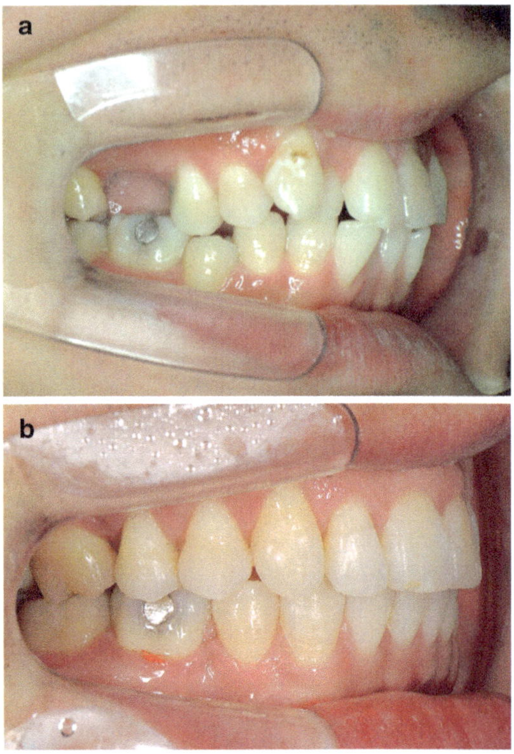

Fig. 8.10 Class III molar and Class I canine relation: missing maxillary first molar and mandibular bicuspid extraction. (**a**) Before treatment. (**b**) After treatment

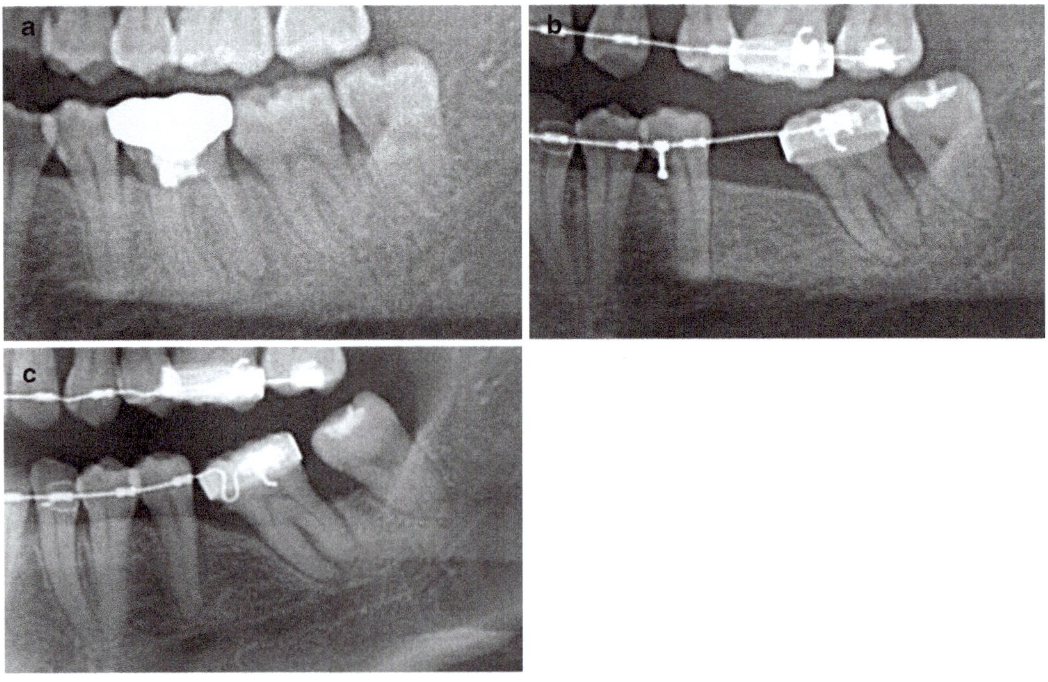

Fig. 8.11 (**a**) Initial, (**b**) during treatment, (**c**) 4 years 6 months after the start of treatment

Fig. 8.12 Protraction force (*B*) produced buccal force (*A*). This swung the posterior dentition into a unilateral crossbite

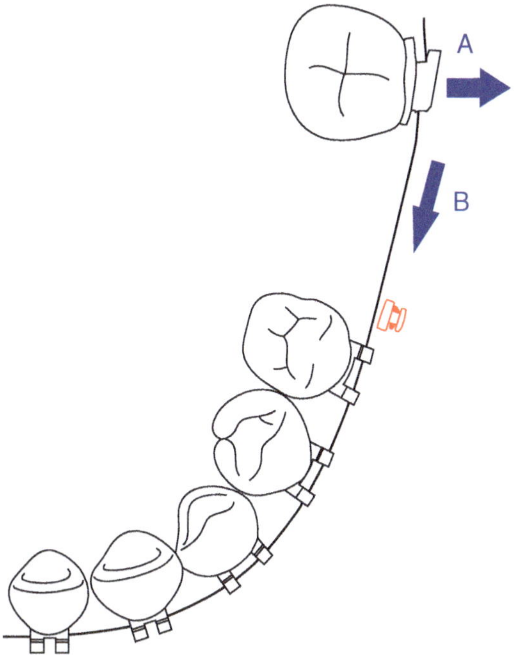

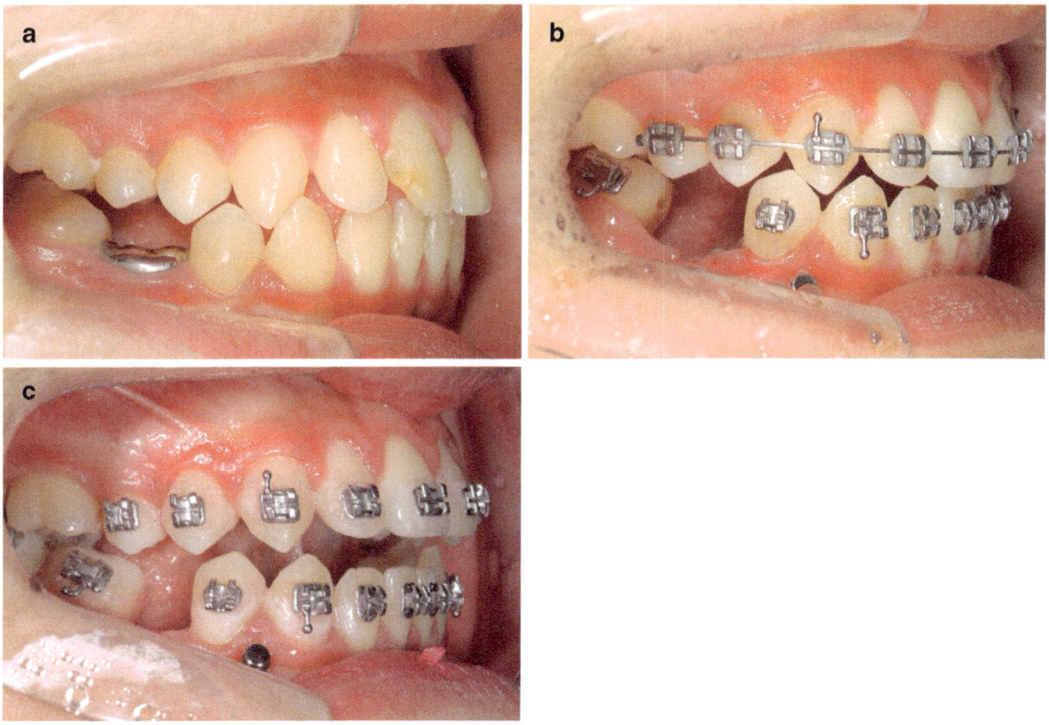

Fig. 8.13 Bite opening during molar protraction (**a**) initial, (**b**) during molar protraction, (**c**) open bite worsened

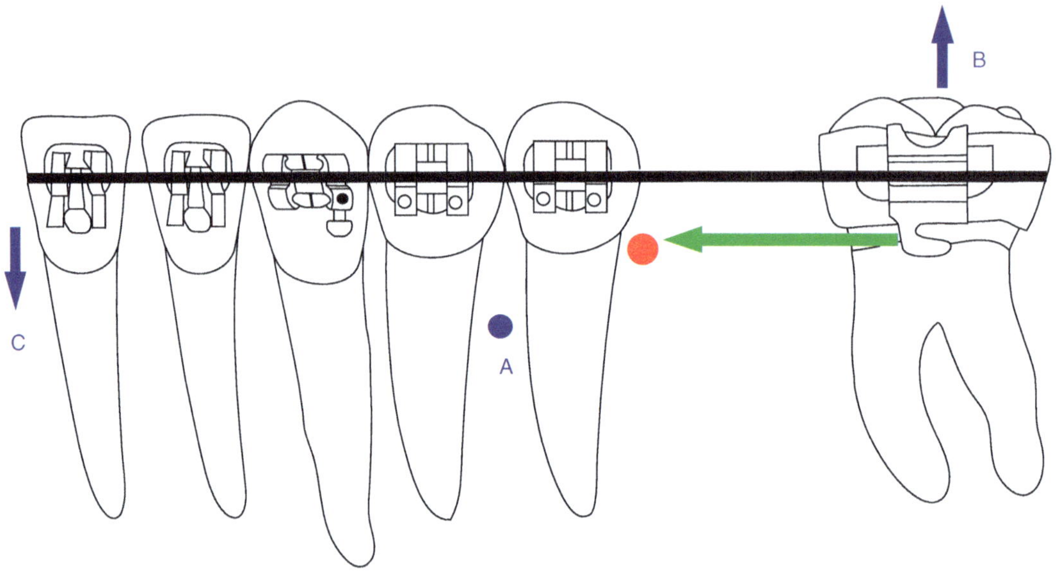

Fig. 8.14 The center of rotation of the entire arch (**a**) is located under the TSAD (*red point*). Protraction of the posterior teeth caused the extrusion of the posterior tooth (**b**) and intrusion of the anterior teeth (**c**)

needed to be extracted that seemed to be intact at earlier stage, then three cases are classified into failure. Success rate was 97.3 %.

Success Rate: 107/110 = 97.3 %

8.7 Mandibular Third Molar

There has not been sufficient research on the issue of the third molar eruption after first molar extraction up to now. TSADs are essential for this type of treatment, but TSADs have only been utilized in the last 10–15 years. After the extraction of the first molars, the second molars move mesially to provide space for the third molar to erupt. The related factors are as follows:

(i) Securing of space
(ii) Age and developmental stage of the root
(iii) Morphology of the tooth germ

Is it possible to predict the morphology of the third molar after eruption in advance? Clear configuration of the impacted stage does not always warrant desired results.

When space for third molar eruption was created by protracting the second molar, the third molar erupted spontaneously without any appliances in even the case of adults [22].

The following cases show the eruption of the third molar after first molar substitution treatment (Figs. 8.26, 8.27, 8.28, 8.29, 8.30, 8.31, 8.32 and 8.33). They were arranged according to the age of the patients. Even in such cases, in which the root formation was slightly insufficient at the initial stage, the root developed well and the tooth erupted. Even among the adults after root development is complete, the third molar also erupted in most cases. This critical issue demands a far better organized research in a very near future.

8.8 Evaluation

Until now, 110 cases of missing posterior teeth were treated. Among these, only three missing mandibular first molar cases have failed, largely

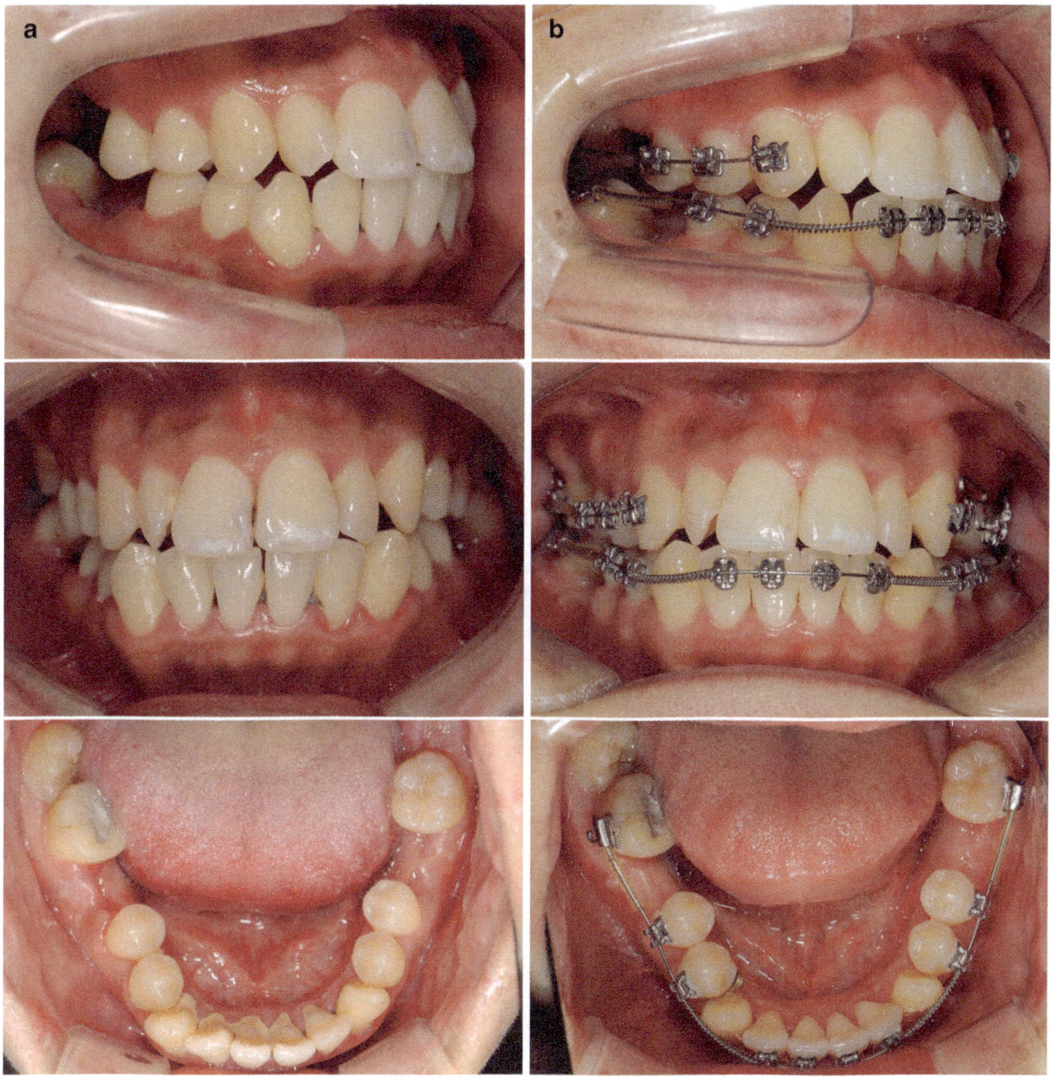

Fig. 8.15 (**a**) Initial, (**b–d**) during treatment, (**e**) debonding. A 26-year, 6-month-old male patient came for correction of crowding and protrusion. He had three missing first molars in total. The left maxillary first bicuspid was extracted, and the missing spaces of the three first molars were closed instead of extracting the bicuspids. During the treatment, the mandibular left third molar emerged into the oral cavity, allowing control of the tooth axis by bracket attachment. At debonding, the spaces closed completely, and the patient had no need for three dental implants

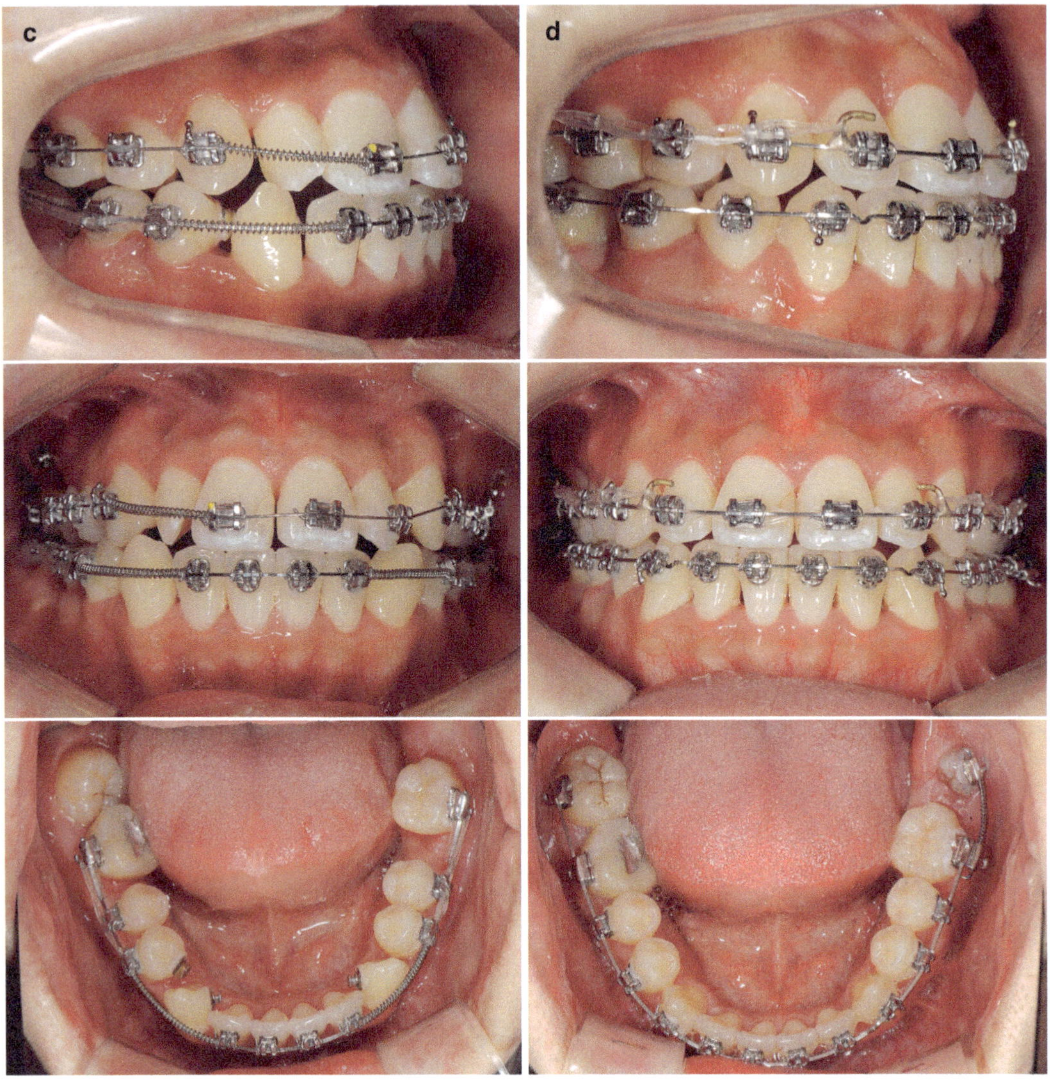

Fig. 8.15 (continued)

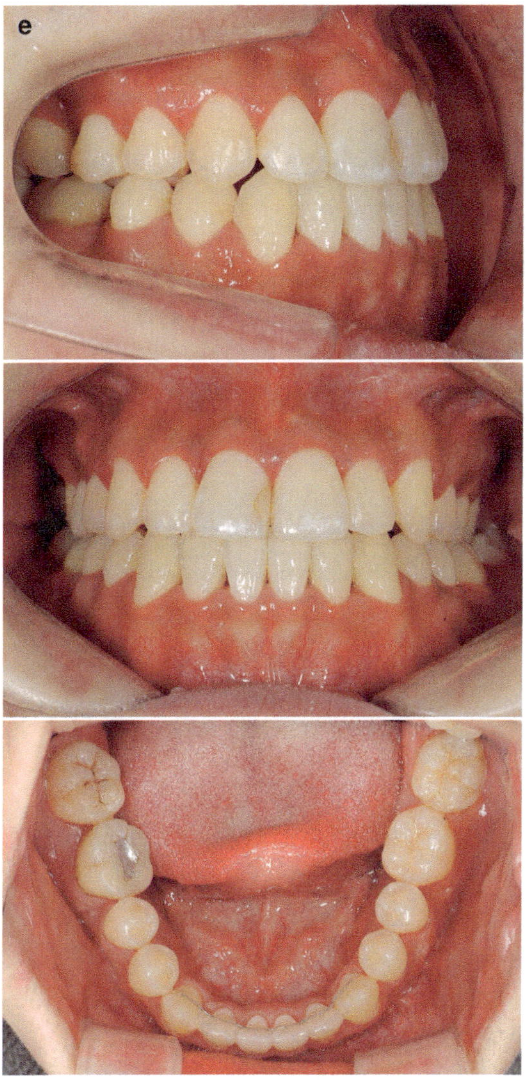

Fig. 8.15 (continued)

due to periodontal problems. In the future, henceforth, all more meticulous selection of cases is expected to lower the rate of failure.

Missing teeth have prompted the traditional treatment method, such as bridges or implants; however, orthodontic substitution treatment suggests another viable option. This is why some patients may choose orthodontic treatment despite lengthy treatment time. When patient has missing tooth, orthodontic evaluation should be done prior to other treatment options, because orthodontic treatment course becomes much more complex and difficult for the cases when implants or bridges are already applied.

It is highly likely that prosthodontists, endodontists, or periodontists may have more opportunities of seeing patients with missing teeth than orthodontists. For this reason, general dentists as well as orthodontists should consider orthodontic treatment as another good option.

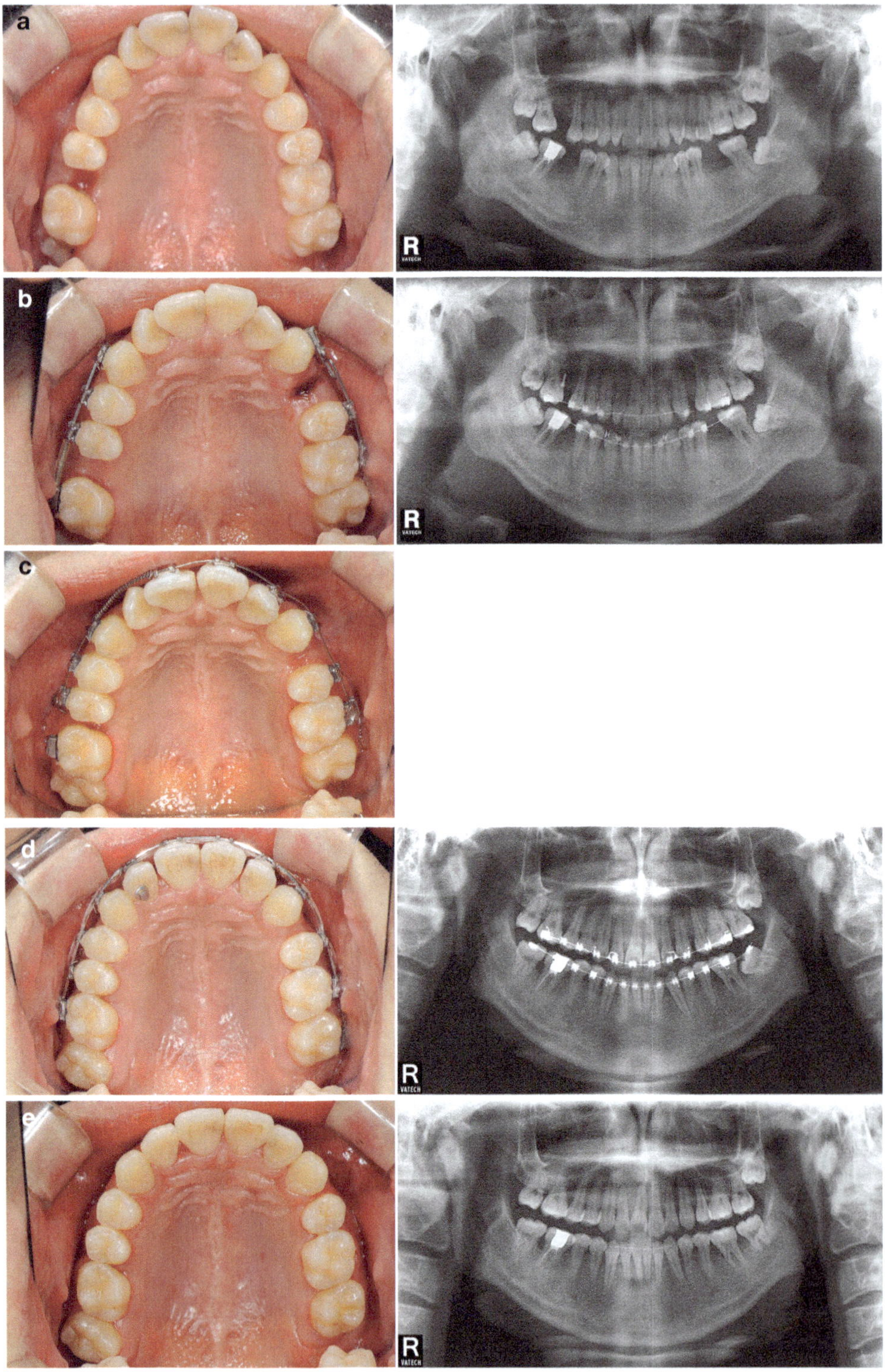

Fig. 8.16 (**a**) Initial, (**b**–**d**) during treatment, (**e**) debonding. Initially, the right and left mandibular third molars were horizontally impacted and uprighted during treatment. At debonding, the maxillary right first molar showed relatively good alveolar bone level, while that of the mandibular right second molar was low due to the horizontal impaction of the third molar at the beginning

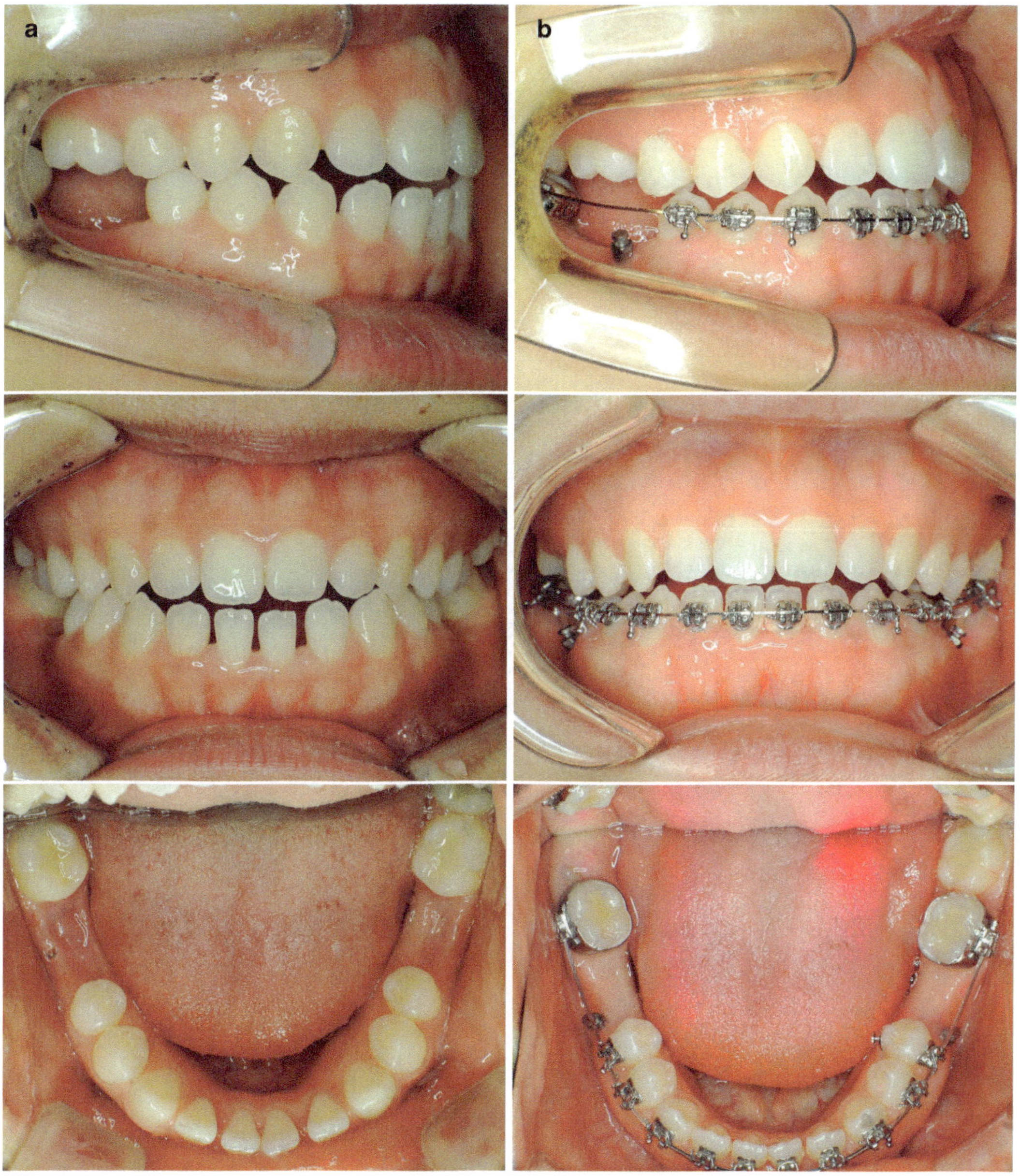

Fig. 8.17 (**a**) Initial, (**b**, **c**) during treatment, (**d**) debonding, (**e**) 1 year after treatment. An 18-year, 8-month-old female patient came for the treatment of an anterior open bite and spacing of the anterior teeth. This is a very difficult case because of the long missing space, pure protraction of the posterior teeth, and open bite problems. After a combination of molar protraction and molar intrusion, the long missing molar space was completely closed and the impacted third molars also erupted. Although the open bite slightly relapsed at 1 year after treatment, it was not severe

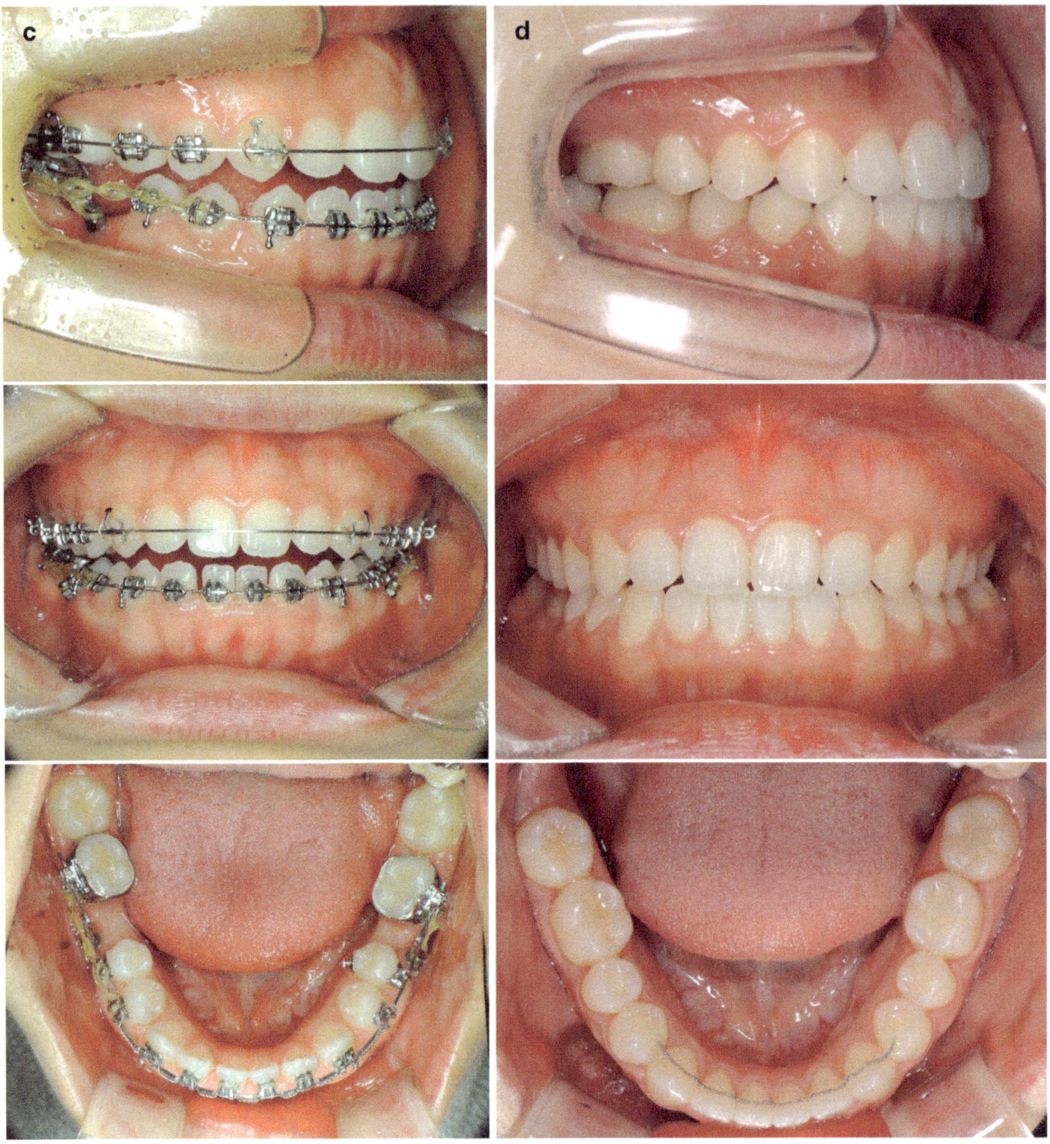

Fig. 8.17 (continued)

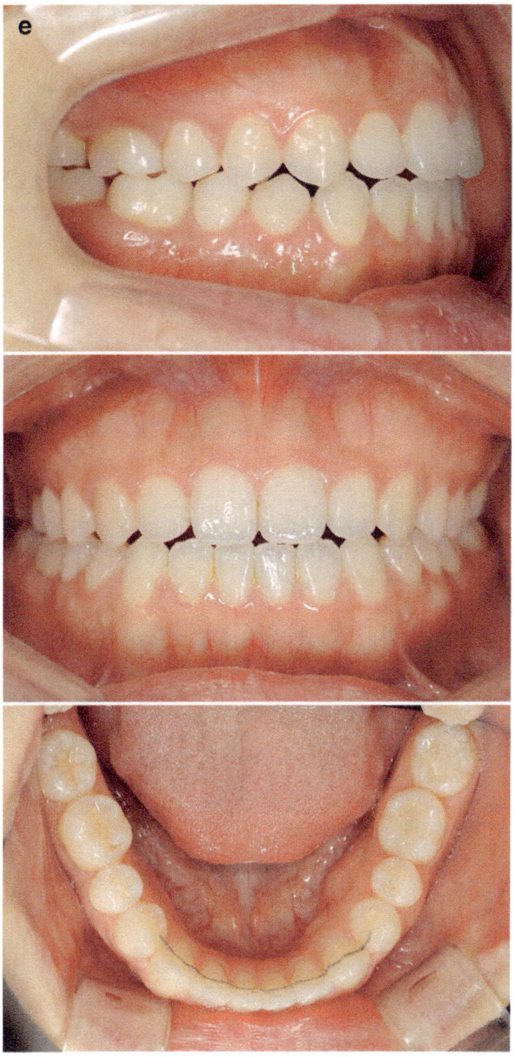

Fig. 8.17 (continued)

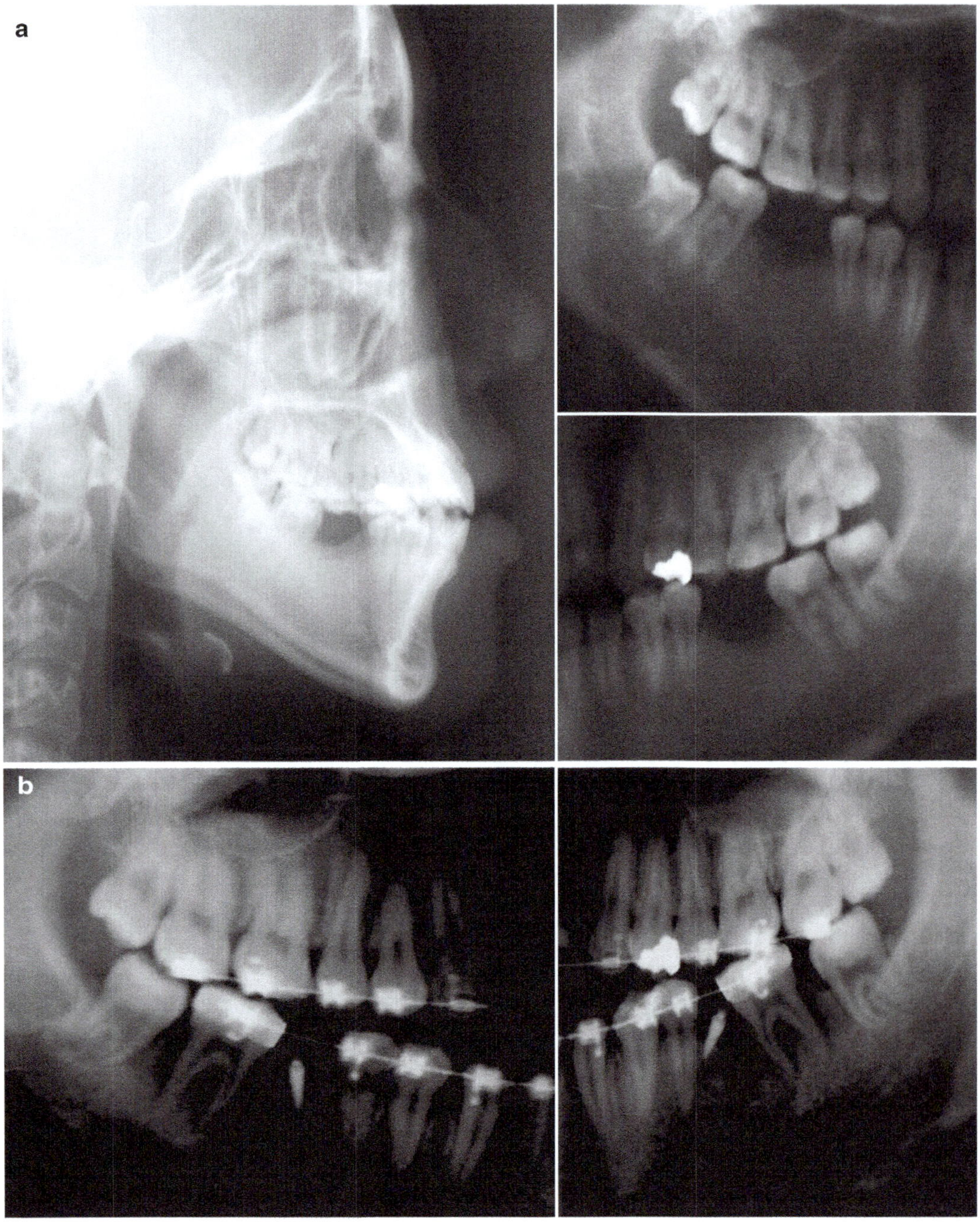

Fig. 8.18 (**a**) Initial, (**b**, **c**) during treatment, (**d**) debonding, (**e**) 1 year after treatment. At debonding, the second and third molars looked like first and second molars. Root paralleling could be seen on the panorama. This case report was selected as a "Case of the Month" in the *American Journal of Orthodontics and Dentofacial Orthopedics*, June, 2012 (From Baik et al. [5])

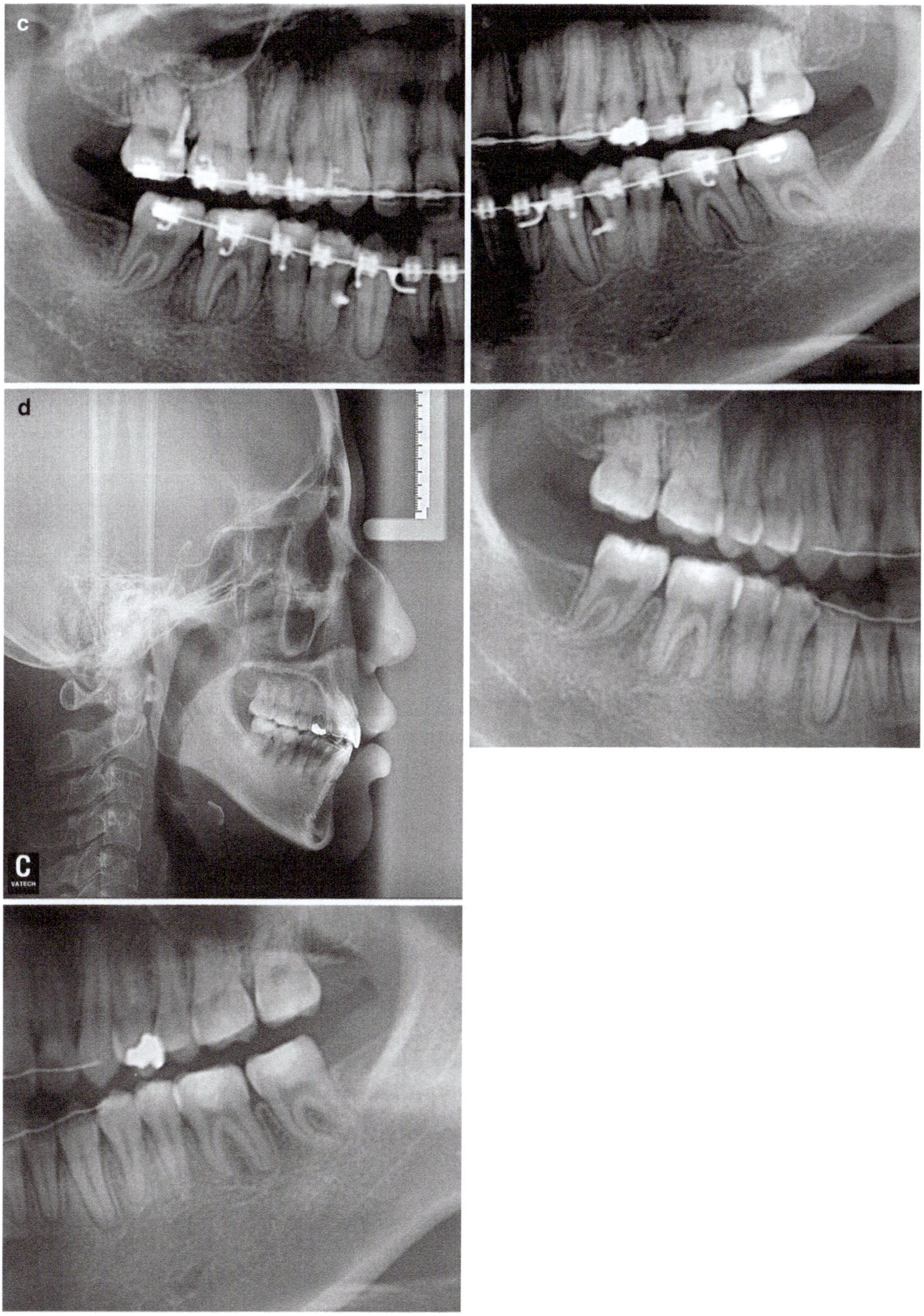

Fig. 8.18 (continued)

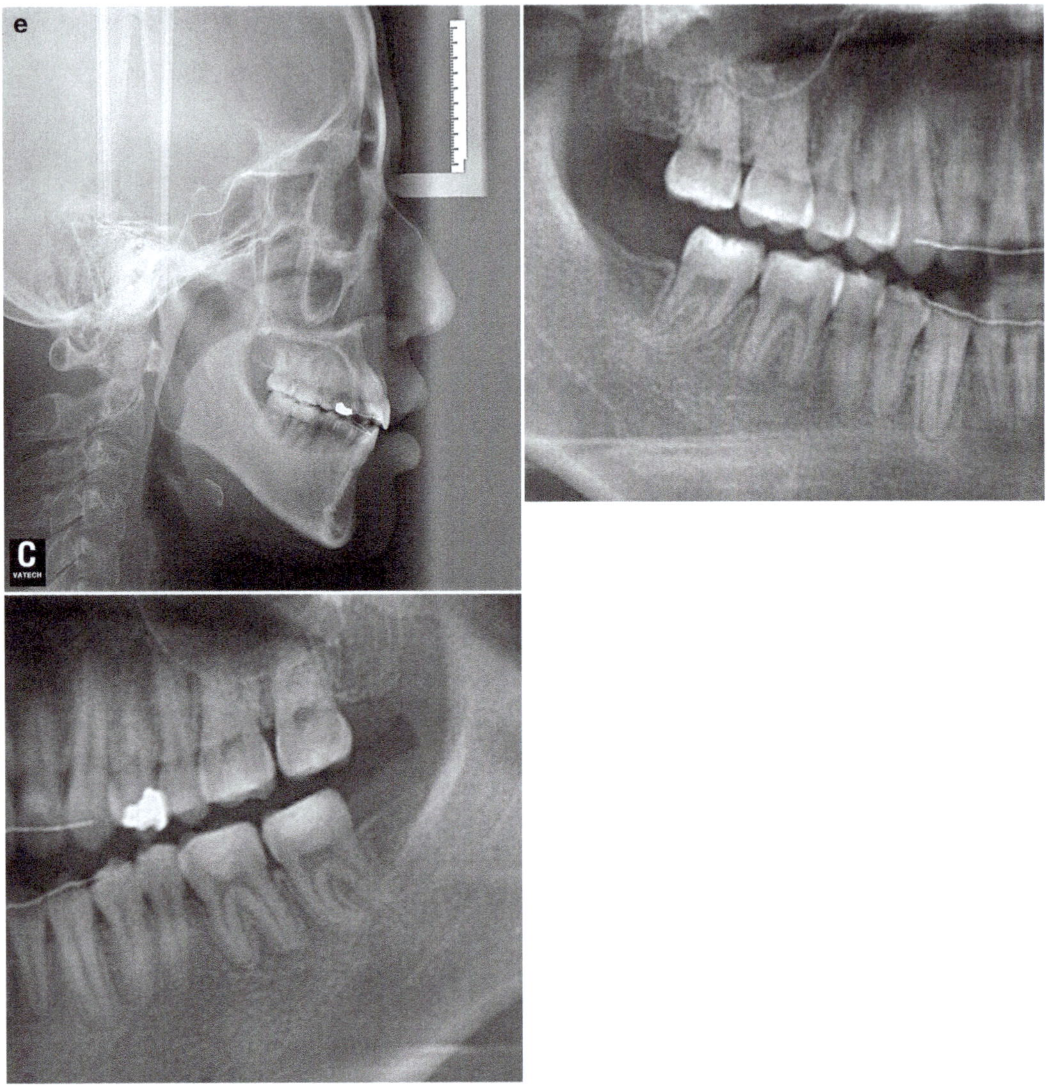

Fig. 8.18 (continued)

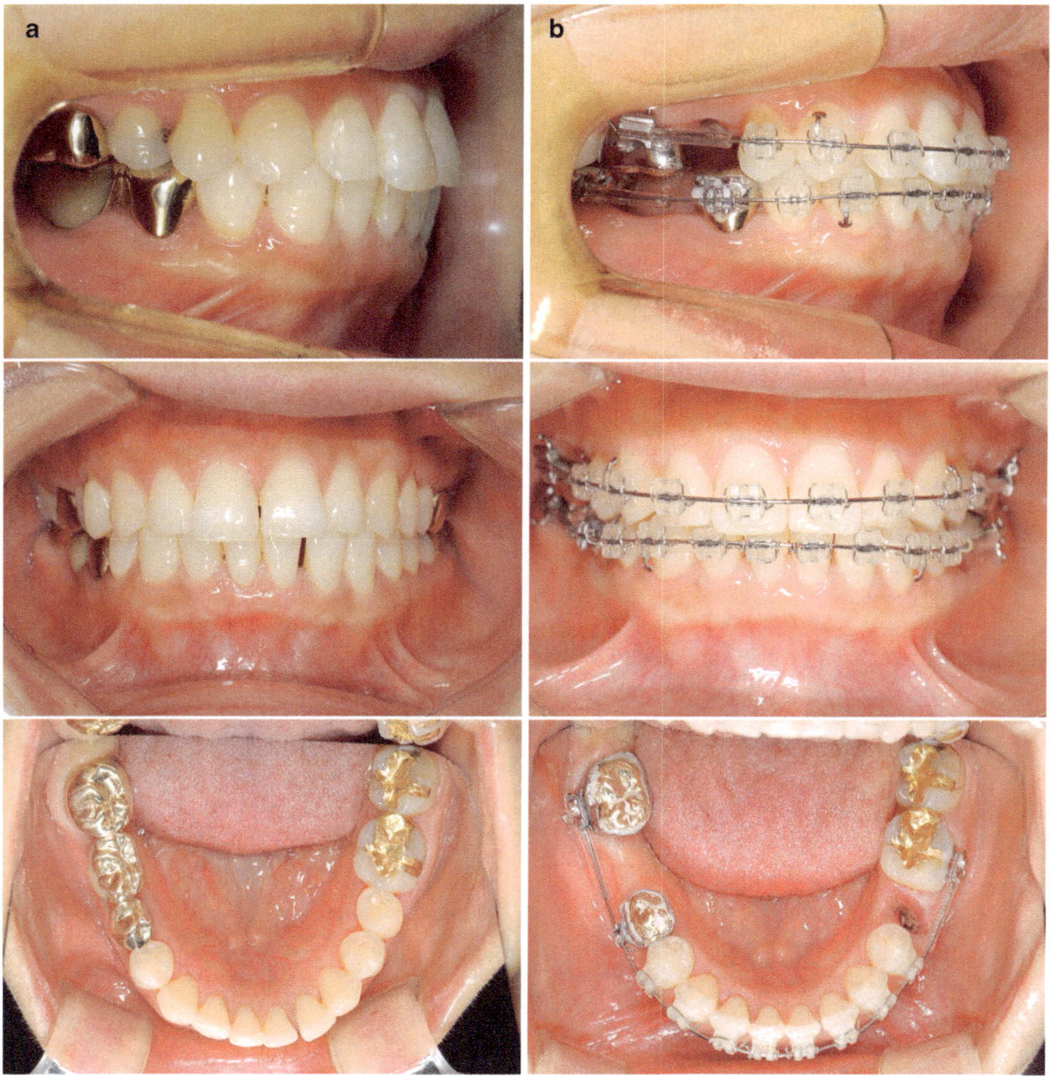

Fig. 8.19 (**a**) Initial, (**b**, **c**) during treatment, (**c**) debonding, (**e**) X-ray. A 22-year, 4-month-old female patient came for the correction of anterior protrusion. On the mandibular right side, the missing first molar space that was created by the removal of the pontic was used, and on the other side, three bicuspids were extracted. During the treatment, the periodontal pocket on the mesial side of the mandibular right second molar deepened and mobility had increased. At debonding, the other spaces were closed, but the periodontium of the mandibular left second molar was destroyed. That tooth would be extracted soon afterward. As a substitution treatment, this case is a failure; however, because the protrusion was improved, the treatment was not meaningless

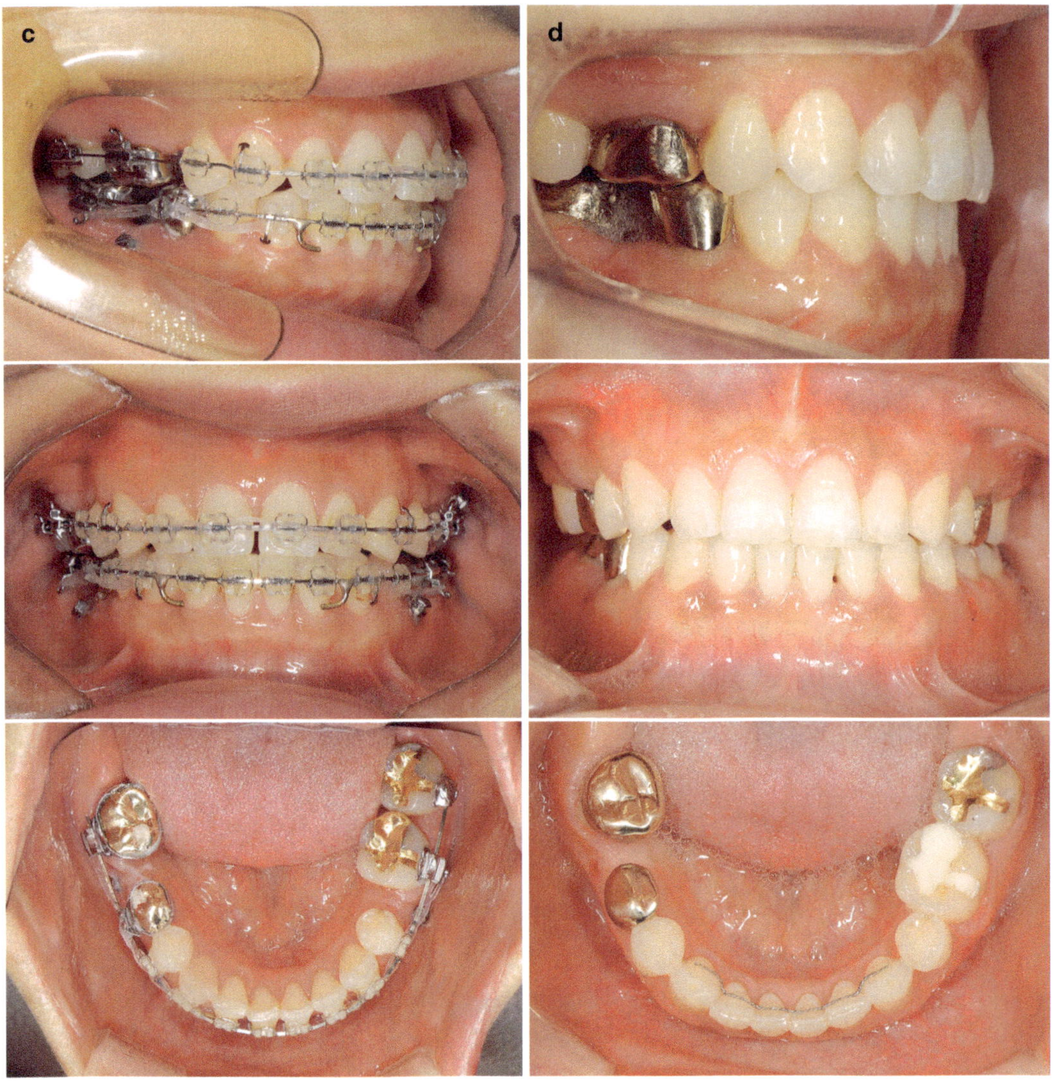

Fig. 8.19 (continued)

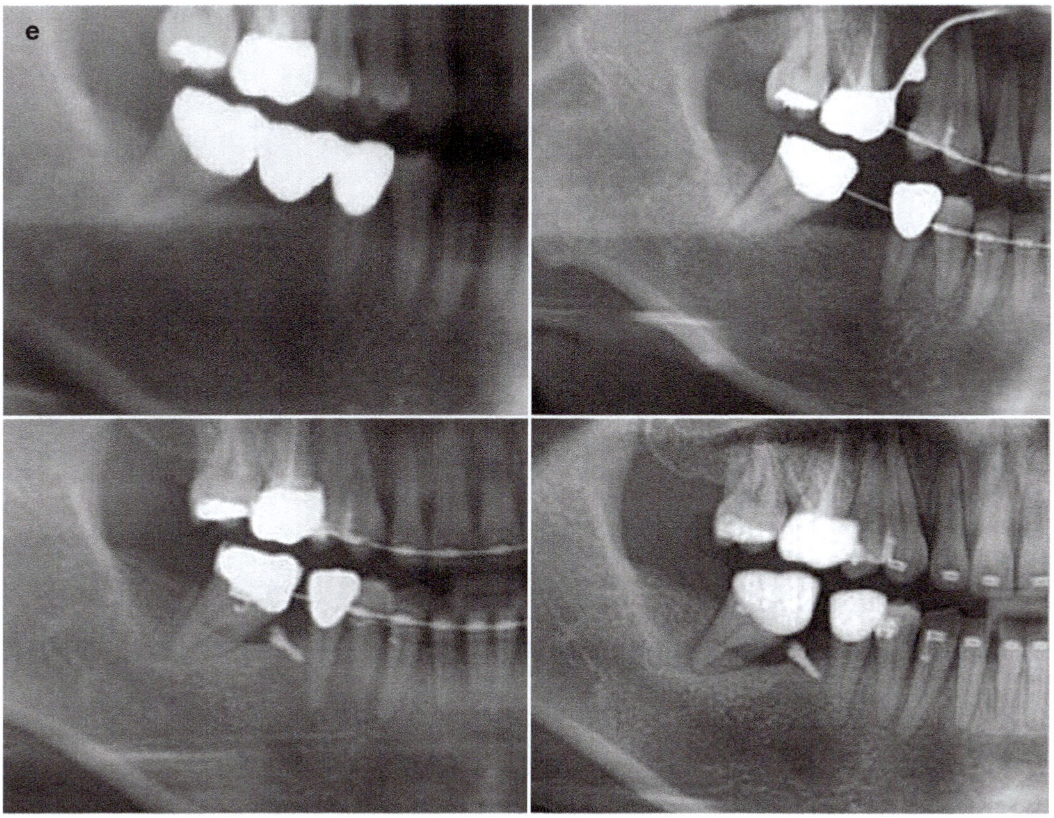

Fig. 8.19 (continued)

Table 8.1 Number of teeth

	Male	Female	Total
Upper-6	10	17	27
Lower-6	14	49	63
Lower E	12	6	20
Sum	36	72	110

Table 8.2 Number of patients

	Male	Female	Total
Upper-6	8	15	23
Lower-6	11	41	52
Lower E	8	4	12
Sum	27	60	87

Table 8.3 Age distribution

	Age
Upper-6	23.4
Lower-6	23.9
Lower E	15.3
Average	20.8

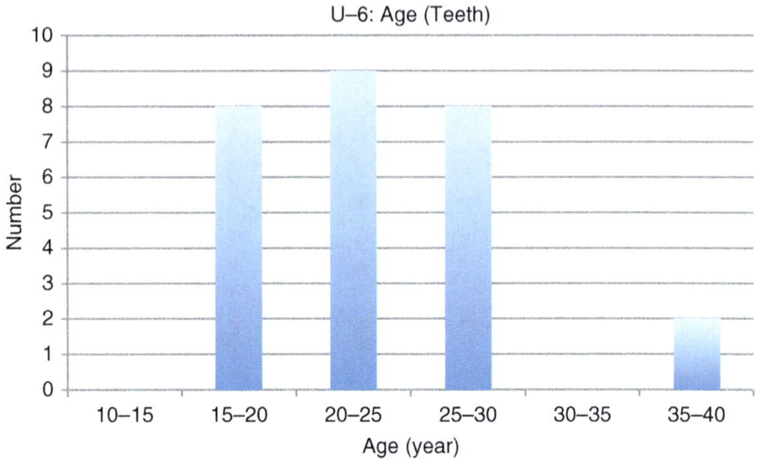

Fig. 8.20 Age distribution (U-6)

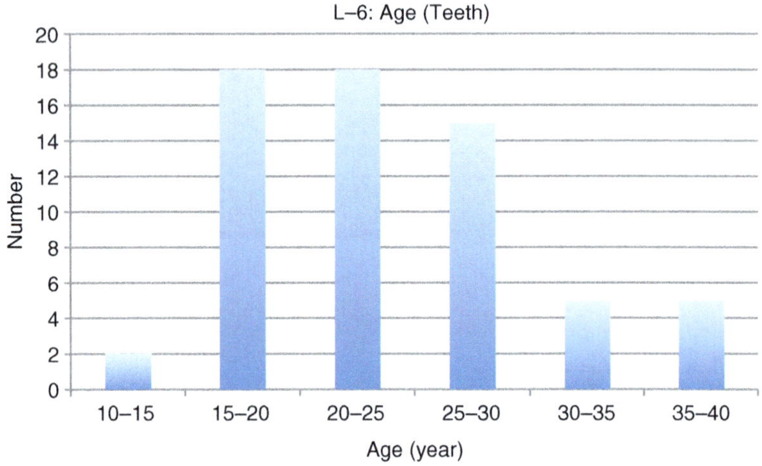

Fig. 8.21 Age distribution (L-6)

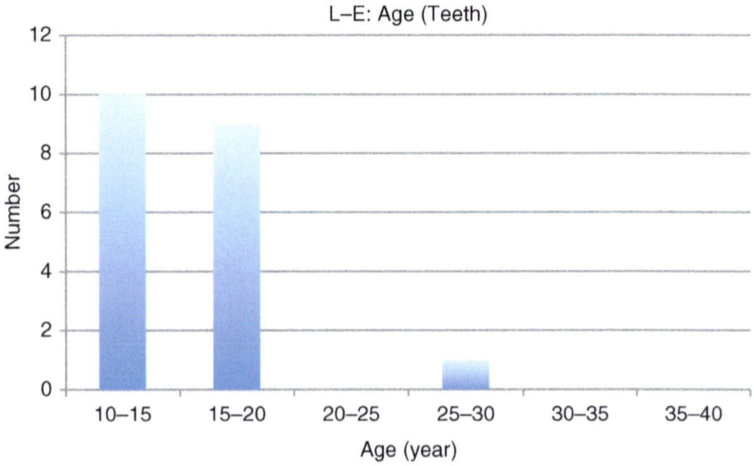

Fig. 8.22 Age distribution (L-E)

Table 8.4 Treatment time (months)

	Treatment time
Upper-6	34.1
Lower-6	34.5
Lower E	33
Average	33.9

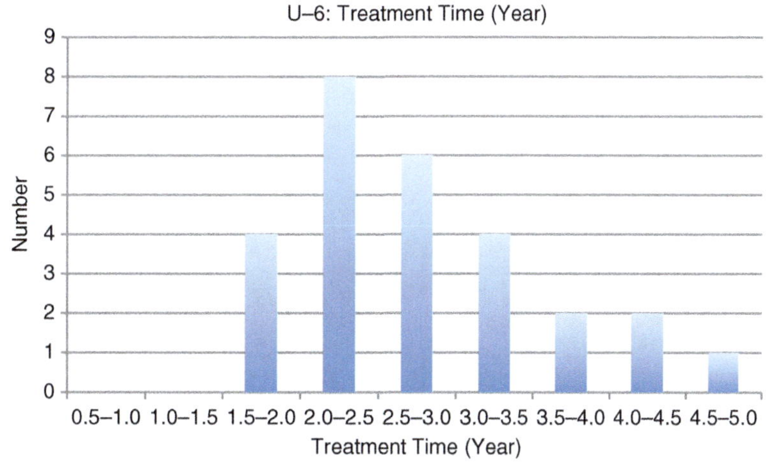

Fig. 8.23 Treatment time (U-6)

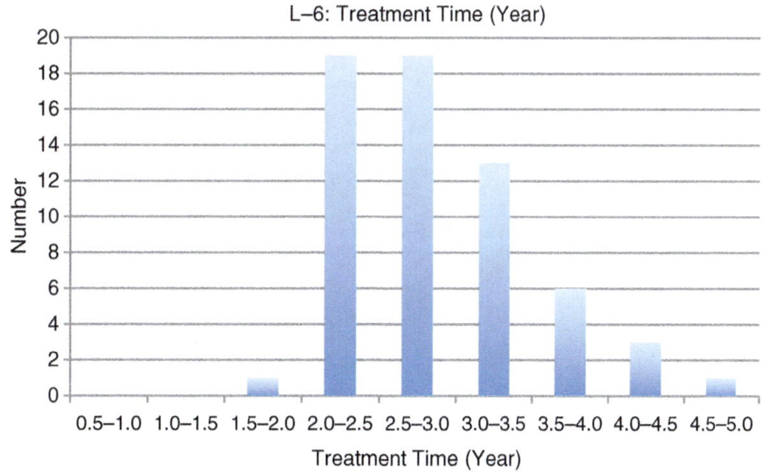

Fig. 8.24 Treatment time (L-6)

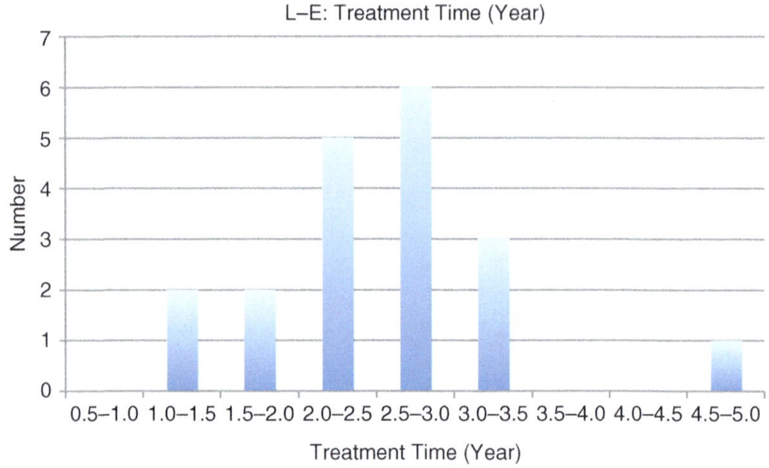

Fig. 8.25 Treatment time (L-E)

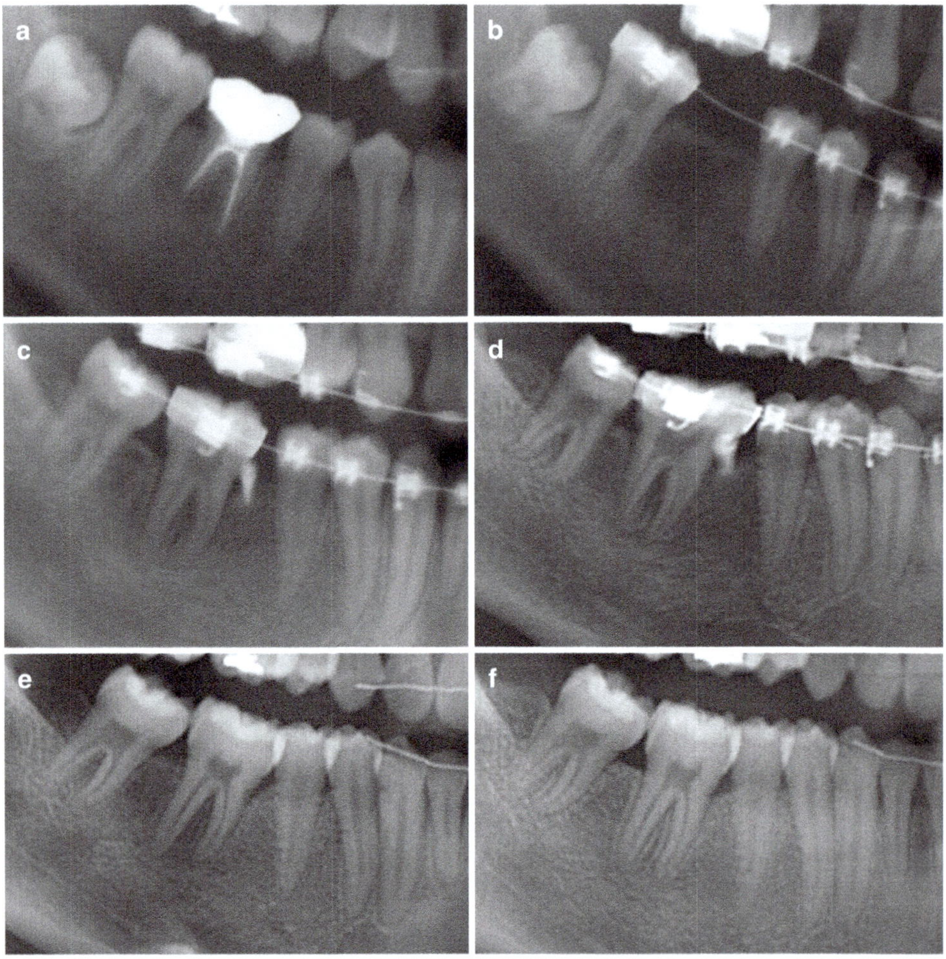

Fig. 8.26 (**a**) Initial, (**b–d**) during treatment, (**e**) debonding, (**f**) 3 years and 1 month after treatment. A 15-year, 1-month-old male patient. The long space of the missing right first molar was successfully closed. At the initial stage, the third molar was impacted and the root had not yet developed. As the second molar was protracted, the root of the third molar developed. At debonding, the root developed completely. Three years and 1 month after the treatment, there was no space relapse

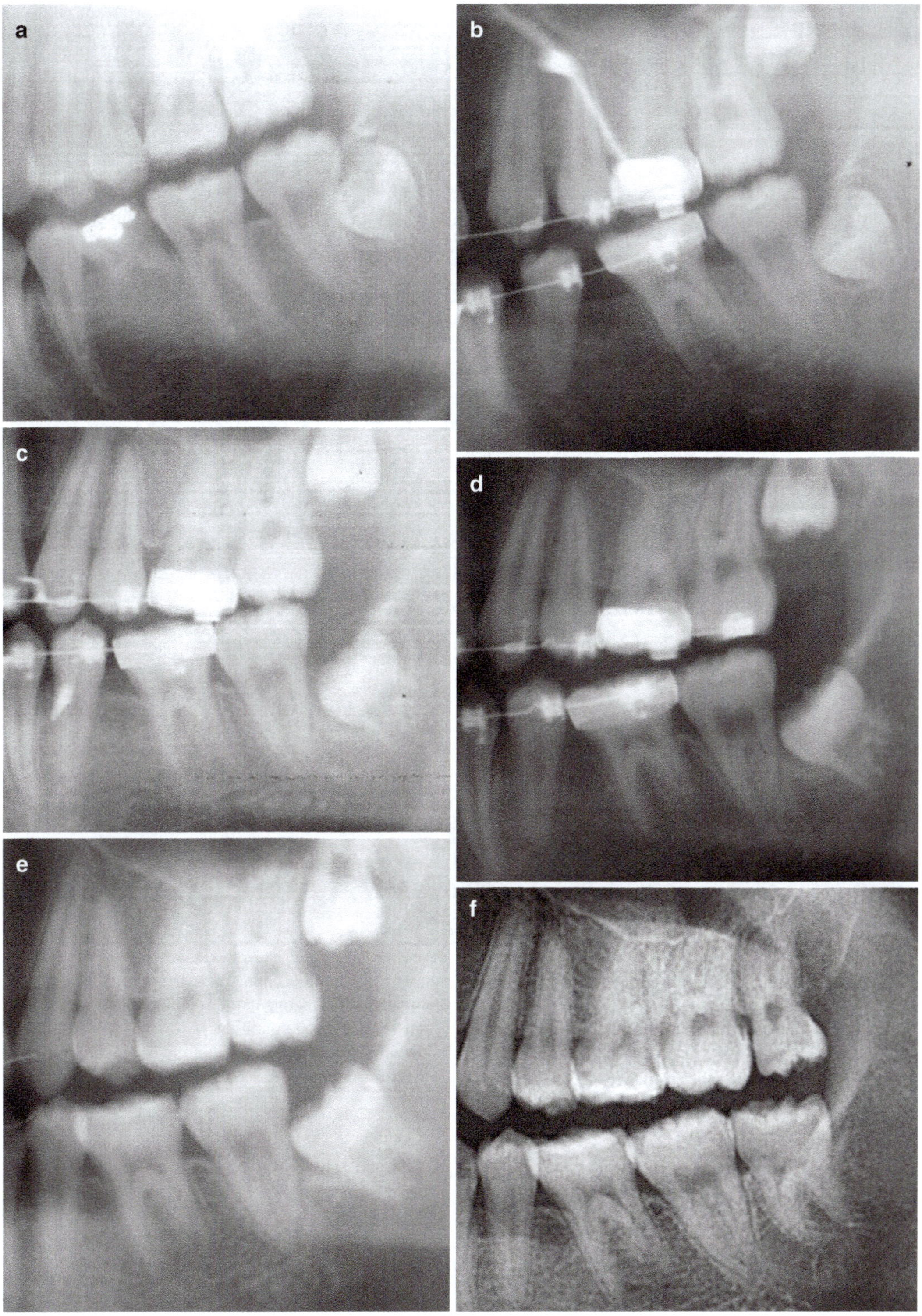

Fig. 8.27 (**a**) Initial, (**b–d**) during treatment, (**e**) debonding, (**f**) 4 years and 9 months after treatment. A 15-year, 11-month-old male patient. At the beginning, the root of the third molar had not formed. During the treatment, the third molar grew considerably, but at debonding, it had not yet erupted. Four years and 9 months after the treatment, it had fully erupted with completed formation of the root

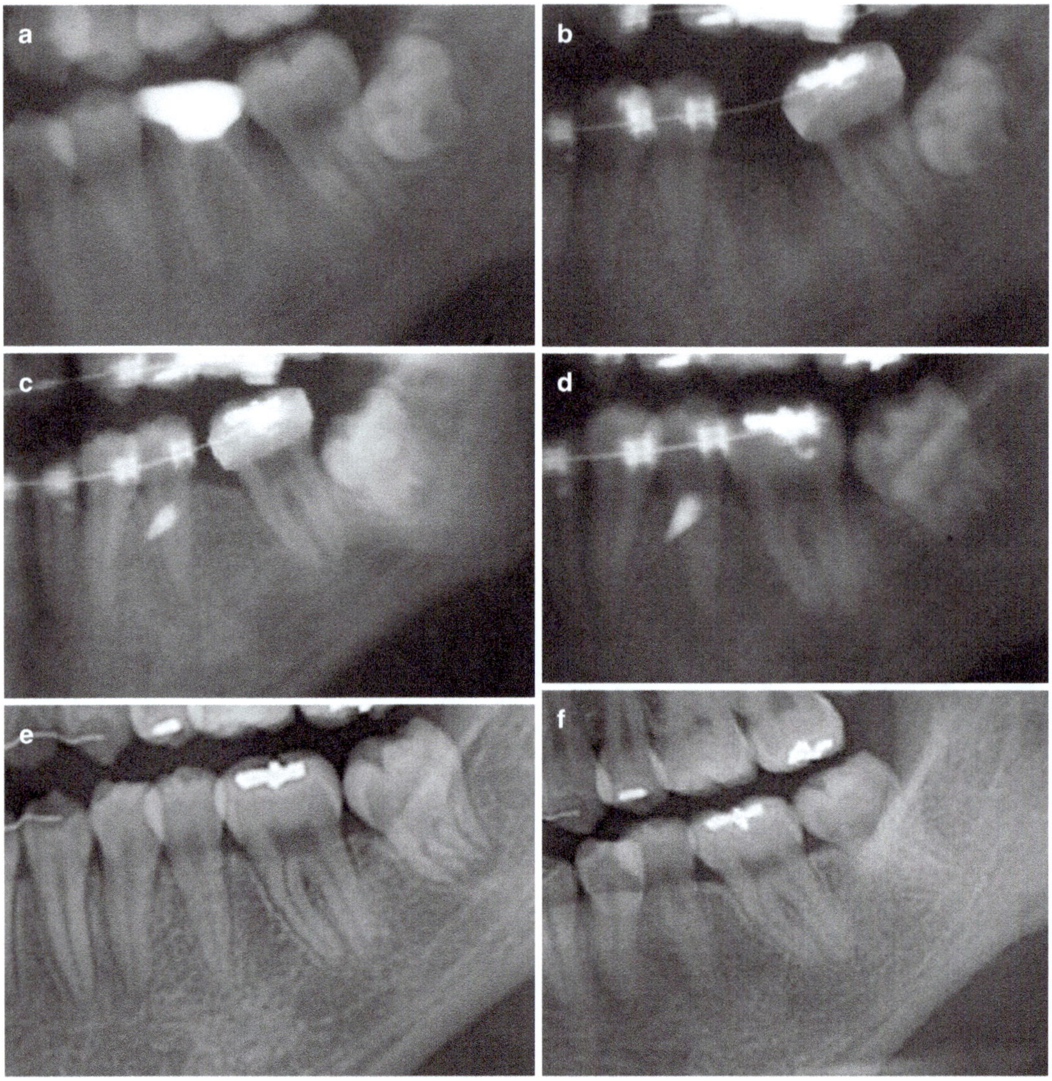

Fig. 8.28 (**a**) Initial, (**b–d**) during treatment, (**e**) debonding, (**f**) 5 years and 8 months after treatment. A 16-year, 11-month-old female patient. At the beginning, the development of the root was very primitive. However, at debonding, the impacted third molar erupted well even though the configuration was not good. At 5 years and 8 months after treatment, the alveolar bone and periodontium were in good condition. It will be usable for a considerable amount of time without major problems

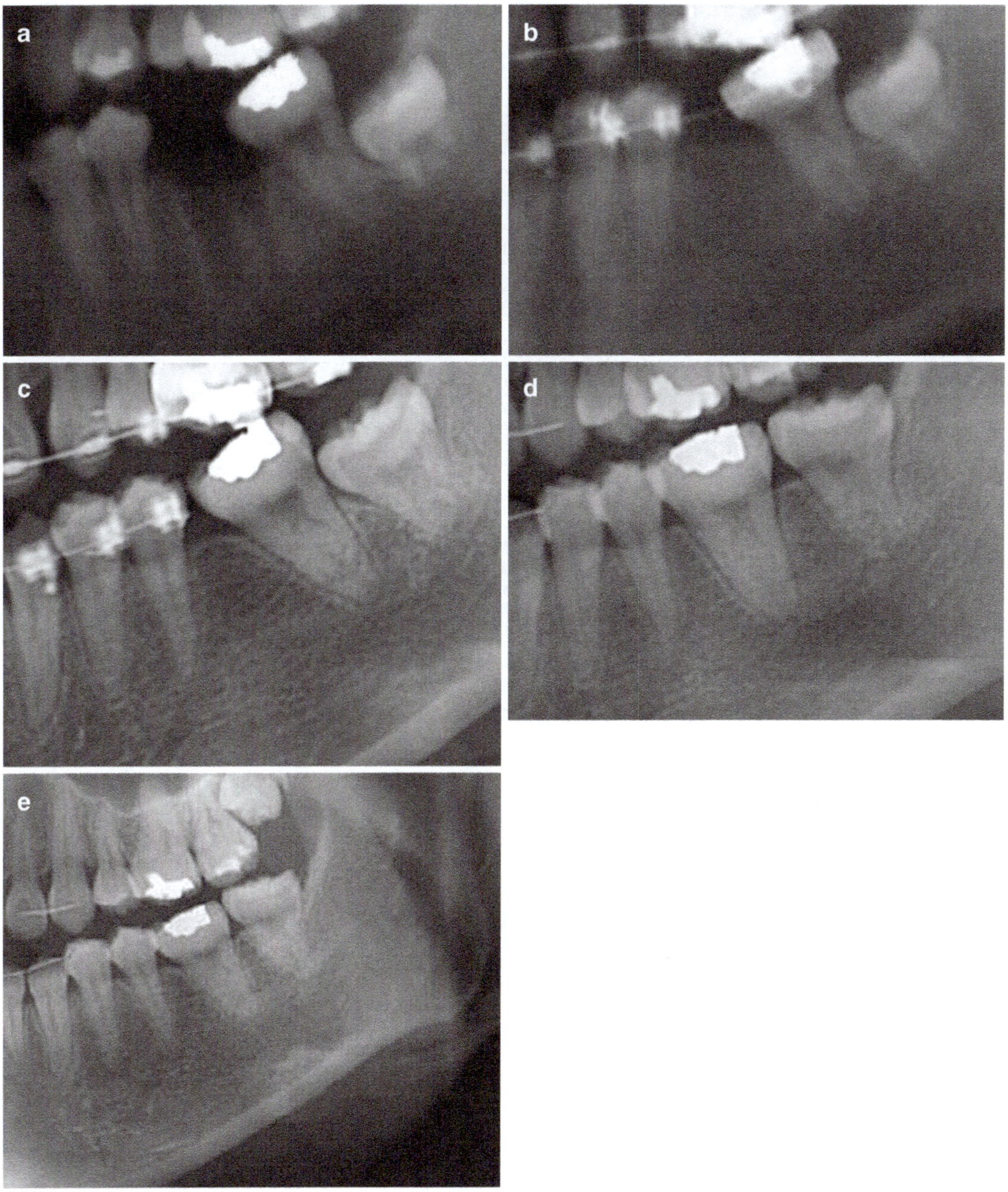

Fig. 8.29 (**a**) Initial, (**b**–**c**) during treatment, (**d**) debonding, (**e**) 3 years after treatment. A 17-year, 3-month-old female patient. Even with this patient whose physical growth was finished, the root of the third molar developed well. At 3 years after treatment, there were no problems and the third molar functioned well

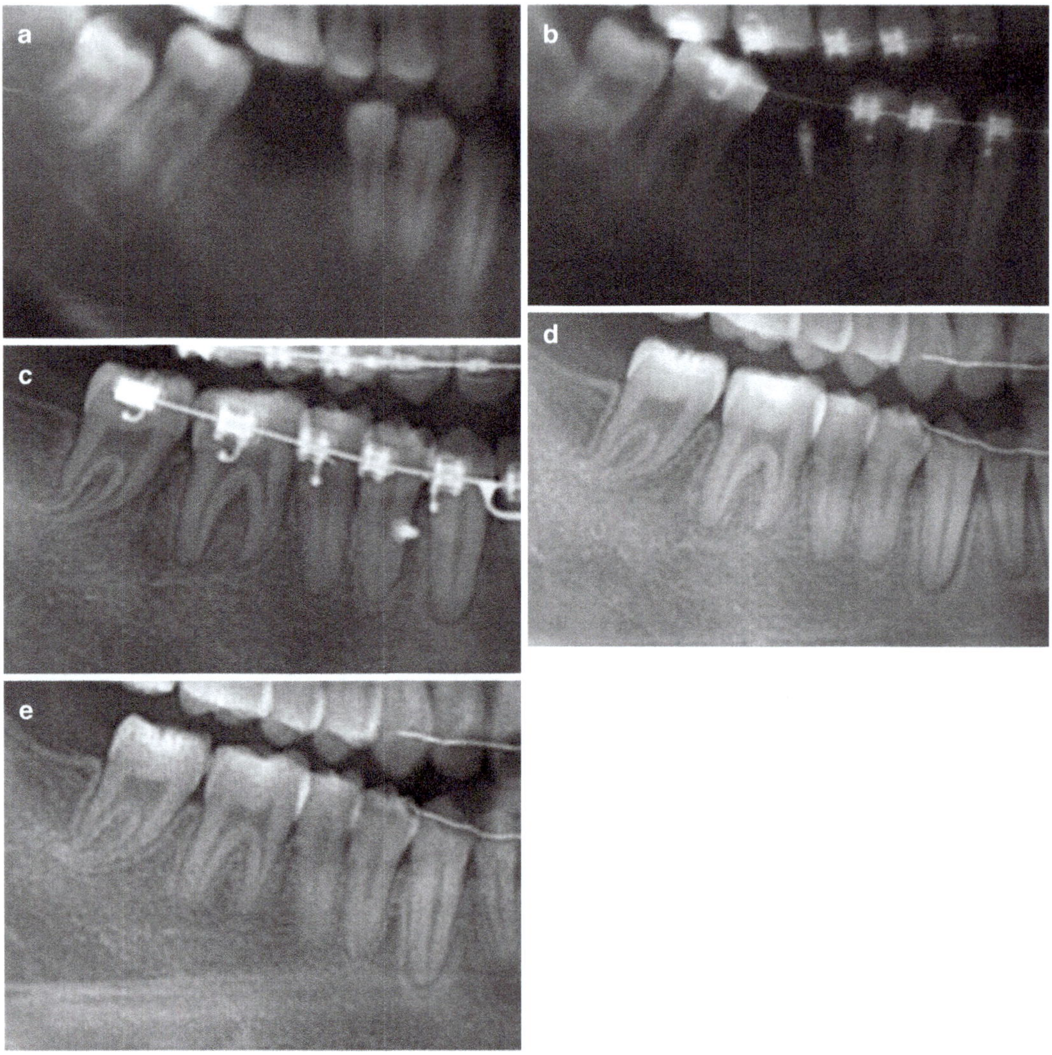

Fig. 8.30 (**a**) Initial, (**b**–**c**) during treatment, (**d**) debonding, (**e**) 1 year after treatment. An 18-year, 8-month-old female patient. Pure protraction of the second and third molar was conducted. An initially underdeveloped root apex formed completely at debonding. The second and third molars showed very good root parallelism despite moving a long distance

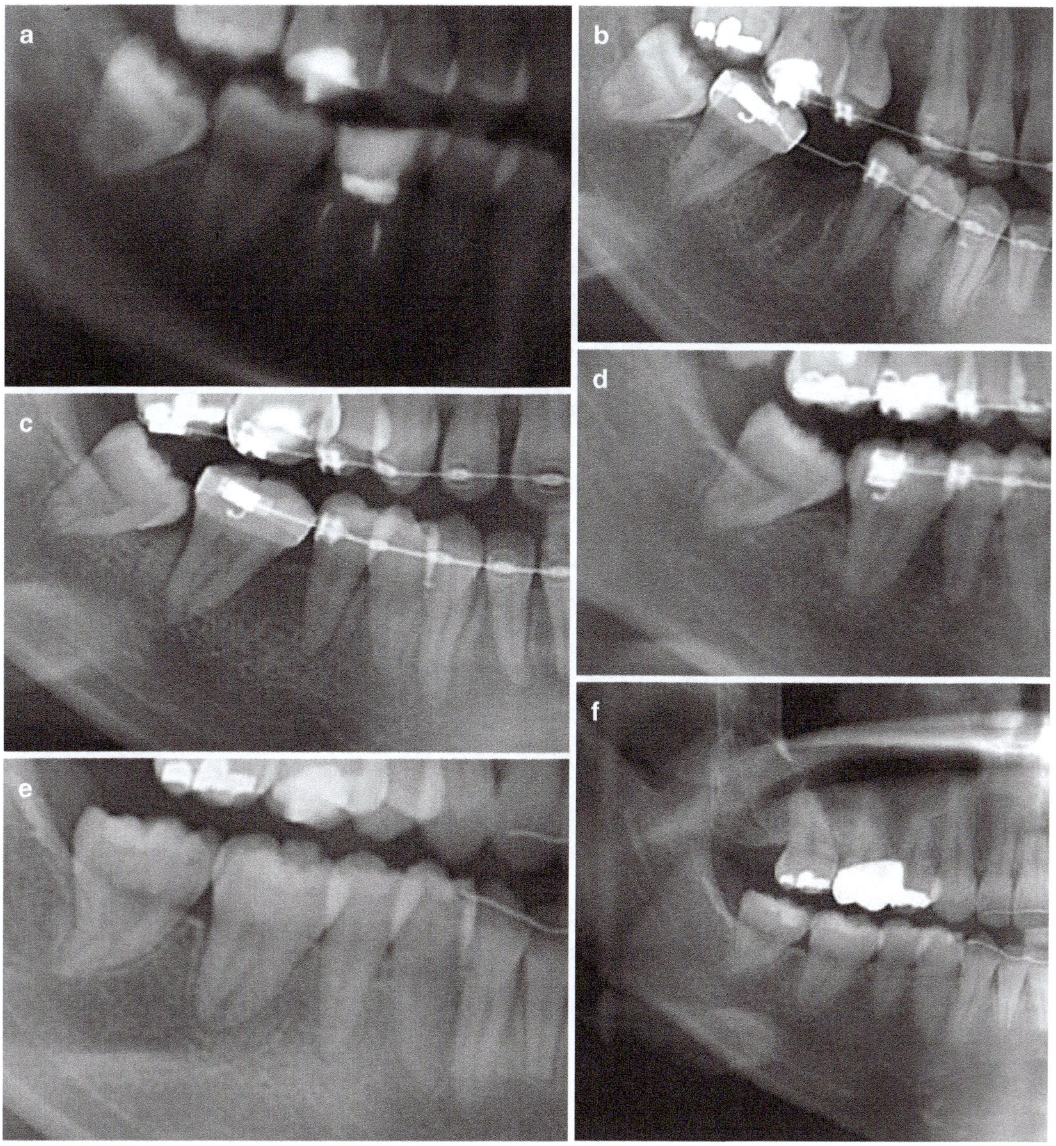

Fig. 8.31 (**a**) Initial, (**b–d**) during treatment, (**e**) debonding, (**f**) 2 years and 8 months after treatment. A 21-year-old female patient. The impacted third molar fully erupted and showed good root parallelism. Good alveolar bone support can be seen around the third molar

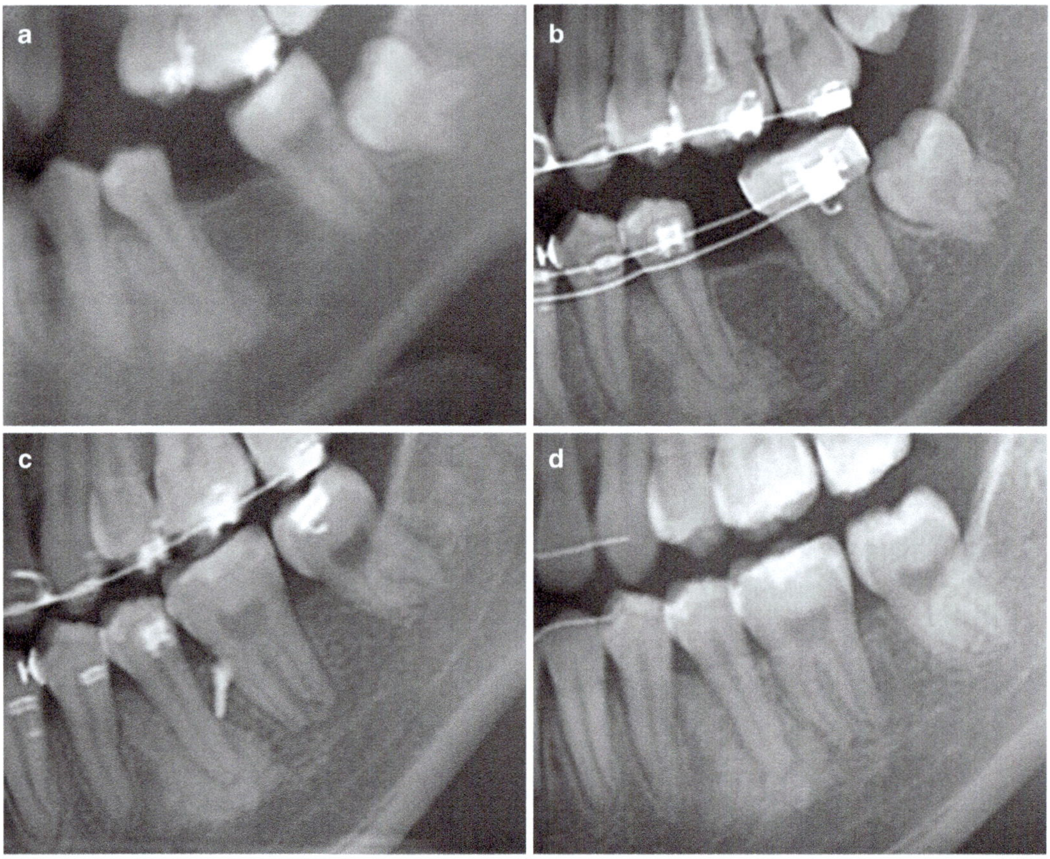

Fig. 8.32 (**a**) Initial, (**b**–**c**) during treatment, (**d**) debonding. A 24-year-old female patient. This patient was an adult, but root development had not yet been completed. During the orthodontic treatment, the root of the third molar developed and functioned well

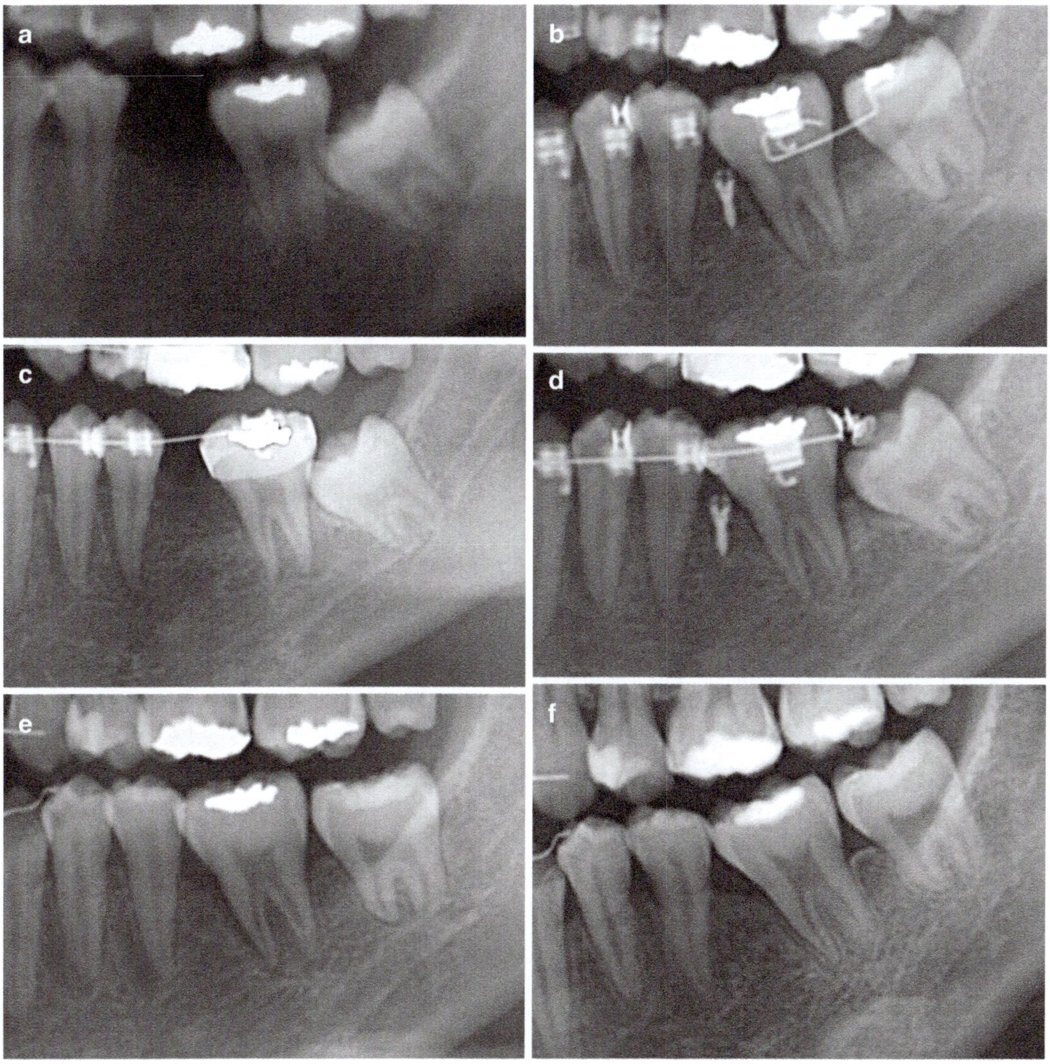

Fig. 8.33 (**a**) Initial, (**b–d**) during treatment, (**e**) debonding, (**f**) 1 year and 9 months after treatment. A 25-year, 10-month-old female patient. The third molar was deeply impacted. In this patient, the root of the third molar was almost developed. Even though this patient was an adult, the third molar was able to erupt and function well. One year and 9 months after debonding, there were no problems

References

1. Roberts WE, Marshall KJ, Mozsary PG. Rigid endosseous implant utilized as anchorage to protract molars and close an atrophic extraction site. Angle Orthod. 1990;60(2):135–52.
2. Roberts WE, Nelson CL, Goodacre CJ. Rigid implant anchorage to close a mandibular first molar extraction site. J Clin Orthod. 1994;28(12):693–704.
3. Nagaraj K, Upadhyay M, Yadav S. Titanium screw anchorage for protraction of mandibular second molars into first molar extraction sites. Am J Orthod Dentofacial Orthop. 2008;134(4):583–91.
4. Kravitz ND, Jolley T. Mandibular molar protraction with temporary anchorage devices. J Clin Orthod. 2008;42(6):351–5. quiz 340.
5. Baik U-B, Chun Y-S, Jung M-H, Sugawara J. Protraction of mandibular second and third molars into missing first molar spaces for a patient with an anterior open bite and anterior spacing. Am J Orthod Dentofacial Orthop. 2012;141(6):783–95.
6. Bechtold TE, Kim J-W, Choi T-H, Park Y-C, Lee K-J. Distalization pattern of the maxillary arch depending

on the number of orthodontic miniscrews. Angle Orthod. 2013;83(2):266–73. doi: 10.2319/032212-123.1. Epub 2012 Sep 12.
7. Huanca Ghislanzoni LT, Piepoli C. Upper molar distalization on palatal miniscrews: an easy to manage palatal appliance. Prog Orthod. 2012;13(1):78–83.
8. Kinzinger GSM, Gülden N, Yildizhan F, Diedrich PR. Efficiency of a skeletonized distal jet appliance supported by miniscrew anchorage for noncompliance maxillary molar distalization. Am J Orthod Dentofacial Orthop. 2009;136(4):578–86.
9. Kyung S-H, Lee JY, Shin JW, Hong C, Dietz V, Gianelly AA. Distalization of the entire maxillary arch in an adult. Am J Orthod Dentofacial Orthop. 2009;135(4 Suppl):S123–32.
10. Kinzinger G, Gülden N, Yildizhan F, Hermanns-Sachweh B, Diedrich P. Anchorage efficacy of palatally-inserted miniscrews in molar distalization with a periodontally/miniscrew-anchored distal jet. J Orofac Orthop. 2008;69(2):110–20.
11. Carano A, Velo S, Incorvati C, Poggio P. Clinical applications of the Mini-Screw-Anchorage-System (M.A.S.) in the maxillary alveolar bone. Prog Orthod. 2004;5(2):212–35.
12. Byloff FK, Kärcher H, Clar E, Stoff F. An implant to eliminate anchorage loss during molar distalization: a case report involving the Graz implant-supported pendulum. Int J Adult Orthodon Orthognath Surg. 2000;15(2):129–37.
13. Grec RH, Janson G, Branco NC, Moura-Grec PG, Patel MP, Castanha Henriques JF. Intraoral distalizer effects with conventional and skeletal anchorage: a meta-analysis. Am J Orthod Dentofacial Orthop. 2013;143(5):602–15.
14. Jacobs C, Jacobs-Müller C, Luley C, Erbe C, Wehrbein H. Orthodontic space closure after first molar extraction without skeletal anchorage. J Orofac Orthop. 2011;72(1):51–60.
15. Lai EH-H, Yao C-CJ, Chang JZ-C, Chen I, Chen Y-J. Three-dimensional dental model analysis of treatment outcomes for protrusive maxillary dentition: comparison of headgear, miniscrew, and miniplate skeletal anchorage. Am J Orthod Dentofacial Orthop. 2008;134(5):636–45.
16. Antonarakis GS, Kiliaridis S. Maxillary molar distalization with noncompliance intramaxillary appliances in Class II malocclusion. A systematic review. Angle Orthod. 2008;78(6):1133–40.
17. Liddle DW. Second molar extraction in orthodontic treatment. Am J Orthod. 1977;72(6):599–616.
18. Rindler A. Effects on lower third molars after extraction of second molars. Angle Orthod. 1977;47(1):55–8.
19. Mimura H. Protraction of mandibular second and third molars assisted by partial corticision and miniscrew anchorage. Am J Orthod Dentofacial Orthop. 2013;144(2):278–89.
20. Giancotti A, Greco M, Mampieri G, Arcuri C. The use of titanium miniscrews for molar protraction in extraction treatment. Prog Orthod. 2004;5(2):236–47.
21. Kyung S-H, Choi J-H, Park Y-C. Miniscrew anchorage used to protract lower second molars into first molar extraction sites. J Clin Orthod. 2003;37(10):575–9.
22. De-la-Rosa-Gay C, Valmaseda-Castellón E, Gay-Escoda C. Spontaneous third-molar eruption after second-molar extraction in orthodontic patients. Am J Orthod Dentofacial Orthop. 2006;129(3):337–44.

C-Tube Plate: Less Hardship and More Treatment Options

9

Kyu-Rhim Chung, Kyung-Won Seo, and Seong-Hun Kim

Abstract

With introduction of mini-implants in orthodontic treatment, the anchorage control became a less of challenge and enabled orthodontic tooth movement once believed to be too difficult to be achieved with conventional anchorage control. With introduction of C-implant, the stability issues of mini-implant were solved with osseointegration potentials to resist multidirectional orthodontic forces. Nevertheless, there were remaining obstacles that placing C-implants was limited due to the anatomical limitations on recipient site. In order to solve this problem, C-tube plate was invented to overcome the anatomical limitations. The C-tubes are fixated with 4 mm fixation screws to overcome the placement limitations, and it has high survival rate. C-tube plate can bring less hardship in anchorage control and open more treatment options to clinicians.

An orthodontic miniplate is a reliable alternative to conventional orthodontic mini-implants. The miniplate system has been reported to achieve greater stability compared with orthodontic mini-implant systems. The high success rate and the availability of force application independent of the adjacent teeth have made the miniplate anchorage system increasingly popular. Miniplates are used as temporary anchorage device by exposing the occlusal end of the plate. The miniplate design has been modified by Sugawara et al. [1] to act as a hook, and De Clerk and Cornelis introduced Bollard miniplate [2]. However, conventional miniplates have drawbacks such as complicated design, need of aggressive surgical procedures, and risk of damaging adjacent roots or penetration of the sinus [3, 4].

Chung et al. [5, 6] designed C-tube with a fixation part, neck portion, and a head part to utilize the miniplate for orthodontic usage (Fig. 9.1). At the end of head part, rolling the end of a titanium miniplate neck, which can accommodate an archwire, forms a 0.036 in.-diameter tube. Two hooks on either side of the tube head

K.-R. Chung, DMD, MSD, PhD
Division of Orthodontics, School of Medicine, Ajou University, Wonchun-dong 5, Youngtong-Ku, Suwon 443-380, South Korea
e-mail: speedor@hotmail.com

K.-W. Seo, DDS • S.-H. Kim, DDS, MSD, PhD (✉)
Department of Orthodontics, School of Dentistry, Kyung Hee University, #1 Hoegi-dong, Dongdaemun-gu, Seoul 130-701, South Korea
e-mail: kwseo01@gmail.com; bravortho@gmail.com, bravortho@khu.ac.kr

K.B. Kim (ed.), *Temporary Skeletal Anchorage Devices*,
DOI 10.1007/978-3-642-55052-2_9, © Springer-Verlag Berlin Heidelberg 2014

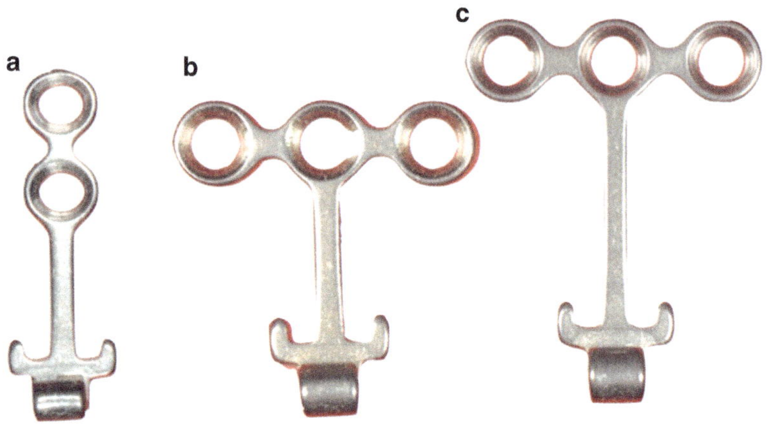

Fig. 9.1 Design of C-tube. (**a**) I-type. (**b**) T-type C-tube with short neck. (**c**) T-type C-tube with long neck

enable the elastic to be applied. The different neck lengths give options for clinician to choose depending on the location of placement and expected movement as shown in Fig. 9.1. There are two kinds of C-tube: I-type and T-type. I-type C-tube is a titanium miniplate with two anchoring holes for fixation miniscrews and a tube-shaped head serving as the point of orthodontic force application. T-type C-tube has three horizontal fixation holes and the neck and the head part are perpendicular to the plane of the fixation holes. I-type or T-type C-tubes can be selected on the recipient site morphology. In Fig. 9.2a, there are modifications of the C-tube design; multiple hooks on T-type C-tube, L-type C-tube with multiple hooks, modified T-type C-tube without side hooks, and I-type C-tube without hook. The modification of miniplate's design accommodates the same biomechanics for the C-therapy and also achieves high stability during orthodontic treatment application.

In the recent research of Lee et al., the C-tube showed excellent data of 96 % survival rates [7]. Even with minor complications, C-tube resulted in high success ratio. The versatile C-tube possesses many advantages for clinicians and patients with minimum invasive minor surgical placement. For the successful survival rate, maintenance of good oral hygiene is most important, and experiences of clinicians rank in the second place. Kim et al. suggested in a journal that C-tube placement is very safe with the miniplate anchoring screws (MPAS) and the stability is maintained even with less-than-ideal placement by MPAS [8]. Due to the small size of MPAS, close proximity of the root contact and root perforated MPAS posed no harm to dentition and served as stable temporary skeletal anchorage devices (TSADs). Cautions to avoid these complications are necessary, but C-tube is definitely a good option of TSADs for patients and clinicians.

C-tube is useful in places where placement of conventional TSAD faces difficulty such as extremely narrow interradicular space, extended maxillary sinus space, severe alveolar bone loss, and dilacerated root (Fig. 9.3). The total length of fixation screw is 4 mm, which means it will actually penetrate about 2–3 mm into the alveolar bone for anchorage, but strong enough to resist orthodontic force application. As in Fig. 9.4, in cases of very narrow interradicular space and pneumatization of sinus floor to the roots of posterior teeth, C-tube placement certainly can be a legible option to replace the mini-implant. Figure 9.3c shows the fixation screw penetration into the sinus wall, and it is clearly shorter than the C-implant placement on the other side, Fig. 9.3b.

Narrow interradicular space is common findings in the anterior area of both the upper and lower jaws, and the C-tubes can be successfully

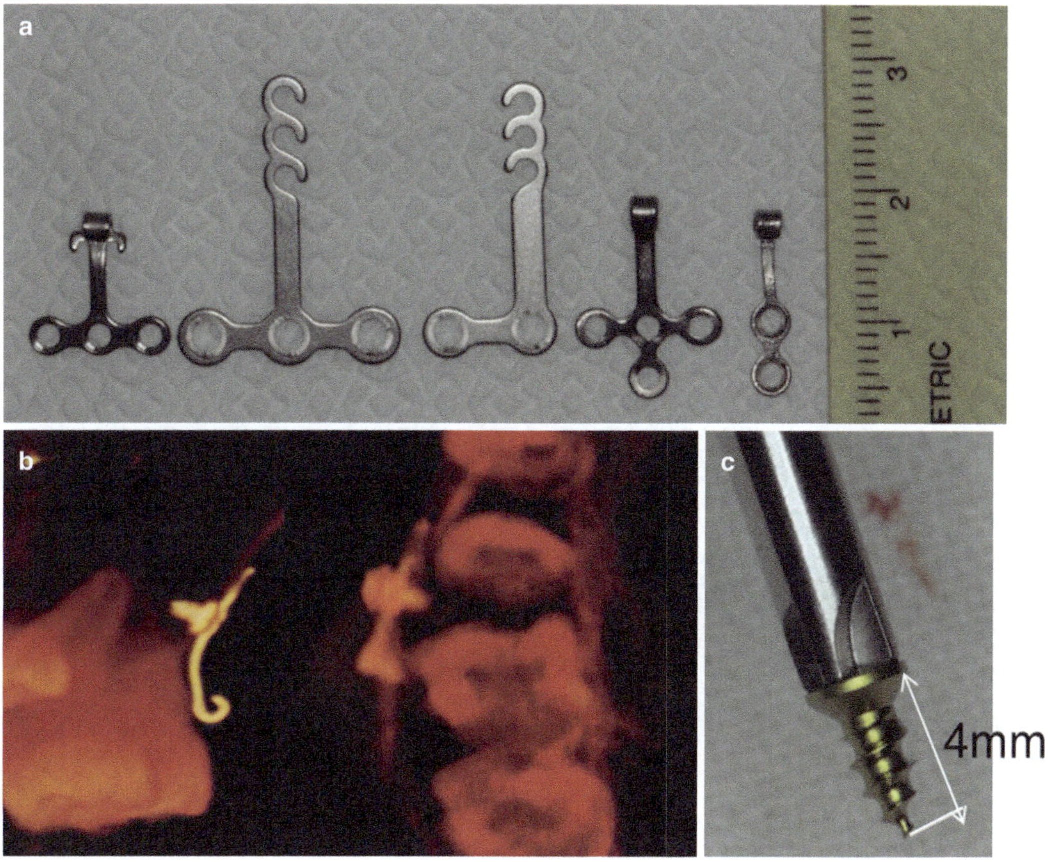

Fig. 9.2 (**a**) Modifications of the design. (From *left* to *right*) Basic T-type, T-type SAS system, L-type SAS system, hookless T-type, and hookless I-type. (**b**, **c**) Although miniplate anchoring screws penetrated into the sinus space, C-tube was successfully stabilized and exerted sufficient absolute anchorage without any complications due to the short length (less than 4 mm)

placed into these particular areas to apply intrusive orthodontic forces (Figs. 9.4 and 9.5). When patients have stable posterior occlusion but with deep overbite, intrusion of the anterior teeth can solve the problem. However, finding the wide-enough interradicular space for conventional mini-implants is very rare in the anterior legion, and additionally, the buccal frenums often interfere with the placement. The C-tube can be anchored underneath the movable mucosa, and the neck and head portion can be exposed through the attachable gingiva or the junction of the movable and attached gingiva to control gingival inflammation. Also, this allows bypassing the frenums during placement. With these absolute skeletal anchorages, the intrusive orthodontic force of the anterior teeth can be achieved, and with extension of a hook, midline discrepancy correction can be achieved in Fig. 9.4d.

Another advantage of C-tube is easy adjustment of the tube according to the location of insertion. The titanium possesses enough rigidity to withstand orthodontic force application without distortion, but moldable enough to fit the curvatures of recipient bone contour. It is easily bent with a plier and clinicians can adapt to different locations with no trouble. Notice the curvature of the C-tube in Fig. 9.5b that is following the mandibular symphysis contour. When attempting to achieve intrusion of the teeth, the replacements of the TSADs are often needed to achieve the expected amount of intrusion. But with a C-tube,

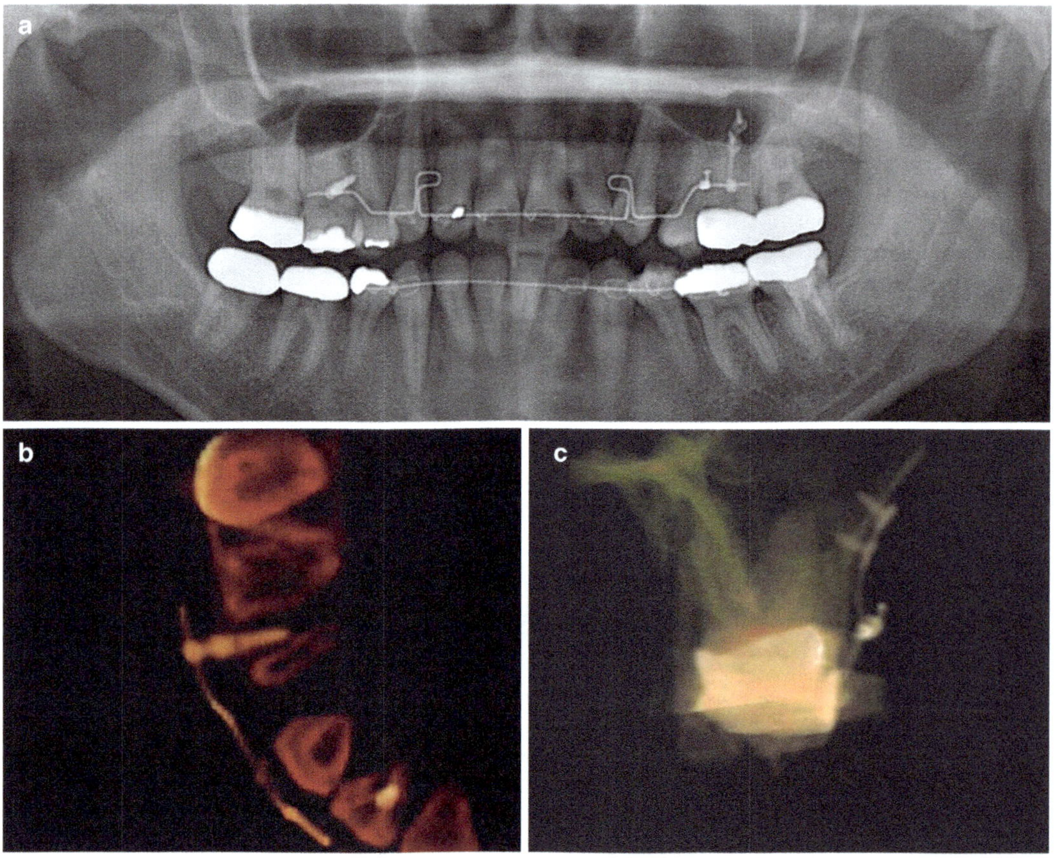

Fig. 9.3 It is very difficult to safely place conventional mini-implant in this patient where interradicular space is extremely narrow and maxillary sinus had extended (**a**). C-implant was placed between the upper right second premolar and first molar (**b**) and I-type C-tube was placed between the mesiobuccal and distobuccal root of the upper left first molar (**c**). Sufficient stability of the C-tube was obtained from cortical bone of the sinus wall

the drawbacks can be solved with just a weingart plier to bend the C-tube neck portion to gain more length for the intrusion force [9]. Furthermore, the C-tube neck portion can be twisted off to get detached from the anchoring portion leaving the fixation portion in place [10].

C-tube also serves as an excellent alternative for immediately replacing loosened TSADs. C-tube acts as a stable anchorage device enabling en masse retraction. Miniscrew loosening occurred before planned retraction of the upper arch completed, and for the immediate replacement of TSAD, C-tube was performed (Fig. 9.6). First, check where the fixation screws should be placed and one horizontal incision made on movable mucosa. By stretching the movable mucosa, enough access for the two fixation screws was made. By connecting the removed screw hole to the incision line by a tunneling technique, the C-tube head can be placed out of the screw hole in attached gingiva (Fig. 9.7). Simple sutures are placed for the closure of horizontal incision, and C-tube placement is completed (Fig. 9.8). The C-tube placement is minimally invasive and pain medication will alleviate the discomfort with a procedure.

For the removal of the C-tube, it is exact reversal of the insertion process. When you are removing the C-tube after usage, first estimate where the fixation screws are located according to the shape of it (Fig. 9.9) or palpate the location with an explorer under local anesthesia (Fig. 9.11a). Then, make a vertical incision or horizontal incision to access and remove the fixation screws. For I-type C-tube, connecting the incision from the fixation screw to the neck is

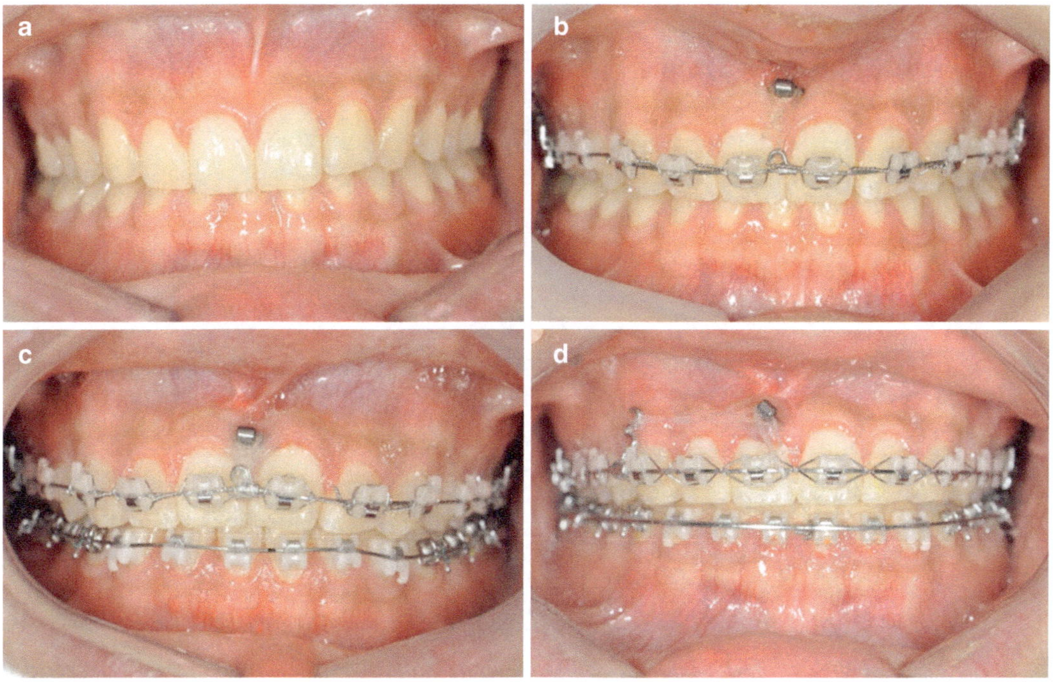

Fig. 9.4 Intrusion of upper dentition with C-tube. (**a**) Initial photo. (**b**) C-tube was placed between the right and left upper central incisor. (**c**) Intrusion mostly occurred on central incisors. (**d**) After upper dentition was sufficiently intruded, dental midline was corrected by connecting elastics between C-tube and extension hook on the distal of the upper right canine

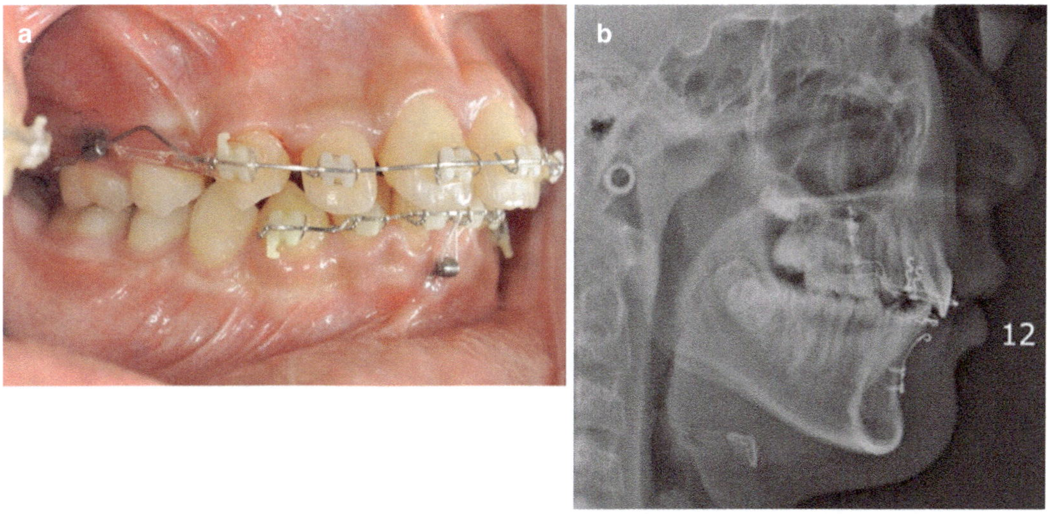

Fig. 9.5 (**a**) Intrusion of the lower six anteriors and en masse retraction of the upper six anteriors with C-tubes after extraction of the upper first premolars. (**b**) Lower C-tube was adapted to the curvature of the symphysis

not necessary as seen in Fig. 9.10 because the fixation portion can be easily pulled out through the hole of the C-tube neck part. However, for the T-type or modified T-type C-tube, it is rather easier to extend the incision to the neck to ease the removing process of the C-tube (Figs. 9.10 and 9.11). Finally, simple sutures can close the incision.

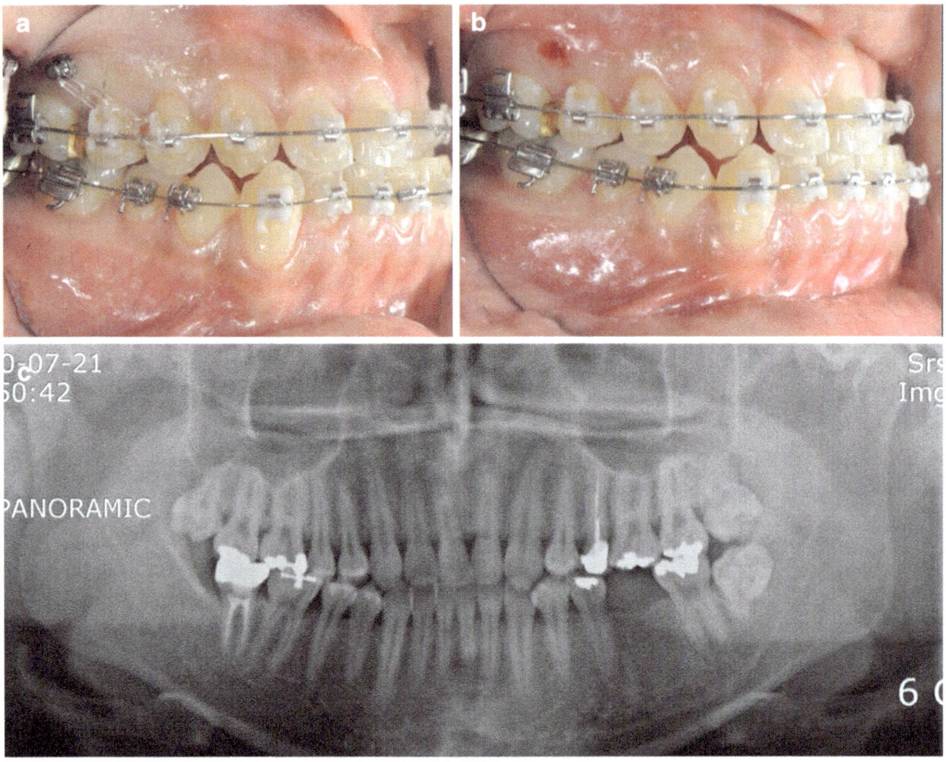

Fig. 9.6 Immediate replacement of loosened TSAD with C-tube. (**a**) Loosened TSAD between the upper right second premolar and first molar. (**b**) TSAD was removed. (**c**) Panoramic x-ray

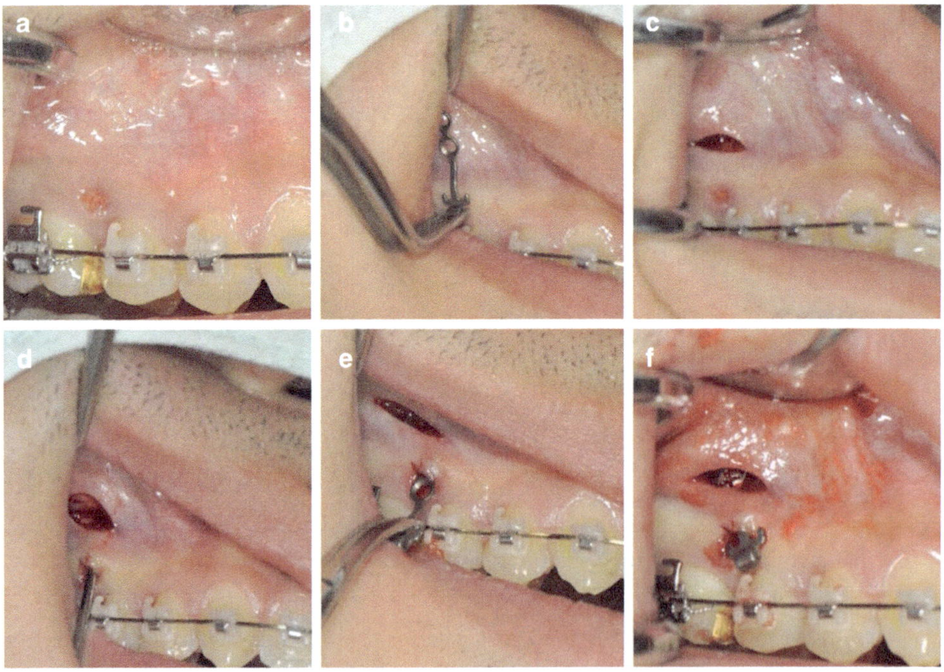

Fig. 9.7 Replacement protocol. (**a**) Minor incision for entry to embed screw holes. (**b**) Preoperative try-in of C-tube. (**c**) Horizontal incision for placing fixation screws. (**d**) Tunneling through the entry incision to the horizontal incision. (**e**) Insertion of C-tube to the entry incision. (**f**) After placing fixation screws

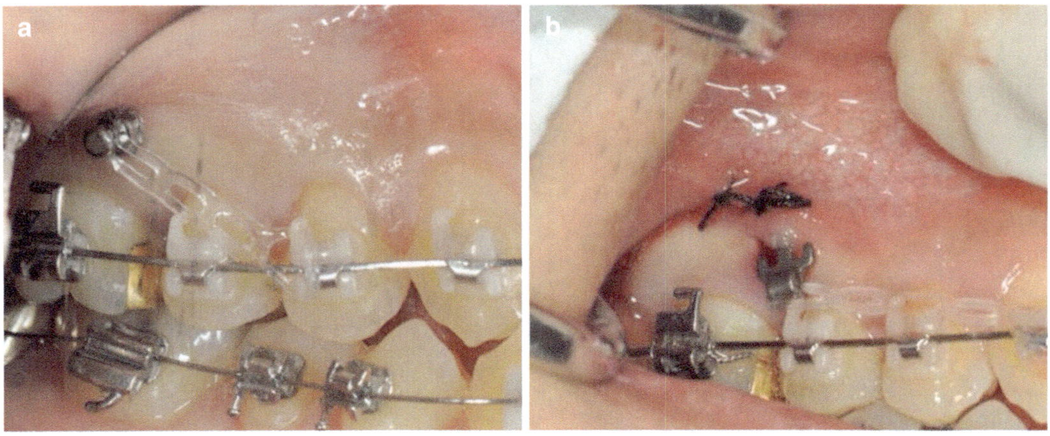

Fig. 9.8 (Continued) (**a**) Before removing loosened TSAD. (**b**) Replacing with C-tube

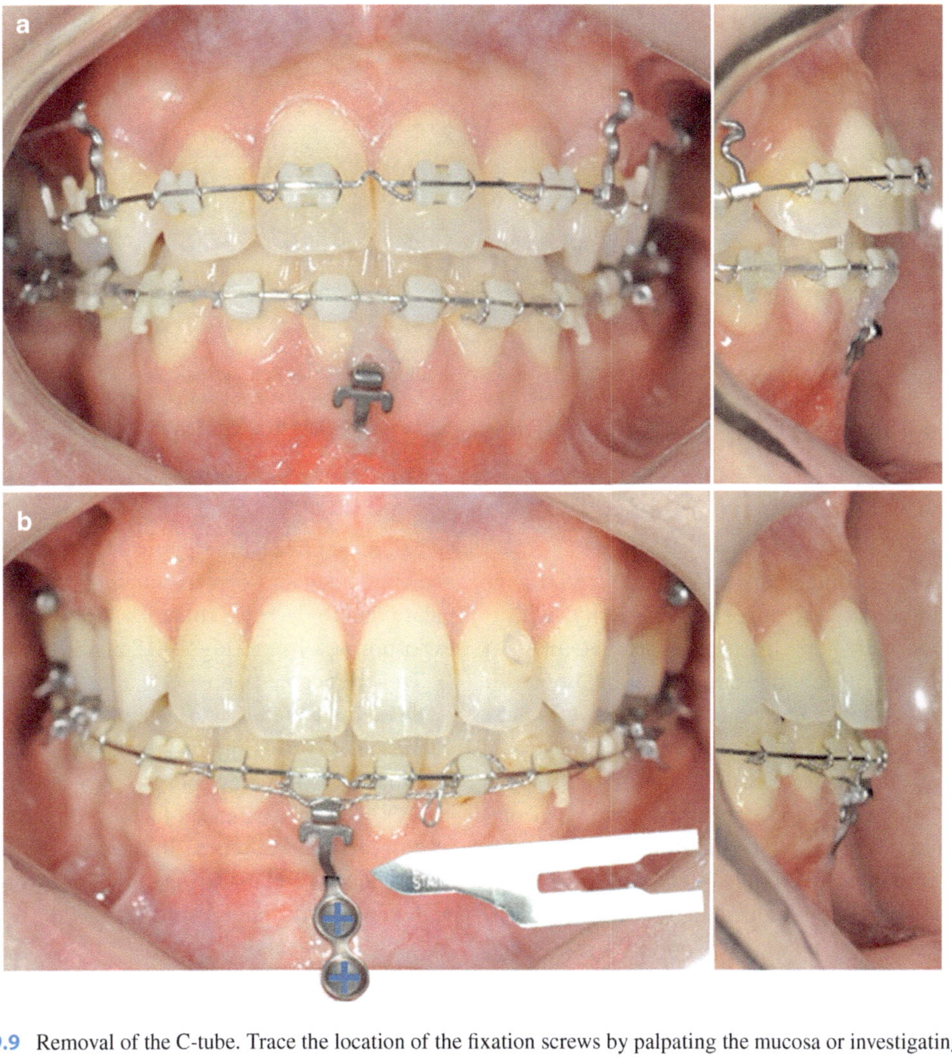

Fig. 9.9 Removal of the C-tube. Trace the location of the fixation screws by palpating the mucosa or investigating the shape of the screw

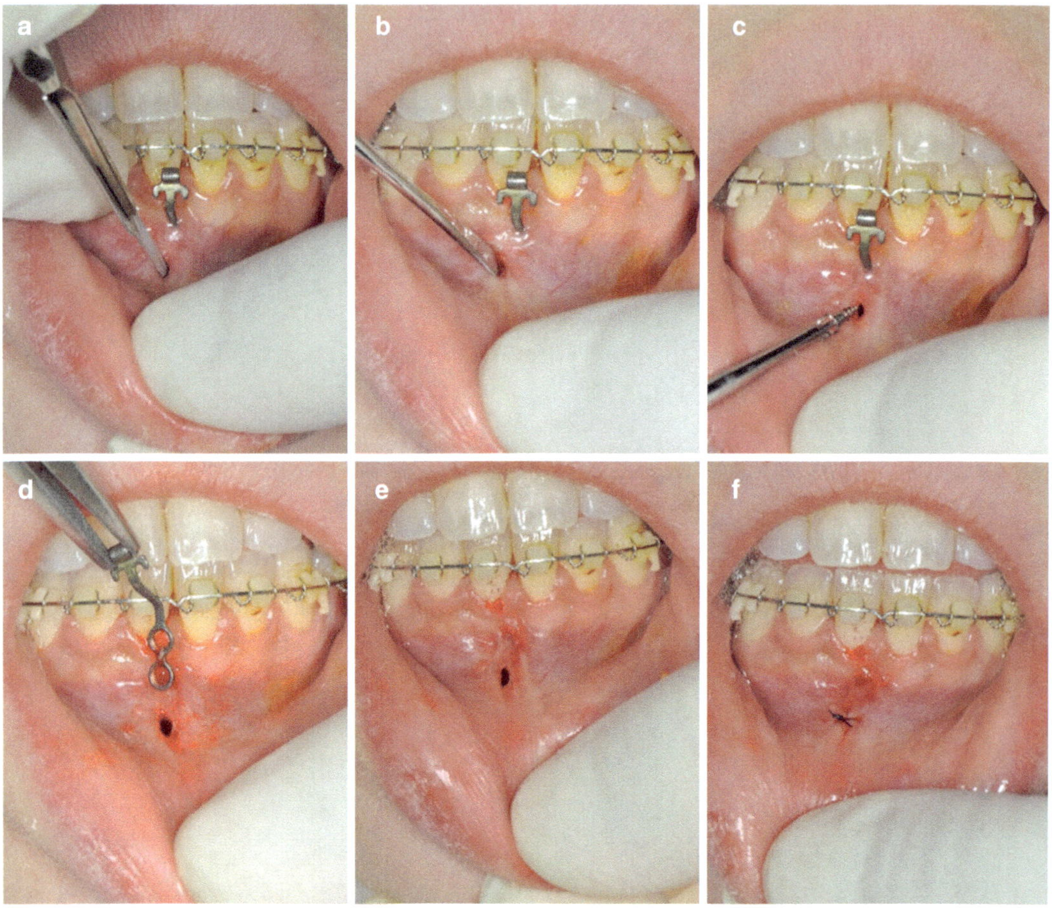

Fig. 9.10 Removal of I-type C-tube. (**a**) Making a short incision on the expected location of the fixation screw. (**b**) Blunt dissection with periosteal elevator. (**c**) Removing fixation screw. (**d**) Pulling the C-tube out of the mucosa. (**e**) After removal of the C-tube. (**f**) Single interrupted suture is sufficient to close the incision

Case 1

A 27-year-old male presented to the department of orthodontics, Kyung Hee University, with a chief complaint of lip protrusion. Patient's lip was incompetent and protrusion of the upper lip was prominent. Intraoral exam showed large overjet (20 mm), exaggerated curve of Spee, Class I molar relationship, constricted upper arch, protruded upper centrals, and crowded lower dentition. The temporomandibular joints were within normal limits. He had dentoalveolar Class II Division 1 malocclusion with an impinging deep bite. Upper dental midline was shifted 2 mm to the right and lower dental midline coincided with facial midline. The lower four incisors and alveolar bone were significantly over-erupted and the lower incisor was touching the anterior palate due to deep overbite. The upper incisors' exposure was 1 mm (Figs. 9.12 and 9.13).

Treatment goals were to [1] align and level the teeth in both arches and establish a functional occlusion, [2] obtain Class I canine and molar relationship [3], achieve normal overjet and overbite, [4] obtain a balanced facial profile, and [5] improve facial esthetics. Intrusion of the four lower incisors and extrusion of the upper incisors with controlled tipping were planned to achieve the treatment goals.

Periapical radiographs showed extremely narrow interradicular spaces between the central

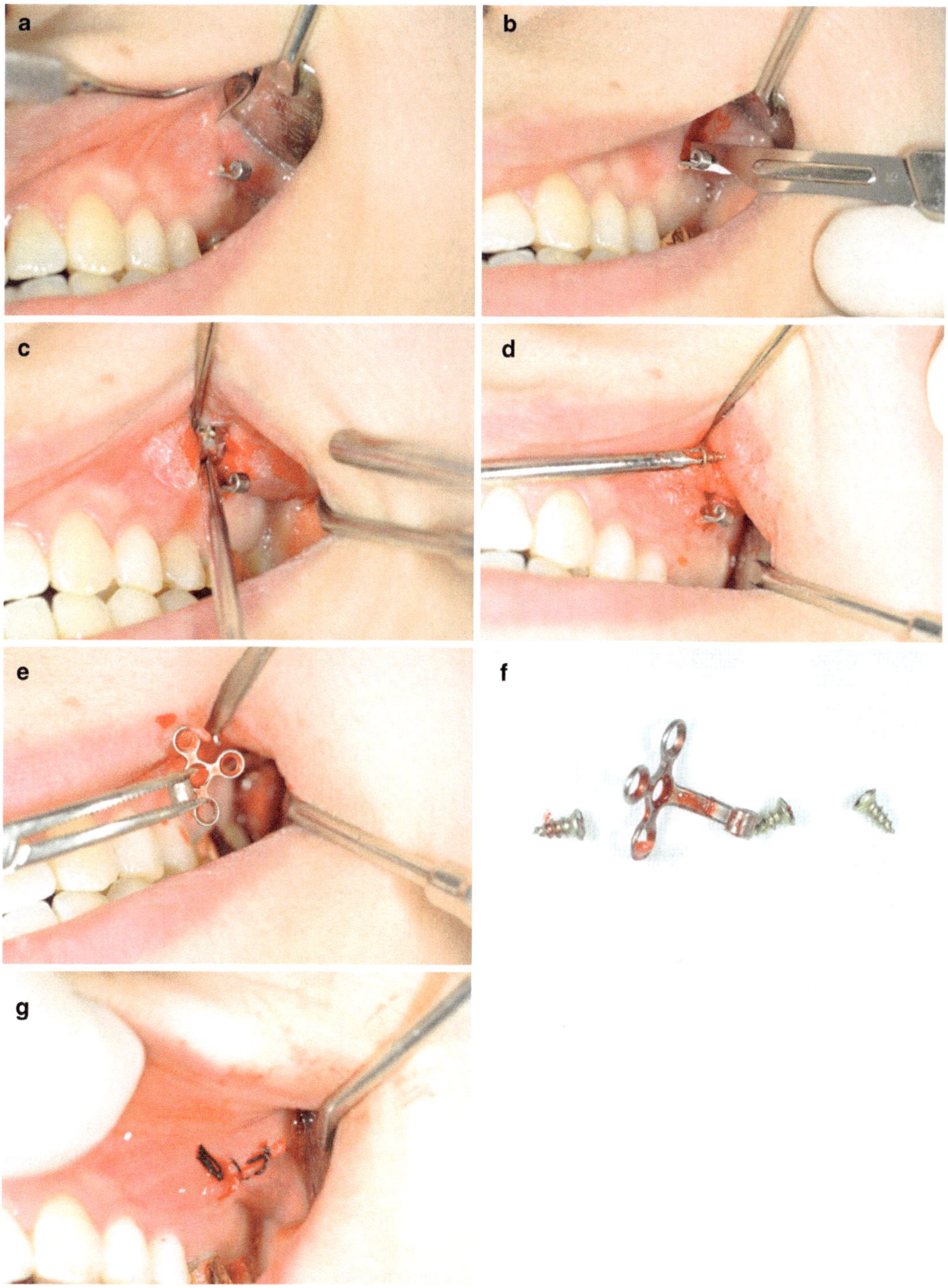

Fig. 9.11 Removal of T-type C-tube. (**a**) Initial photo. (**b**, **c**) Incisions were made to disclose fixation screws. (**d**) Fixation screws were unscrewed. (**e**, **f**) T-type C-tube was removed. (**g**) Sutured

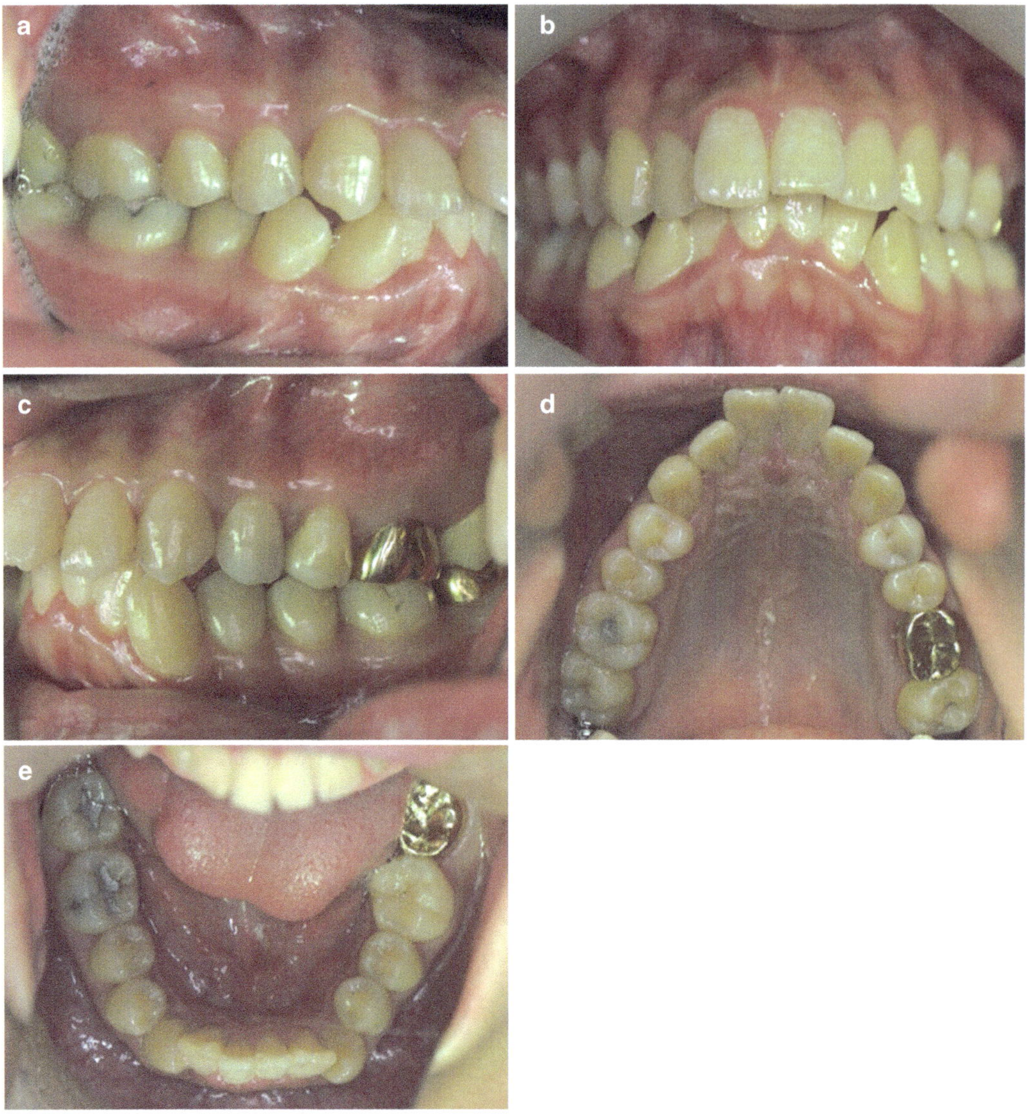

Fig. 9.12 Case 1. Intraoral photos (**a**–**e**). Excessive curve of Spee and over-erupted lower incisors are notable

and lateral lower incisors due to distal tipping of the lateral incisor crowns. The I-type C-tube was chosen as a choice of TSADs primarily because of noticeably narrow interradicular space. Brackets were bonded on the lower dentition. Four first premolars were extracted and I-type C-tube was placed in the apical region of the lower anteriors. Intrusion of the lower anteriors was accomplished out by connecting elastic thread between the C-tube head and lower incisors (Fig. 9.14). After adequate amount of intrusion was obtained, four incisors were ligated to the C-tube head to retain vertical position of the incisors (Fig. 9.15). With successful intrusion of the lower anterior teeth, the C-tube is no longer needed in the mandibular anterior legion. But, it could be replaced in the upper left posterior for the midline correction (Fig. 9.16). The C-tube can be reused in same patient, but the fixation screw loses the sharp edge once used. So, using new fixation screws, the C-tube is repositioned and the elastics are activated for midline correction (Fig. 9.17). The sequential lateral cephalograms (Fig. 9.18a–d) demonstrate

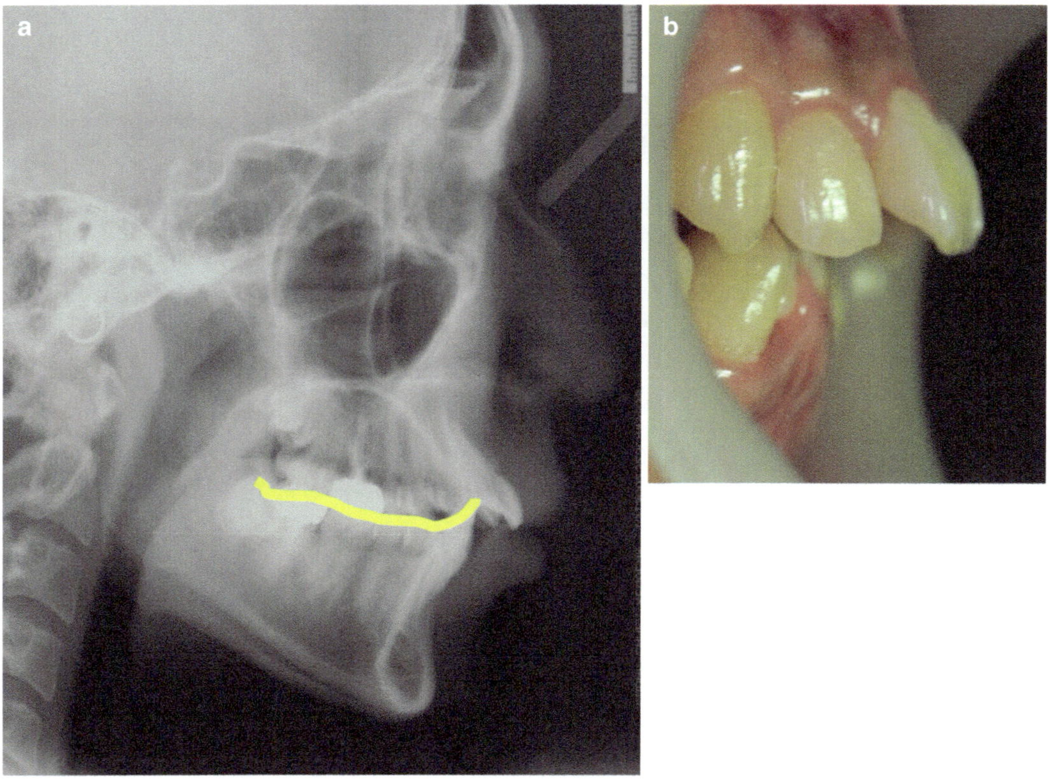

Fig. 9.13 (Continued) Lateral cephalogram (**a**) and photograph (**b**) show exaggerated curve of Spee and extreme amount of overjet

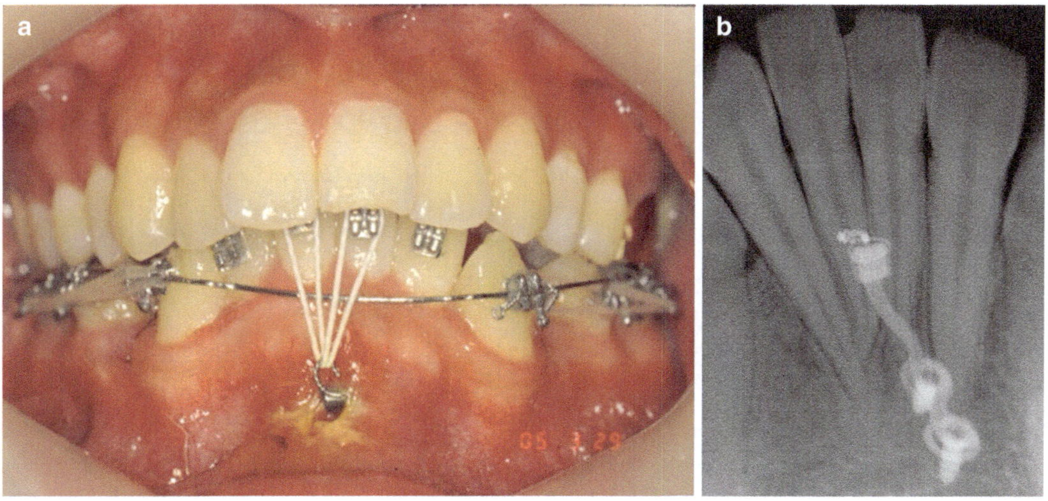

Fig. 9.14 (Continued) I-type C-tube was placed apically to the lower incisors and elastic thread was connected between the C-tube and incisor brackets (**a**). Note close proximity of roots in the lower anteriors (**b**)

the treatment progress and final intraoral pictures (Fig. 9.19) show the accomplishment of the treatment goals. Before and after the treatment, panoramic radiographs compare the root alignment especially on the lower anterior teeth (Fig. 9.20). With a selective use of single C-tube, the patient's chief complaint was solved with a duration of 15 months.

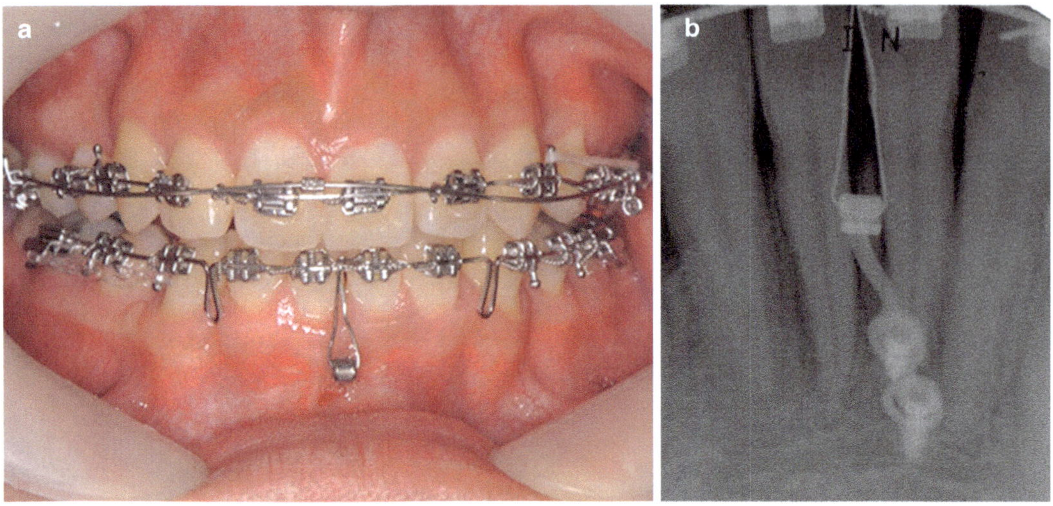

Fig. 9.15 (Continued) After sufficient amount of intrusion was achieved, the incisors were stabilized with steel ligature wire

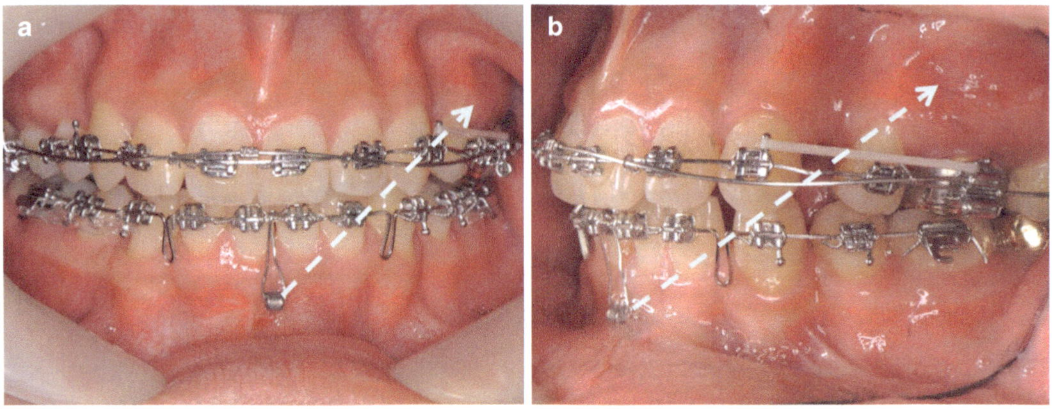

Fig. 9.16 (Continued) Mandibular C-tube was relocated to the posterior upper left area for midline correction

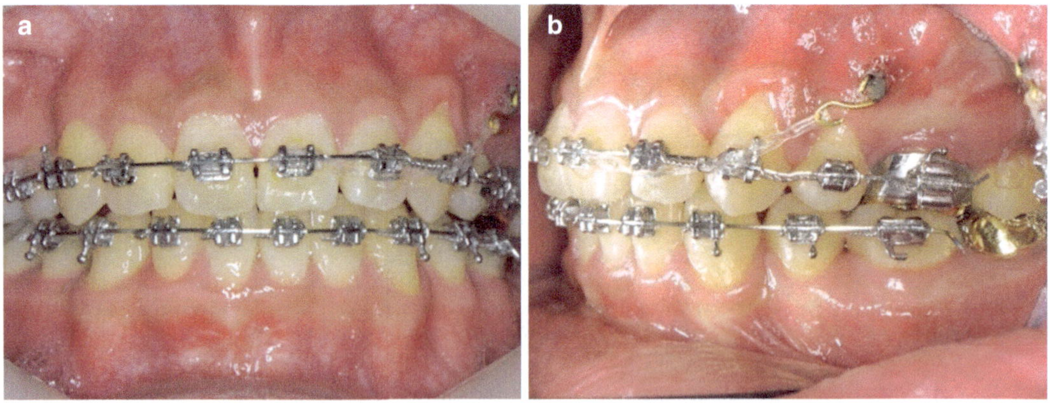

Fig. 9.17 (Continued) C-tube was placed on the interradicular space between the second premolar and first molar, and power chain was connected between the upper left central incisor and C-tube

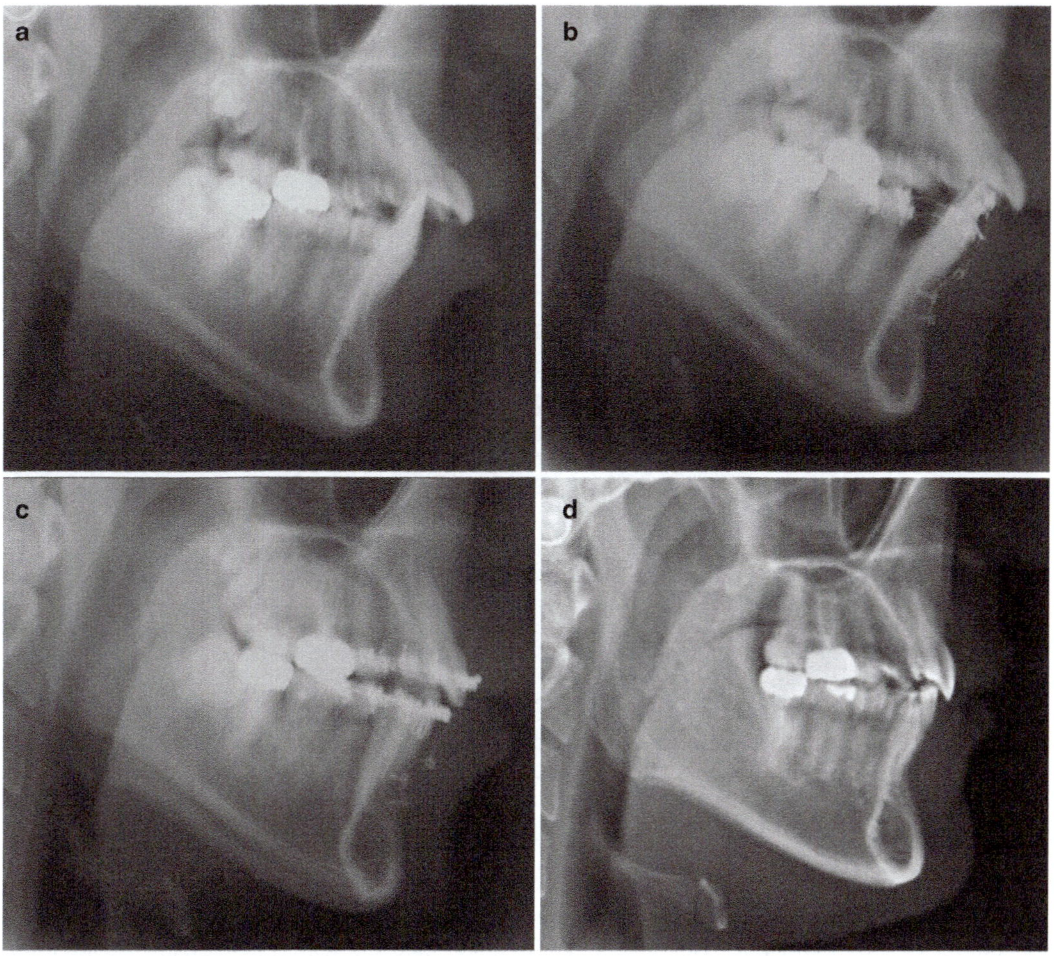

Fig. 9.18 (Continued) Treatment progress. (**a**) Initial cephalogram. (**b**) Beginning of lower incisor intrusion. (**c**) Completion of space closure. (**d**) After debonding

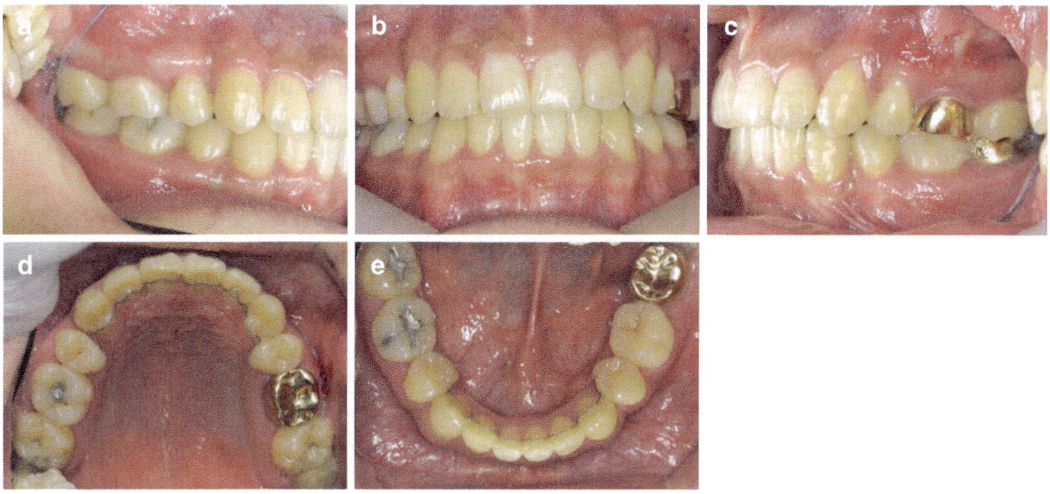

Fig. 9.19 (Continued) Final intraoral photos (**a**–**e**)

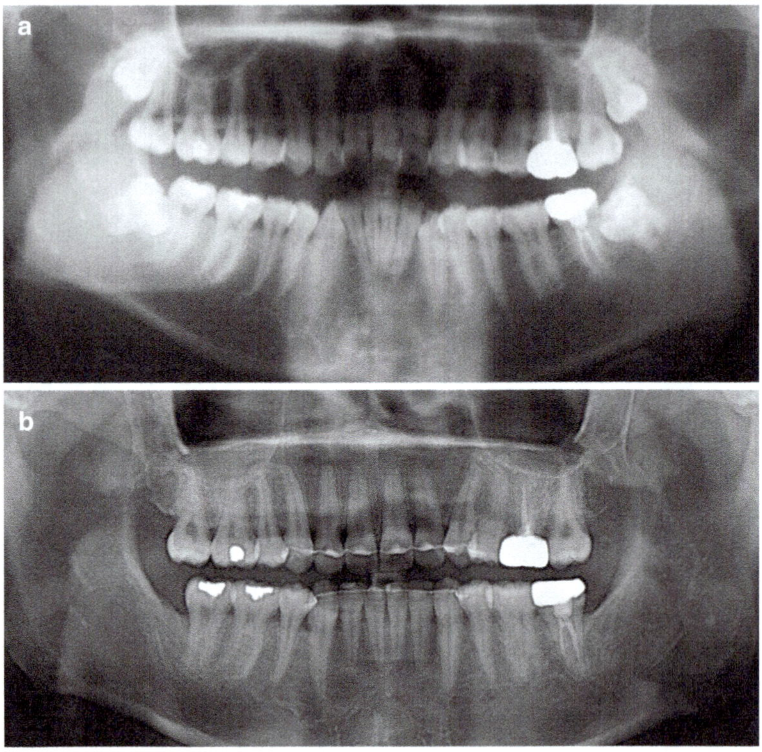

Fig. 9.20 (Continued) Panoramic radiographs of before (**a**) and after treatment (**b**). Note the root alignment especially on the lower anterior teeth

Case 2

A 39-year-old female patient presented with complaint of lip protrusion. The patient had obtuse nasolabial angle, slight lip protrusion, bimaxillary dentoalveolar protrusion, and hyperactive mentalis muscle activity. Intraoral exam revealed Class I molar relationship and generalized black triangles (Fig. 9.21a–c). Panoramic x-ray showed severe vertical bone loss in the right upper and lower second molar and pneumatization of maxillary sinus floor on the upper molars (Fig. 9.21d). In lateral cephalogram, interincisal angle was 110°. Periodontal diagnosis was localized severe chronic periodontitis and generalized moderate chronic periodontitis.

For a treatment plan, distalization of entire dentition without extraction was planned. To exert significant amount of force, two C-tubes were placed on the right and left upper posterior quadrants.

Thickness of the maxillary sinus wall was 2 mm at the apical area of the upper posterior teeth and no pathologic change was found inside the sinus space in the CT scan. Because 2 mm penetration of the sinus membrane with prosthetic implant is spontaneously healed without any complications, C-tube positioning was planned on the cortical bone of the lateral sinus walls. After placement of the modified T-type C-tube with two or three fixation screws, CBCT evaluation of the left and right sinus walls revealed minimum penetration into the sinus floor noticed without complications (Figs. 9.22 and 9.23). Brackets were bonded only on the anterior teeth and lower second premolars because the posterior teeth had acceptable occlusion. Upper archwire was inserted on six anterior teeth and inserted to the C-tube. Power chain was connected from the upper canine to the C-tube and elastics were inserted from the lower canine to the C-tube. In

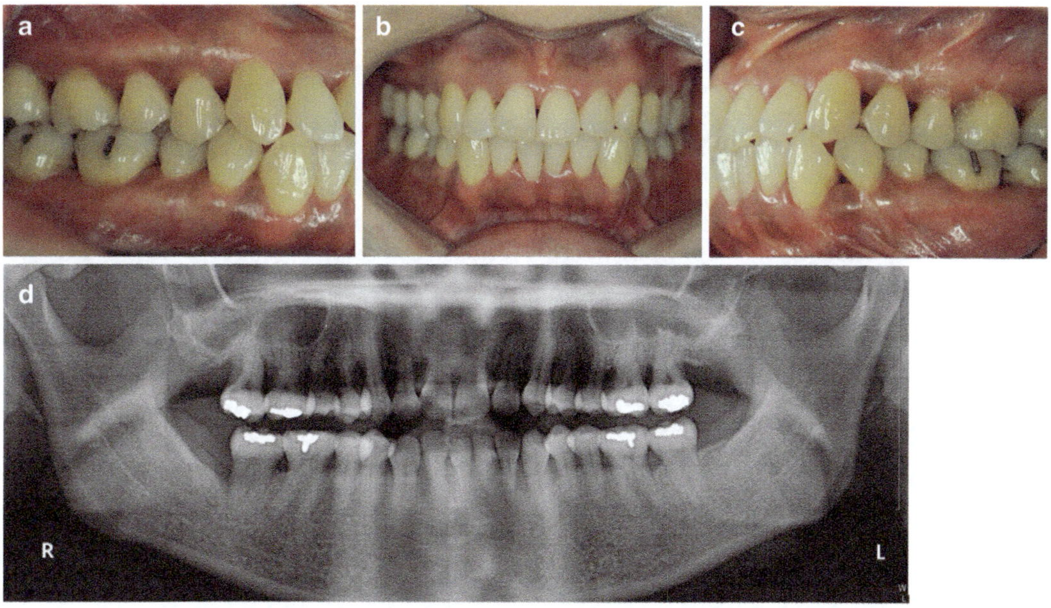

Fig. 9.21 Case 2. Initial photographs (**a–c**) and panoramic x-ray (**d**) of a 39-year-old female patient. Loss of interdental papilla, pneumatization of the maxillary sinus floor on upper molars, and generalized alveolar bone loss are observed

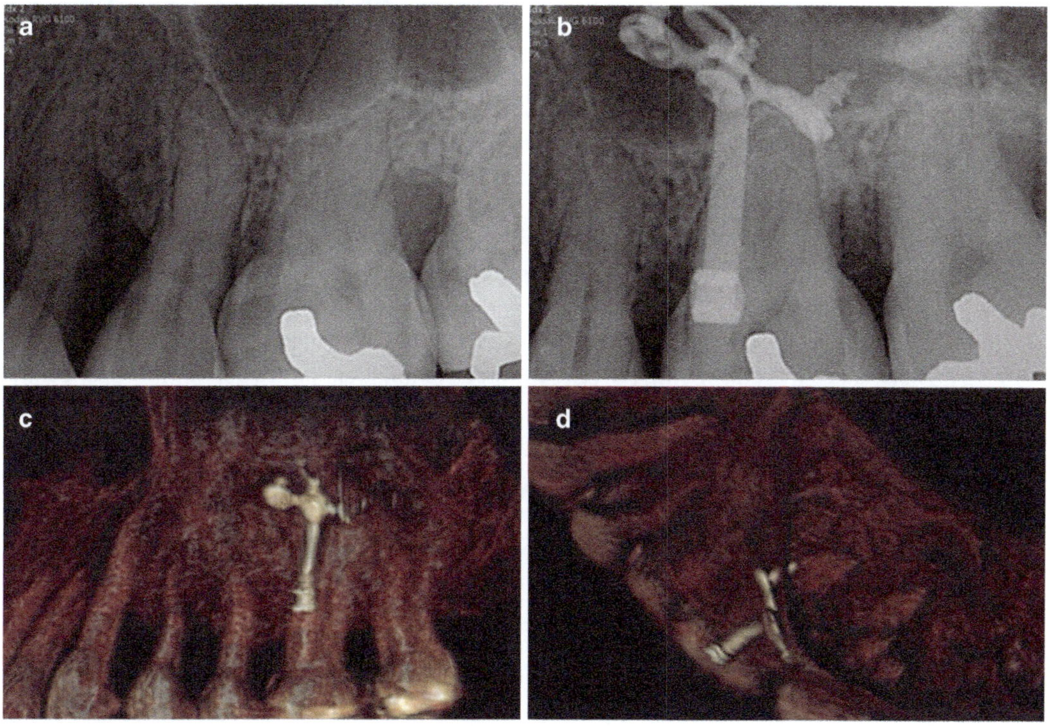

Figs. 9.22 (Continued) T-type C-tube was placed on the sinus wall on the left posterior region (**a–c**). Stability of the C-tube was obtained on the cortical bone of the sinus wall. Slight penetration into the sinus membrane of the fixation screw is seen (**d**)

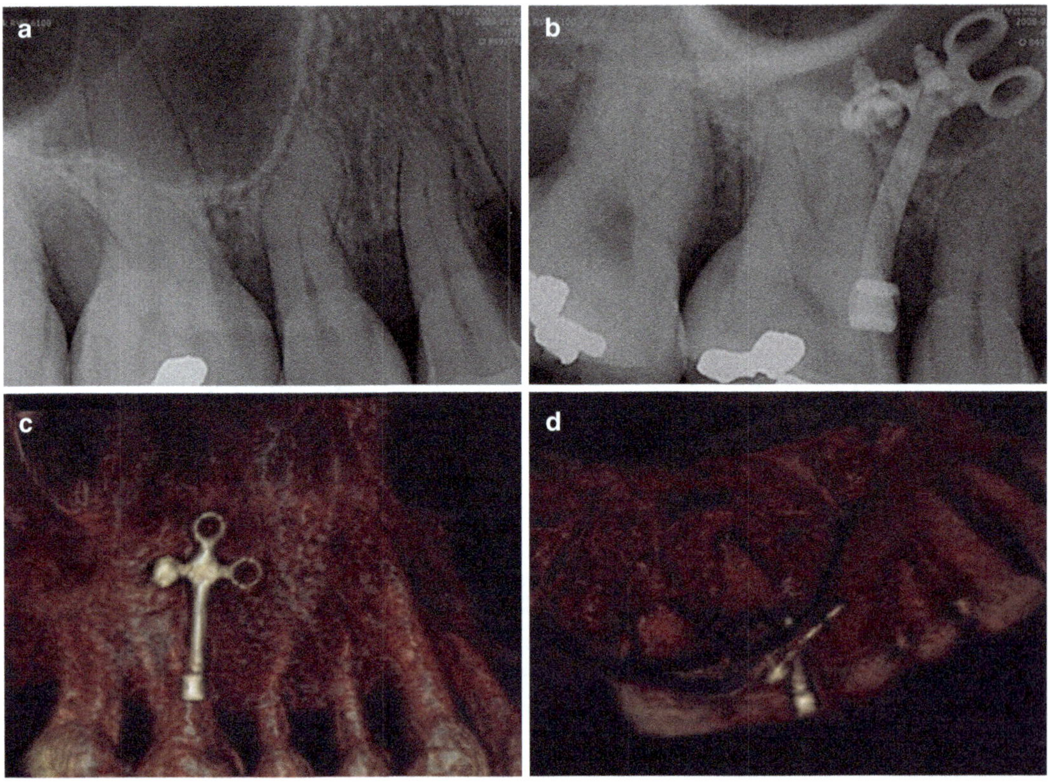

Fig. 9.23 (Continued) T-type C-tube was placed on the sinus wall on the right posterior region (**a**–**c**). Stability of the C-tube was obtained on the cortical bone of the sinus wall. Slight penetration into the sinus membrane of the fixation screw is seen (**d**)

5 months, 3 mm and 2 mm of space were obtained distal to the upper and lower canines, respectively, due to distalization of the posterior teeth (Fig. 9.24).

In 13 months, space was closed with retraction of the anterior teeth, and in 2 years, retention intraoral pictures show well-maintained stable occlusion (Fig. 9.25). Before and after, panoramic radiographs demonstrate the root parallelism and no worsening of periodontal condition after the orthodontic treatment (Fig. 9.26). Interincisal angle increased to 130° with controlled tipping of the upper and lower arch and lip protrusion was significantly improved (Fig. 9.27).

Case 3

A 43-year-old female patient presented to the clinic for correction of irregular anteriors and difficulty of chewing on the left side. Upon intraoral examination, protrusion of the upper central incisors and open bite were observed on the anteriors and left posterior teeth (Fig. 9.28). Moderate amount of crowding was found on the lower dentition. Patient's profile showed mild amount of lip protrusion and Class I skeletal pattern was observed (Fig. 9.29). Treatment objective was to solve crowding in lower dentition and improve alignment of upper dentition without compromising profile. Because the patient did

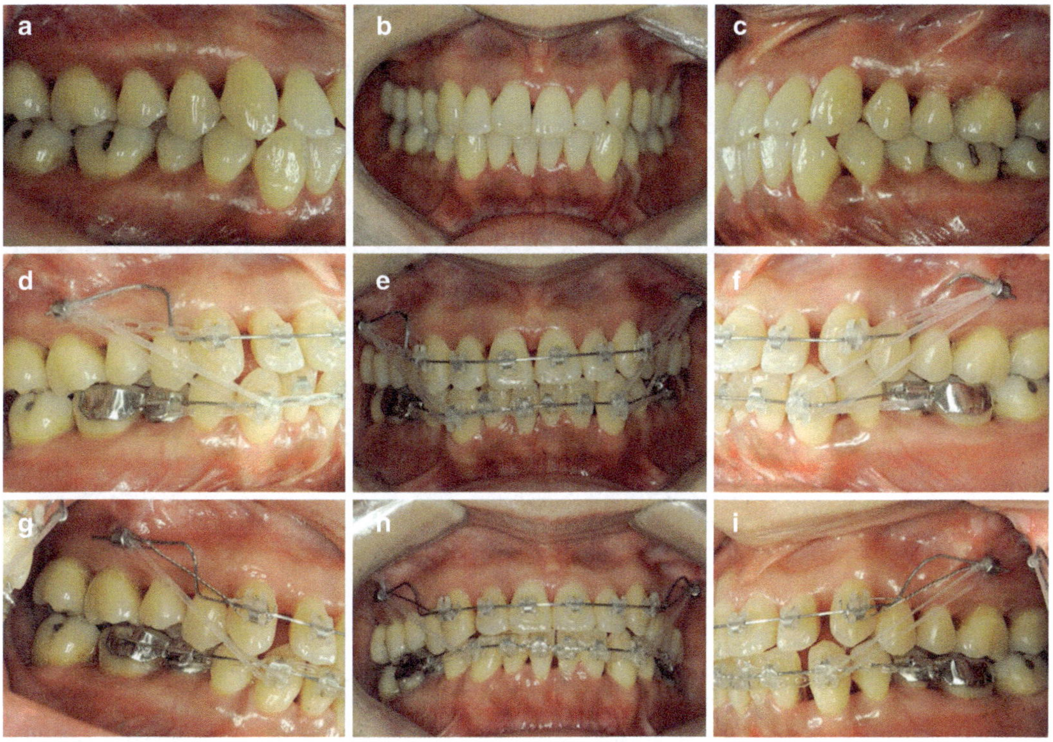

Fig. 9.24 (Continued) Treatment progress. (**a**–**c**) Initial photos. (**d**–**f**) At 1 month. (**g**–**i**) At 5 months

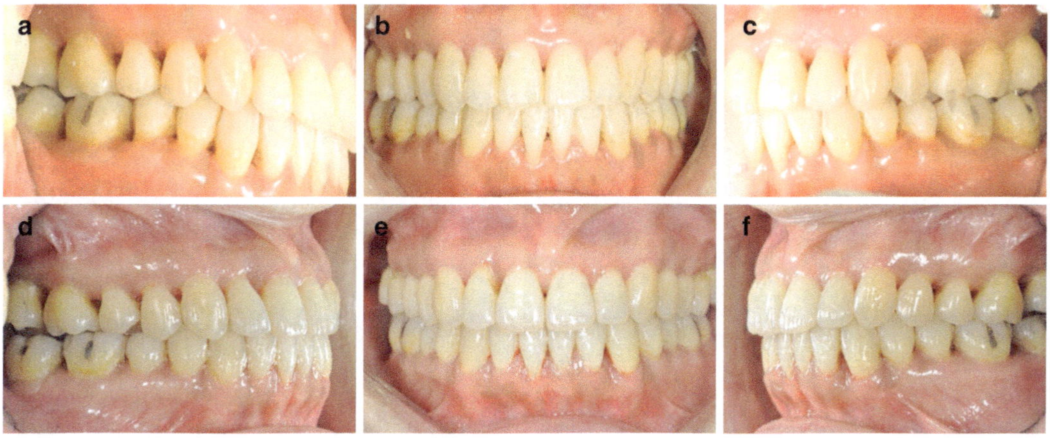

Fig. 9.25 (Continued) (**a**–**c**) After debonding of the fixed appliance (13 months). (**d**–**f**) At 2 years of retention

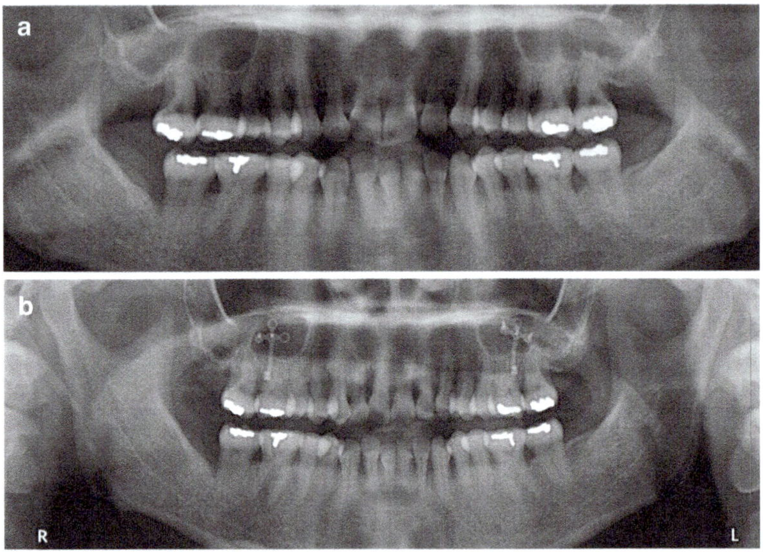

Fig. 9.26 (Continued) Panoramic radiographs of before (**a**) and after treatment (**b**). Note root parallelism and maintenance of periodontal health after the orthodontic treatment

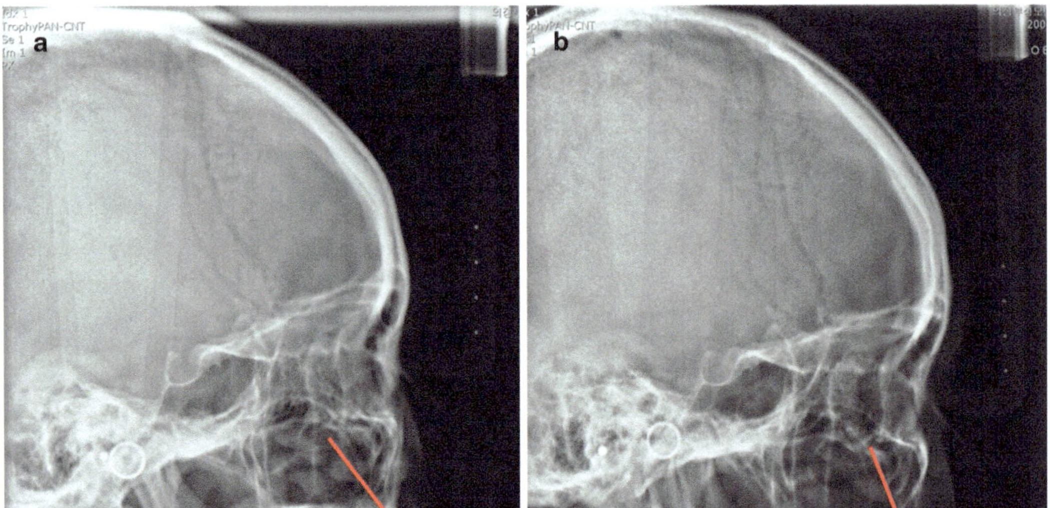

Fig. 9.27 (Continued) Lateral cephalograms of before (**a**) and after treatment (**b**). Interincisal angle was considerably improved after 13 months of treatment period

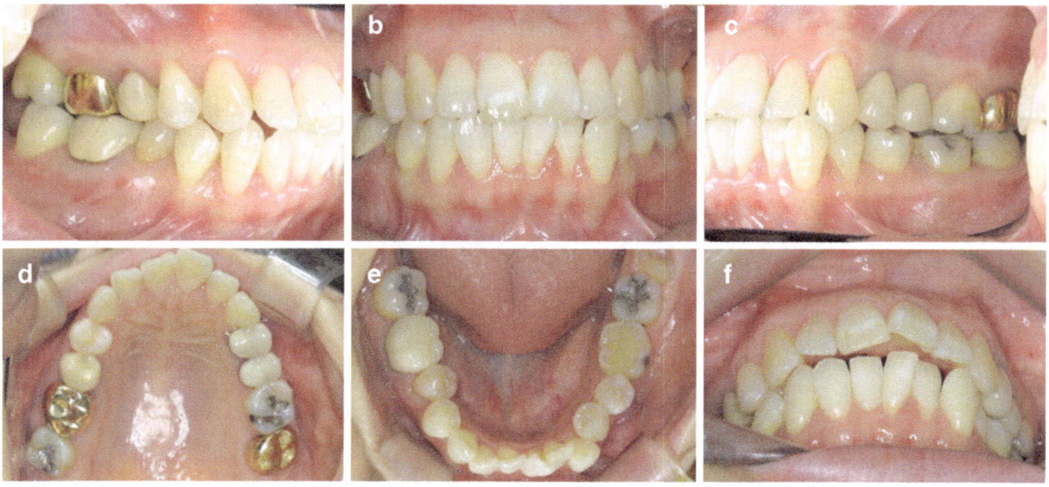

Fig. 9.28 Case 3. Initial photos (**a**–**f**). Moderate amount of crowding was found on the lower dentition. Upper central incisors were protruded and open bite was observed on the anteriors and left posterior teeth

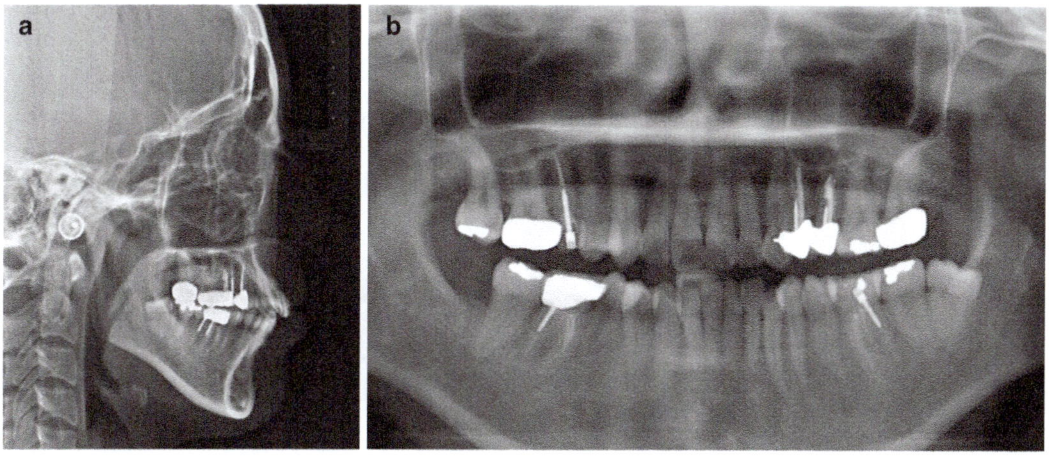

Fig. 9.29 (Continued) Initial lateral cephalogram (**a**) and panoramic x-ray (**b**) showing mild amount of lip protrusion and Class I skeletal pattern

not want premolars extracted, distalization of the entire dentition using C-tube was planned. After extraction of the lower left third molar, C-tubes were placed on the retromolar areas of the lower right and left and extension hooks were connected. Brackets were bonded on canines, first and second premolars, and second molars. The lower second molars were distalized primarily by power chain connected between the C-tube and lower first premolar. Distalization force was augmented with open coil springs inserted between the second premolar and second molar. The upper second molars were initially distalized only with open coil springs between the second premolar and second molar (Fig. 9.30). To prevent counteraction against canines, stabilizing lingual archwires were bonded between the right and left canines of both arches (Fig. 9.30d, e). Later on, Class II elastics were connected between the C-tube hook and upper canine (Fig. 9.31). After 5 months, sufficient amount of second molar distalization was

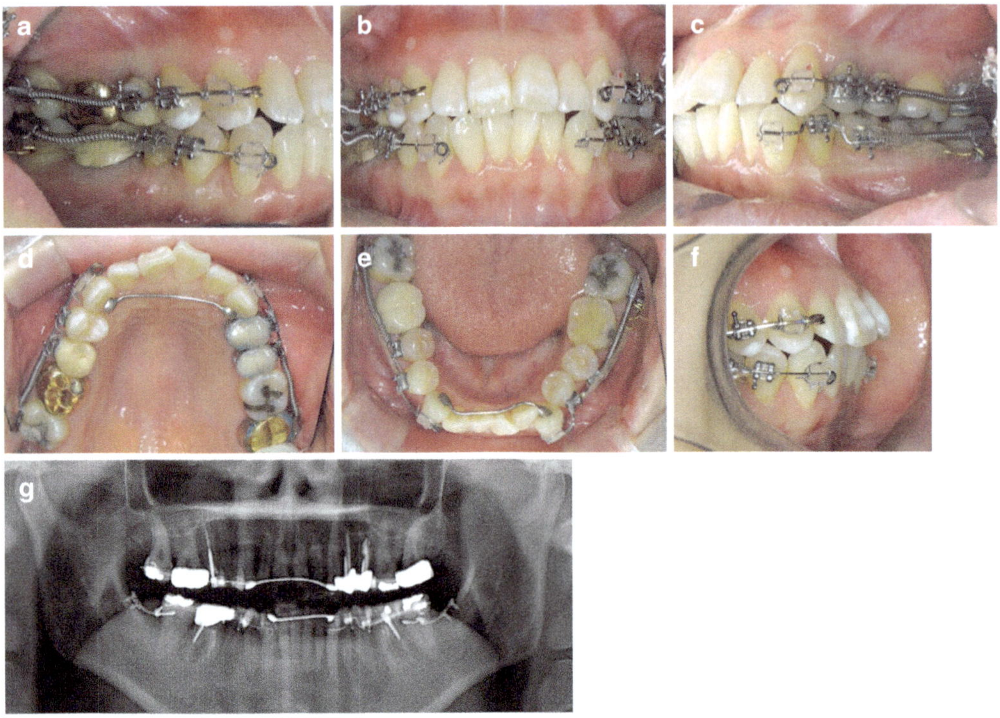

Fig. 9.30 (Continued) Distalization of the entire dentition. Distalization force was augmented with open coil springs inserted between the second premolar and second molar (**a–c**). Lingual arches were bonded on the upper and lower arches to prevent protrusive force against canines (**d**, **f**). C-tubes placed in the right and left retromolar areas are observed (**g**)

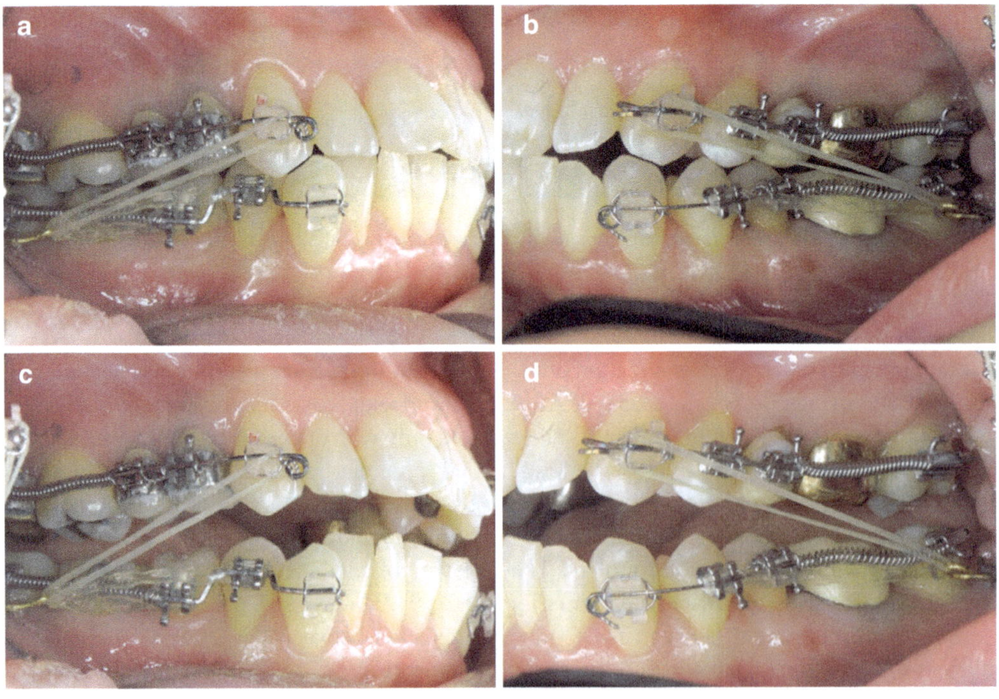

Fig. 9.31 (Continued) Class III elastics were connected between the C-tube hook and upper canine for distalization of the upper second molars. (**a**, **b**) When closed. (**c**, **d**) When opened

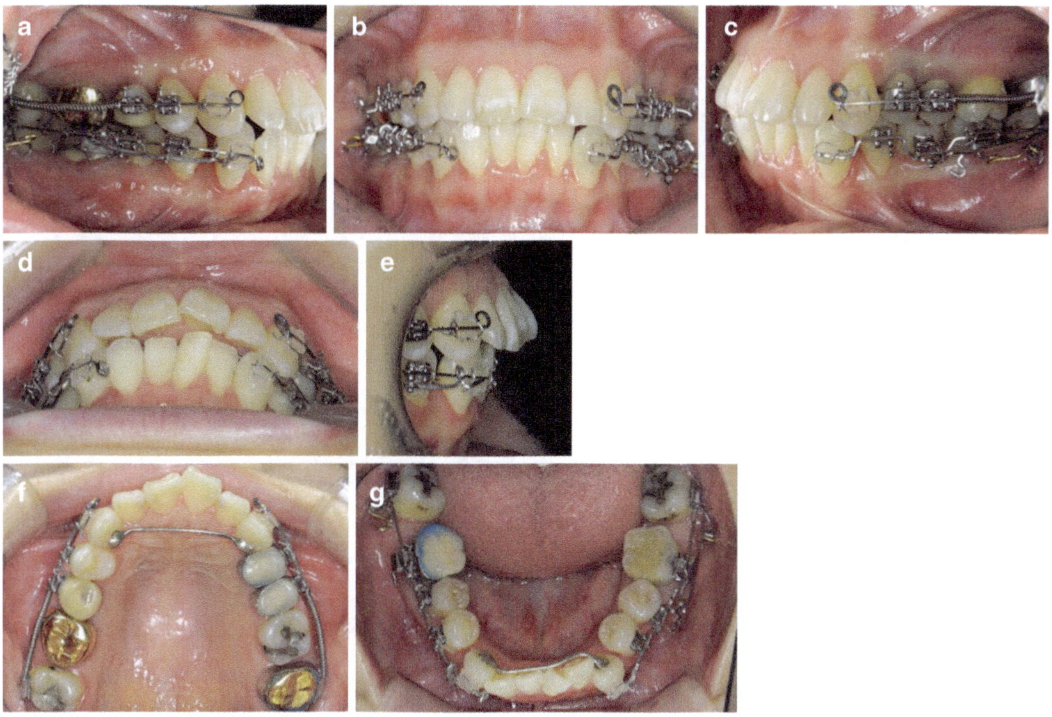

Fig. 9.32 (Continued) (**a–g**) Second molars were sufficiently distalized after 5 months without any change on the upper and lower four incisors

achieved. Interestingly, spaces were also found between the lower canines and first premolars (Fig. 9.32). Brackets were bonded on the remaining incisors and archwires were inserted on both arches. Upper dentition was further distalized with Class II elastics between the C-tube hook and upper lateral incisor (Fig. 9.33) and open coil springs placed between the upper canine and first premolar (Fig. 9.34c). Remaining space was consolidated and finishing completed (Figs. 9.35 and 9.36). After completion of the treatment, smile arc was considerably improved and lower lip protrusion was slightly decreased (Fig. 9.37). As in this case, C-tube can dramatically improve adult patient's acceptance for the treatment because it can shorten the treatment time and efficiently distalized entire dentition without adverse effects.

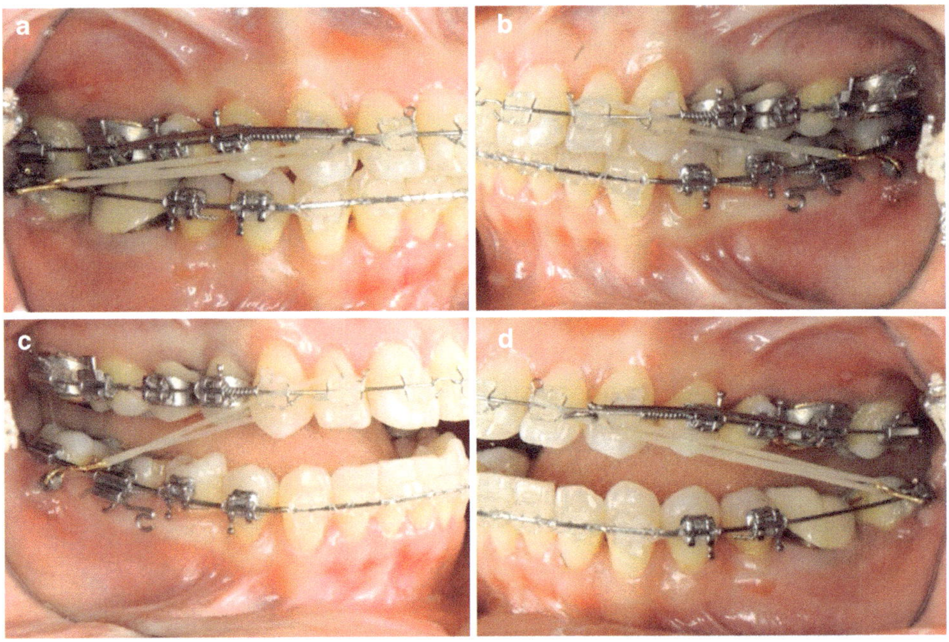

Fig. 9.33 (Continued) Brackets were bonded on the remaining incisors and archwires were inserted on both arches. Upper dentition was further distalized with Class III elastics between the C-tube hook and upper lateral incisor. (**a**, **b**) When closed. (**c**, **b**) When opened

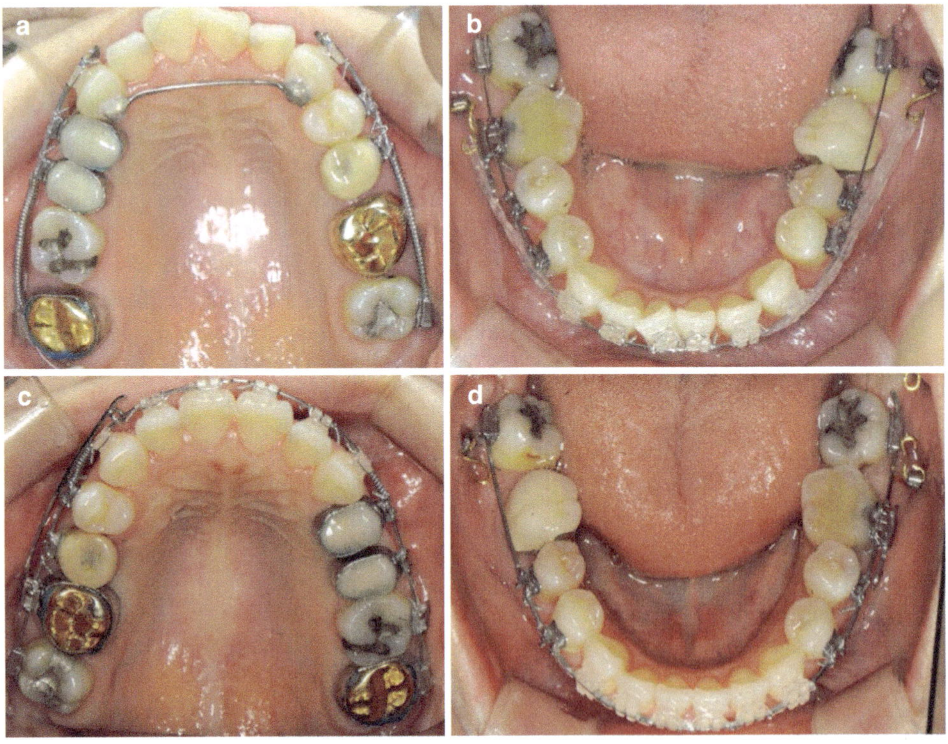

Fig. 9.34 (Continued) (**a**, **b**) After distalization. Space is found between the first and second molars. (**c**, **d**) After consolidation of the space

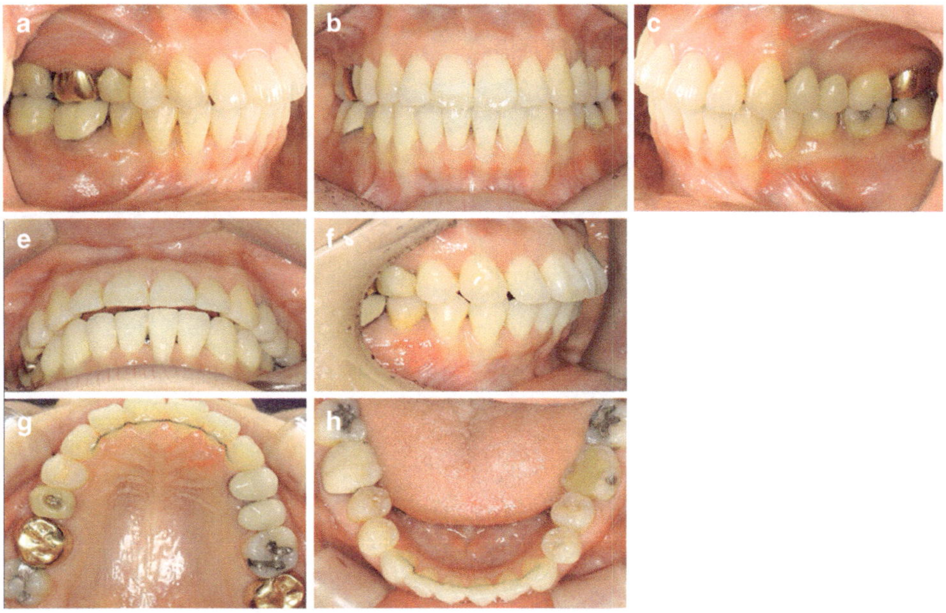

Fig. 9.35 (Continued) (**a–h**) After treatment. Desirable occlusion was achieved on the upper left posterior region where an open bite was present. Periodontal health was also maintained

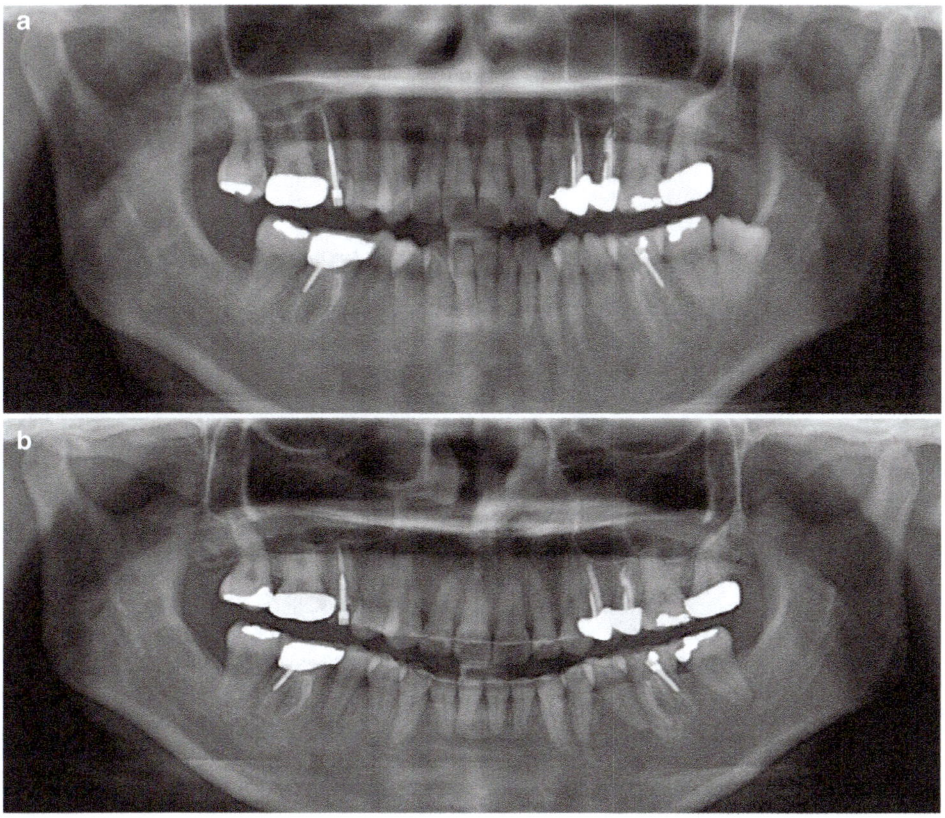

Fig. 9.36 (Continued) Panoramic x-rays of before (**a**) and after treatment (**b**). Note uprighting of the lower molars and amount of the lower molar distalization

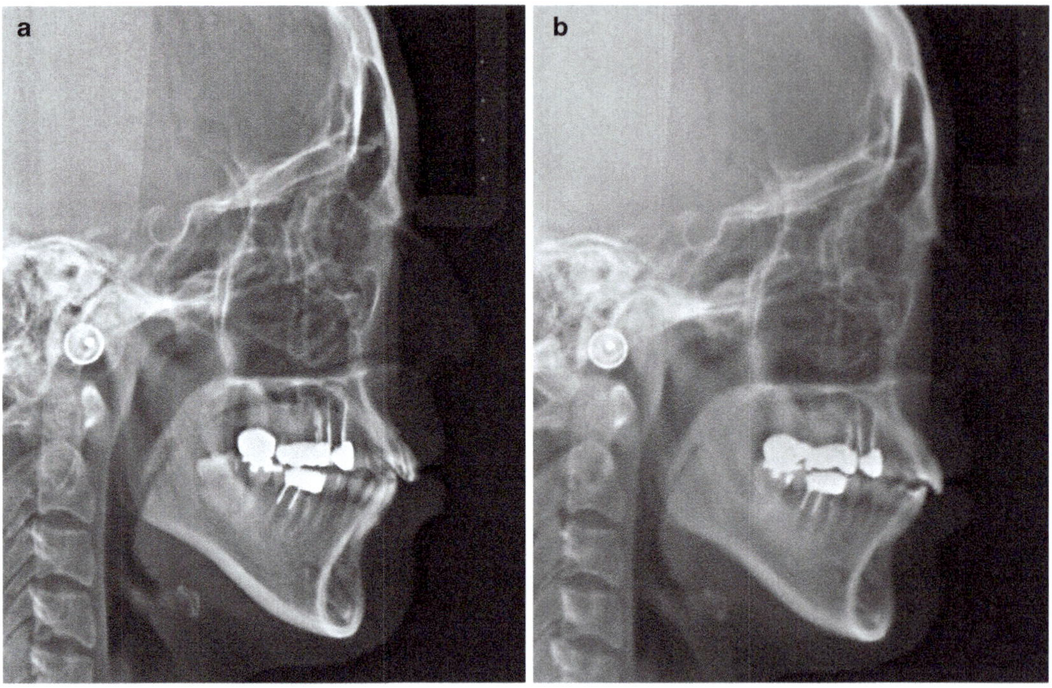

Fig. 9.37 (Continued) Lateral cephalograms of before (**a**) and after treatment (**b**). Lower lip protrusion was slightly decreased

Acknowledgment The authors thank Dr. Yong Kim, Research Assistant of Kyung Hee University School of Dentistry, for manuscript editing.

References

1. Sugawara J, Kanzaki R, Takahashi I, Nagasaka H, Nanda R. Distal movement of maxillary molars in nongrowing patients with the skeletal anchorage system. Am J Orthod Dentofacial Orthop. 2006;129(6):723–33.
2. De Clerck EEB, Swennen GRJ. Success rate of miniplate anchorage for bone anchored maxillary protraction. Angle Orthod. 2011;81(6):1010–3.
3. Chen Y-J, Chang H-H, Huang C-Y, Hung H-C, Lai EH-H, Yao C-CJ. A retrospective analysis of the failure rate of three different orthodontic skeletal anchorage systems. Clin Oral Implants Res. 2007;18(6):768–75.
4. Chung K-R, Kim S-H, Kang Y-G, Nelson G. Orthodontic miniplate with tube as an efficient tool for borderline cases. Am J Orthod Dentofacial Orthop. 2011;139(4):551–62.
5. Chung K-R, Kim Y-S, Linton JL, Lee Y-J. The miniplate with tube for skeletal anchorage. J Clin Orthod. 2002;36(7):407–12.
6. Chung K, Kim S, Kook Y. The C-tube. OrthoTADs book: clinical guideline and atlas. Dallas: Underdog Media; 2007.
7. Lee S-J, Lin L, Kim S-H, Chung K-R, Donatelli RE. Survival analysis of a miniplate and tube device designed to provide skeletal anchorage. Am J Orthod Dentofacial Orthop. 2013;144(3):349–56.
8. Kim S-H, Kang S-M, Choi Y-S, Kook Y-A, Chung K-R, Huang JC. Cone-beam computed tomography evaluation of mini-implants after placement: is root proximity a major risk factor for failure? Am J Orthod Dentofacial Orthop. 2010;138(3):264–76.
9. Seo K-W, Ahn H-W, Kim S-H, Chung K-R, Nelson G. Miniplate with a bendable C-tube head allows the clinician to alter biomechanical advantage without physically moving the skeletal anchorage device. J Craniofasc Surg. 2014;25(2):686–9.
10. Seo K-W, Nahm K-Y, Kim S-H, Chung K-R, Nelson G. Chin plate with a detachable C-tube head serves for both osteotomy fixation and orthodontic anchorage. J Craniofac Surg. 2013;24(4):e424–8.

Application of TADs in Lingual Orthodontics: A Modified Segmented Arch Approach

10

Kee-Joon Lee and Young-Chel Park

Abstract

Lingual orthodontic treatment is indicated for adults who do not want appliance show. Considering the limitation of tissue response in adults, precision tooth movement without round-tripping is crucial. Moreover, in order to camouflage underlying skeletal discrepancies, translation-type tooth movement rather than tipping is essential. For those, adequate segmentation of the dental arch and specific goal-oriented movement of each segment can be helpful. Since maxillary palatal area is characterized by various insertion sites for the miniscrews, combination of the miniscrew position and various lever arms for preliminary segmental movement effectively eliminates the round-tripping, providing a reliable lingual treatment protocol in adults with periodontal complication or temporomandibular joint resorption. A typical inconsistent movement such as total arch displacement is also attainable. The biomechanical backgrounds and applications are explained and demonstrated.

10.1 Introduction

It is evident that the demand for orthodontic treatment among adults has been constantly increasing [1]. While the adults are more motivated for orthodontic treatment than the children, they tend to raise inquiries regarding the pros and cons of the treatment. They are concerned about the specifics, such as possible duration of the treatment, discomfort or pain from the appliance, and overall expense [2]. One of the important issues may be the exposure of the appliance. Therefore, an invisible orthodontic treatment may be very appealing to many of the adults who seek for orthodontic treatment. This chapter will briefly discuss the diagnosis and appliance construction procedure for reliable lingual orthodontic treatment in adults, with the incorporation of miniscrew implants.

K.-J. Lee, DDS, PhD (✉) • Y.-C. Park, DDS, PhD
Department of Orthodontics, Yonsei University, Yonsei-ro 50, Seodaemon-gu, Seoul 120-752, South Korea
e-mail: orthojn@yuhs.ac; ypark@yuhs.ac

10.2 Limitation of Orthodontic Treatment in Adults

What are the characteristics of adults? The limitation of orthodontic treatment in adults has been extensively discussed in the previous literature.

K.B. Kim (ed.), *Temporary Skeletal Anchorage Devices*,
DOI 10.1007/978-3-642-55052-2_10, © Springer-Verlag Berlin Heidelberg 2014

In particular, Melsen classified the limitations into two categories: intrinsic and extrinsic factors [3]. The intrinsic factors include reduced cellular reaction to a mechanical stimulus, age-related changes in the periodontal ligament, age-related bone changes, local age changes, and biological and mechanical interfaces. The extrinsic factor mainly refers to an inability to reproduce the desired stimulus.

For example, reduction in the alveolar bone height caused by marginal bone loss proportionally lowers the position of the center of resistance of a tooth [4]. In order to avoid undesired tipping of the tooth with an apically located center of resistance, an accurate moment-to-force (M/F) ratio is essential and periodontally compromised tooth would require higher M/F ratio at the bracket level for translation. However, the bottom line may be that it is not easy to reproduce the desired M/F ratio at the bracket level. Even though one has successfully calibrated the magnitude of the force and the moment using a particular device, the force system is subject to change according to the minor movement of teeth [5]. Therefore, application of precisely calibrated force system appears to be theoretical and not necessarily practical. This is true when a continuous arch was used, since the continuous archwire tied in two neighboring brackets nearly always creates a statically indeterminate force system, where exact magnitude of the force and/or moment can hardly be calculated [6, 7]. It is conceivable that the treatment goal has to be specified in each quadrant or sextant of each arch, in order to minimize unnecessary round-tripping.

10.3 Selection of Esthetic Appliances According to the Indication

There are various types of "invisible" braces available in the clinical field, such as aligners and lingual brackets. The ceramic or plastic labial brackets are less noticeable than the conventional metal brackets. Shalish et al. studied the patients' perception of recovery following the insertion of respective buccal, lingual, and removable aligner (Invisalign^{TM}) and showed that the fixed lingual appliances were associated with higher initial pain level, greater eating disturbance, and oral dysfunction than the rest appliance types [8]. Recovery time from various oral functional activities was overall longer in fixed lingual patients. Therefore, the use of the lingual fixed appliance is not justified in terms of patients' comfort and adaptation. On the other hand, in spite of the latest improvement, the aligners are not readily indicated in such as moderate crowding, severe rotation, open bite, and severe tipping [9, 10], due to the inherent inability to move teeth precisely. Moreover, one of the major disadvantages of the aligners is that their treatment outcome is entirely dependent upon the patients' compliance, while the result of lingual fixed appliances is mainly dependent upon the way the operator manipulates the appliance [11, 12]. Hence, it is important to understand the strengths and limitations of each appliance or system before appliance selection.

10.4 Need for Selective Tooth Movement

In most orthodontic cases, the planned amount and pattern of tooth movement differ among individual teeth, segments of teeth, and between upper and lower dental arches. In view of the precision tooth movement, one has to remember that aligners always use reciprocal anchorage to move specific tooth since the brace is strained along the overall arch regardless of the intention to move the rest of the teeth, which means arbitrary movement of specific tooth is greatly limited. In other words, undesired tooth movement is largely unavoidable using the aligners. This feature may be critical in adults, considering the limited tissue tolerance [13]. Hence, strategic segmentation of entire arch may help to avoid unnecessary round-tripping [7].

10.5 Need for Translation of Teeth for Camouflage

Another aspect that has to be considered is the skeletal discrepancy. While many adults would naturally have underlying skeletal problems, not

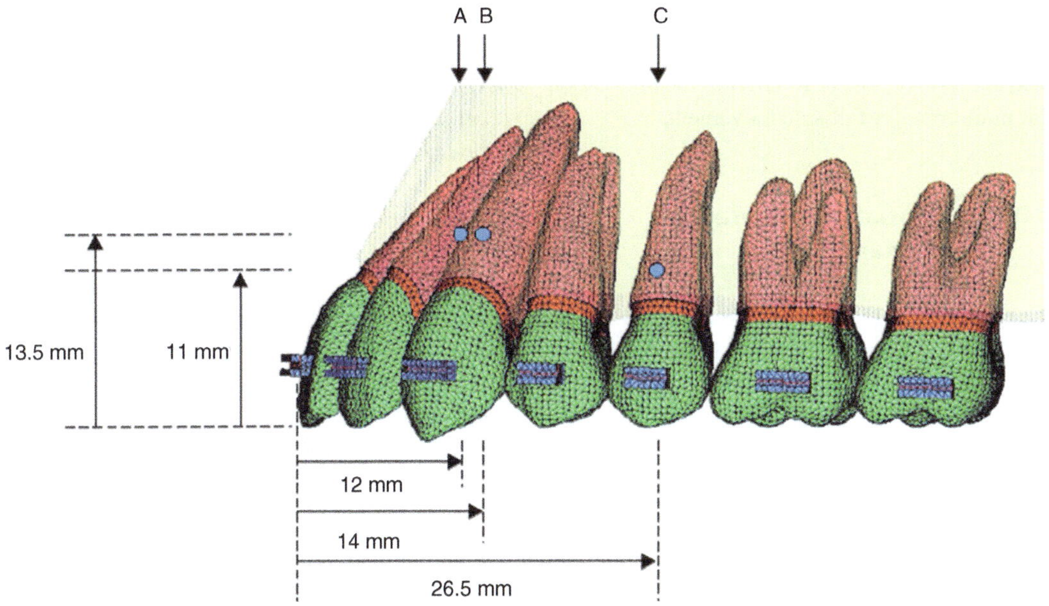

Fig. 10.1 Centers of resistance of maxillary anterior segment and entire arch (Courtesy to Mo S.S.)

all of them would need orthognathic surgery. Since growth modification in any form is not possible in adults, the "camouflage" has to be conducted over underlying basal bones. In spite of the certain degree of skeletal deviation, still main goal of orthodontic treatment is to establish a normal occlusion with appropriate axes of teeth in both buccolingual and mesiodistal direction. In other words, majority of camouflage case would require "translation" of teeth where all points of the object move to the same direction. Translation of teeth is not easily attained with removable-type appliance because they provide the force only to the crowns. Application of adequate M/F ratio at the crown level or any equivalent force system is not possible. This may be the major difference between fixed appliance and removable appliance.

10.6 Centers of Resistance

In order to produce desirable force system for specific type of tooth movement, it is essential to know the position of center of resistance of target segment. According to the recent finite element studies, the centers of respective four incisor segments, six anterior teeth, and entire maxillary arch have been suggested [14]. It is noteworthy that the vertical level of the center of resistance stays nearly same as the segment extends to the distal side. However, the anteroposterior position of the center of resistance varied according to the size of the segment. The information can be reflected in treatment planning and interpretation/revision of appliance design even during treatment (Fig. 10.1).

10.7 How to Induce Translation?

Considering the difficulty in measuring the required moment at the bracket level, it is less technique sensitive to use a single line of force near the estimated center of resistance, which is called as the "equivalent force system."

10.7.1 Translation (Distalization) of Posterior Segment

In order to distalize a single molar, the line of force has to go through the center of resistance. When the posterior teeth are segmented as a unit, they are expected to resistant to tipping, due to the change of the configuration. When distalization of a particular molar segment was indicated, it may be helpful to make the segment into a single unit and use a single line of force from the interradicular miniscrew for fail-safe movement.

10.7.2 Translation of Anterior Segment

Translation of incisors or axis control during retraction using certain combination of retraction force, vertical force, and/or moment at the bracket level is known to be very challenging in lingual orthodontics, because of the lingually positioned vertical force and need for larger moment [15–17]. Moreover, the incisors, unlike the posterior segment, are assumed to be a mesiodistally long segment positioned vertical to the retraction force, which is prone to tipping, like a long single tooth [18]. Instead, one can take advantage of the deep palatal vault to extend a lever arm up to the level of estimated center of resistance or even to the higher level [19].

10.7.3 Lever Arm Design for Incisors

It has been shown that using a lever arm is practical in lingual orthodontics [20], and it appears that long lever arm is able to induce translation or root movement according to the level of the hook. In the three-dimensional model, however, long lever arms are subject to elastic deformation and outward rotation of incisor segment, which can lead to linguoversion of the central incisors and buccoversion of the canine [21, 22].

When using a lever arm, it is therefore conceivable that the long lever arms should be splinted between the two arms, so that transverse bowing in the anterior region can be prevented (Figs. 10.2 and 10.3).

10.7.4 Miniscrew Insertion and Appliance Fabrication

In lingual orthodontics, miniscrews can be inserted on either the buccal side or lingual (palatal) side. Since main appliances are placed on the lingual side, miniscrews on the lingual side would allow direct engagement of elastic chains between the archwire hooks and the miniscrew head. Alternatively, splinting between the buccal miniscrews and the attachment on the tooth may be one solution if buccal miniscrews were to be used.

There can be several combinations of the estimated center of resistance and the miniscrew, each of which leads to differences in line of force and resultant tooth movement (Fig. 10.4a). It is noteworthy that the midpalatal miniscrews can change not only the angulation of the vector but also the presumed point of force application projected at the incisor, due to the distance between the lever arm hooks and the incisor body. Resultant type of tooth movement has to be carefully estimated and interpreted based on the findings in the cephalogram.

Maxillary buccal and/or palatal miniscrews can be used for molar distalization and incisor retraction. Since maxillary buccal areas exhibit around 3 mm of interradicular space, vertical angulation of the insertion path is recommended to avoid possible root damage [23]. In contrast, palatal sides display larger interradicular area due to the presence of palatal single root of molar (Fig. 10.4b). Midpalatal areas exhibit sufficient bone thickness near the midline. However, the parasagittal area is supported by a thin cortical bone and is not considered as an insertion site [19]. Mandibular interradicular and retromolar areas are also considered as reliable insertion sites. The root surface area of mandibular incisors is much smaller than that of the maxillary incisors. The mandibular miniscrews therefore can be useful for the control of posterior segment, either distalization or protraction [24, 25].

10.8 Midline-Based Diagnosis

In order to better understand the etiology of specific malocclusion and to establish a precise plan, a midline-based diagnosis may be helpful. Conventional orthodontic diagnosis using lateral cephalogram provides some information in the

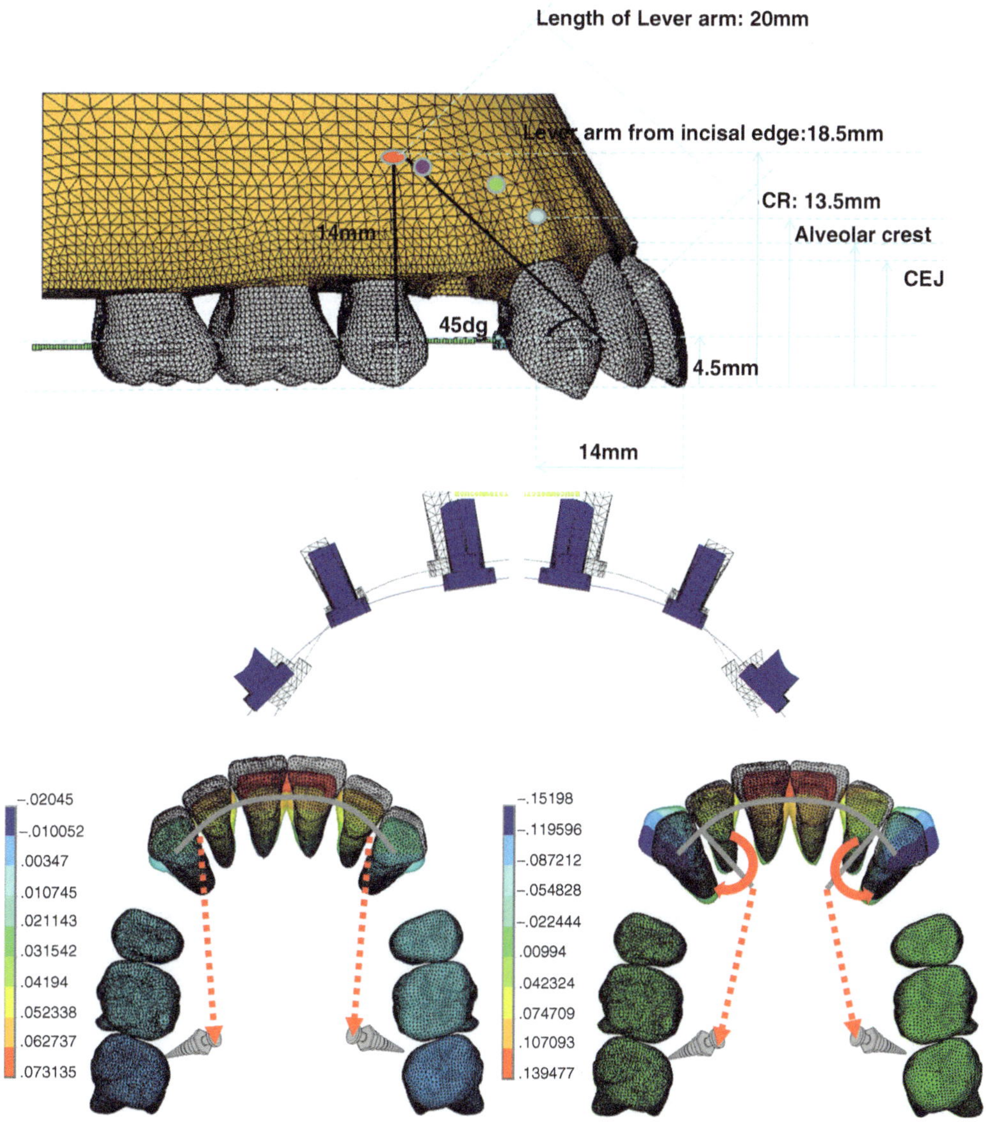

Fig. 10.2 Three-dimensional finite element models and resultant tooth movement. The long lever arm induced anterior transverse bowing and diminished the translation effects of incisors (Modified from Kim et al. [21]. Courtesy to YC Park)

sagittal and vertical planes; however, it hardly gives differential information between right and left sides. For example, in case of denture midline deviation, one has to distinguish whether it comes from asymmetric molar position or simple deviation of incisors. For the former case, asymmetric molar distalization should precede the incisor alignment, and for the latter, symmetric anchorage preparation regardless of the amount of midline deviation has to be made (Fig. 10.5).

Definition of each midline is summarized in Table 10.1. Among the various midline terms, what the patients easily recognize may be the denture midline and soft tissue midline. The orthodontists can further define the skeletal, apical base and geometric midlines, using various radiologic and model analyses. Considering the patients' satisfaction and better communication, the soft tissue midline is well selected as the treatment midline. In terms of treatment planning,

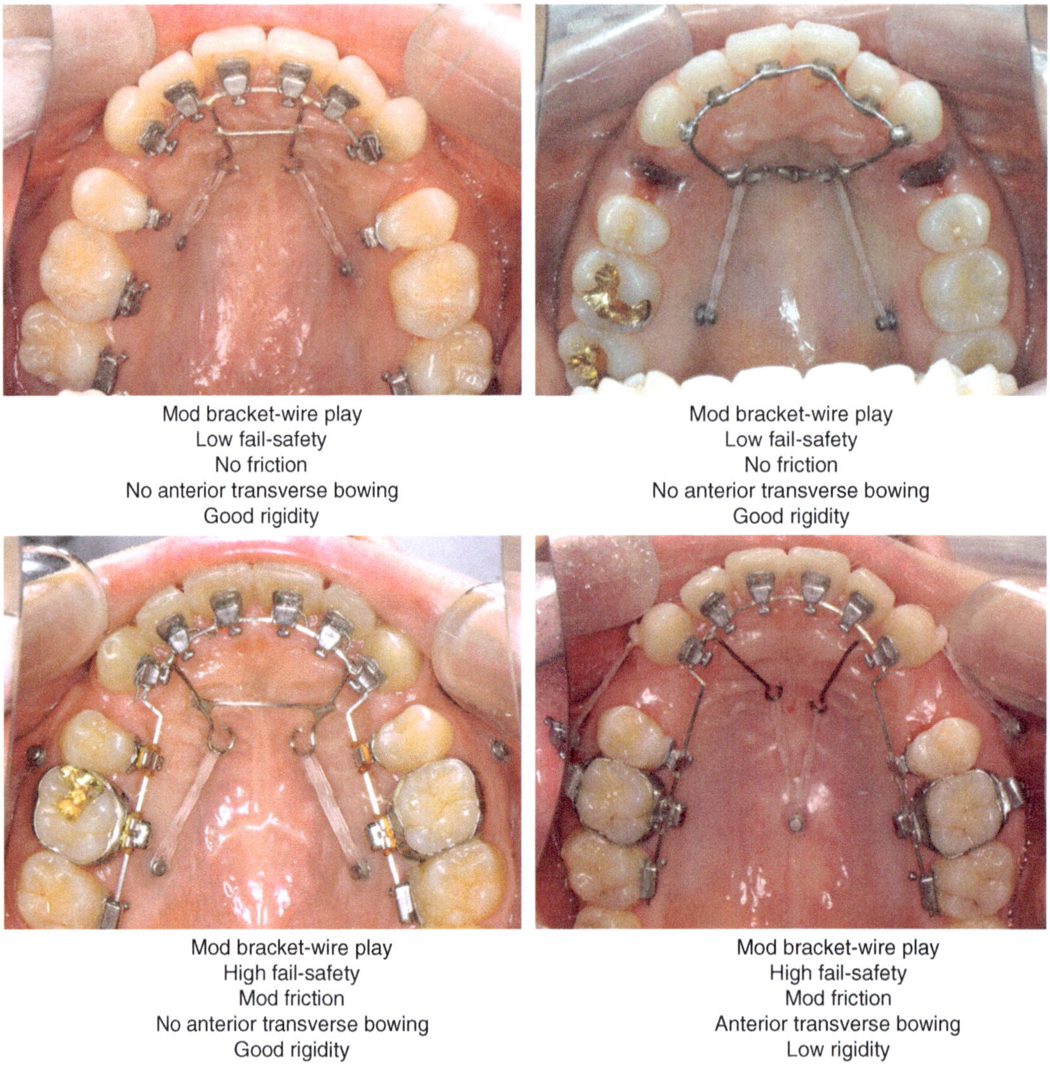

Fig. 10.3 Various lever arm designs and characteristics of each design

the apical base midline rather than denture midline is readily chosen as the representative of the anatomical midline. It is the best if the apical base midline is located on the same line as the soft tissue midline. Then, the treatment should be performed based on the diagnosis. If there is significant discrepancy between the two lines, the anterior segment needs to be translated to either side without "burning" the anchorage. This is important especially in the maxilla since the root surface area of maxillary anterior segment is normally larger than that of the mandibular incisors (Table 10.1).

10.9 Rationale of Miniscrew Application in Lingual Orthodontics

Since orthodontic treatment in adults may demand selective movement of specific tooth or segment of teeth, using a continuous arch is not justified. Along a continuous arch between anchor segment and moving segment, it is not easy to anticipate the amount of anchorage loss. Related to this, strength of the use of miniscrews in lingual orthodontics may be that they enable the precision movement of the specific segment

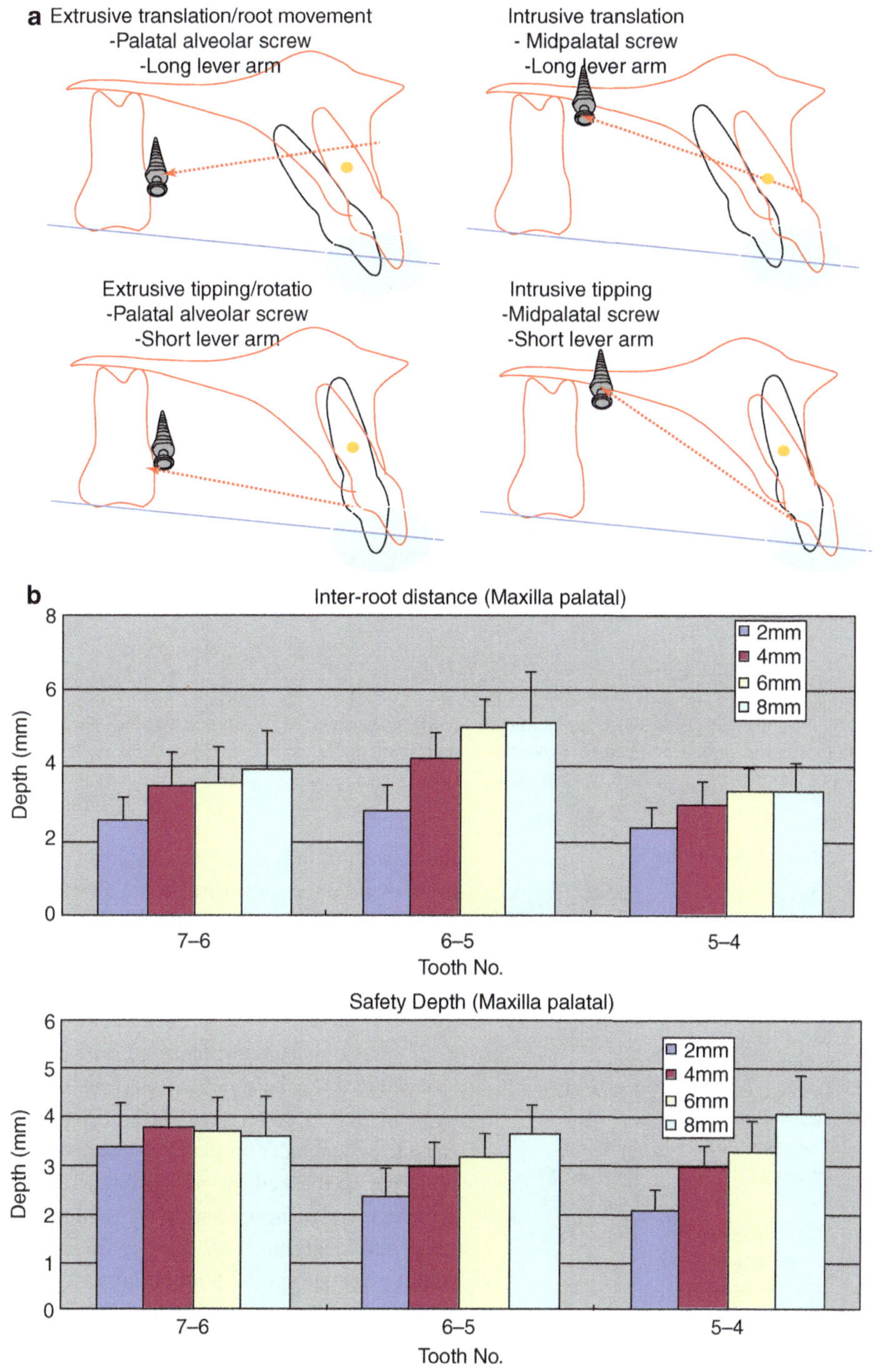

Fig. 10.4 (**a**) Combined use of lever arms and miniscrew positions. (**b**). The interradicular space on the maxillary palatal side (Modified from Lee et al. [23])

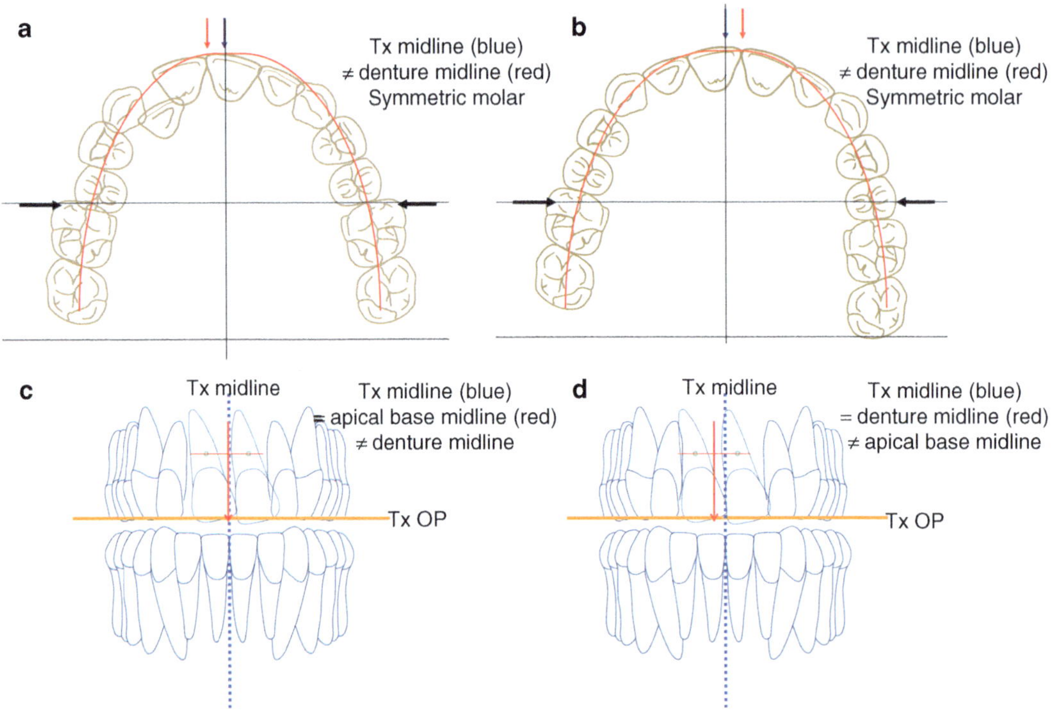

Fig. 10.5 (**a**, **b**) Midline deviation with or without symmetry of the molar, indicating the need for posterior segment control prior to incisor movement or alignment. (**c**, **d**) Assessment of apical base midline. The midline correction on the left side is easier than the right side

Table 10.1 Definition of each midline

	Definition	Source
Skeletal midline	Crista galli – ANS-Me	PA cephalogram
Apical base midline	Midpoint between Cres U1-1 projected onto treatment occlusal plane	PA cephalogram
Facial (soft tissue) midline	Glabella-nose tip-(philtrum)-Me'	Extraoral photograph
Denture midline	Contact point between U1-1 and L1-1	Intraoral photograph Dental cast
Geometric midline	Midpoint between the 1st molars along the arch perimeter	Dental cast

without any movement of anchorage segment via effective combination of the miniscrew position and lingually extended lever arms.

Since miniscrew provides a force vector apart from the dental arch, the segmental movement takes place without the expense of anchorage segment. This implies that the inconsistent movement within the arch, for instance, total arch movement to the same direction, can be achieved. The treatment plan is specifically defined at each segment, with the midline as a major landmark.

Case 1

A 26-year-old woman presented with lip protrusion. Initial cephalometric analysis revealed a skeletal Class I pattern with slight lip protrusion. In spite of her chief complaint, she had a prominent chin, which masked the protrusion of lips to certain degree. The upper and lower denture midline was coincident, but there was significant denture midline deviation by 2.5 mm relative to the facial midline, which was associated with her underlying facial asymmetry. The amounts of crowding in both arches were minimal (Fig. 10.6a).

Retraction of upper and lower incisors was definitely included in the treatment objectives, for which premolar extraction was recruited. However, the midline correction was challenging. Since she did not want appliance show, nor any invasive surgical procedure, a specific consideration for the appliance design for her midline and profile was indispensible. According to the occlusogram, unilateral extraction of premolars on the right side was shown to be able to correct the midline, through the preparation of maximum anchorage on that side. Therefore, instead of bilateral premolar extraction, a unilateral premolar extraction was chosen as a compromised treatment plan. Since her incisor axis was normal to start with, the treatment plan included maximum lateral translation of her upper and lower anterior segment. Since the root surface area is obviously greater in the maxillary anterior region, compared to that of lower anteriors, a splinted lever arm was designed and attached particularly on the maxillary six anterior teeth following the premolar extraction. Full strap of lingual brackets was attached in the mandible. Unilateral retraction was performed through the alternative use of miniscrews (1.8 mm in diameter, 7 mm in length) (Orlus serial #18107, Ortholution, Seoul, Korea) on the midpalate and palatal slope. Following the major movement of the segment, full-strap lingual brackets and continuous archwire were used to finalize the treatment (Fig. 10.6b).

Finally, the midline was coincident with her facial midline, with moderate retraction of her lips. The cephalogram and superimposition view indicate translation of upper incisor segment without significant tipping. She was satisfied with the result since the midline was camouflaged with the use of invisible appliance. This case indicated how a selective segmental movement using miniscrews can effectively lead to the actual treatment goal (Fig. 10.6c).

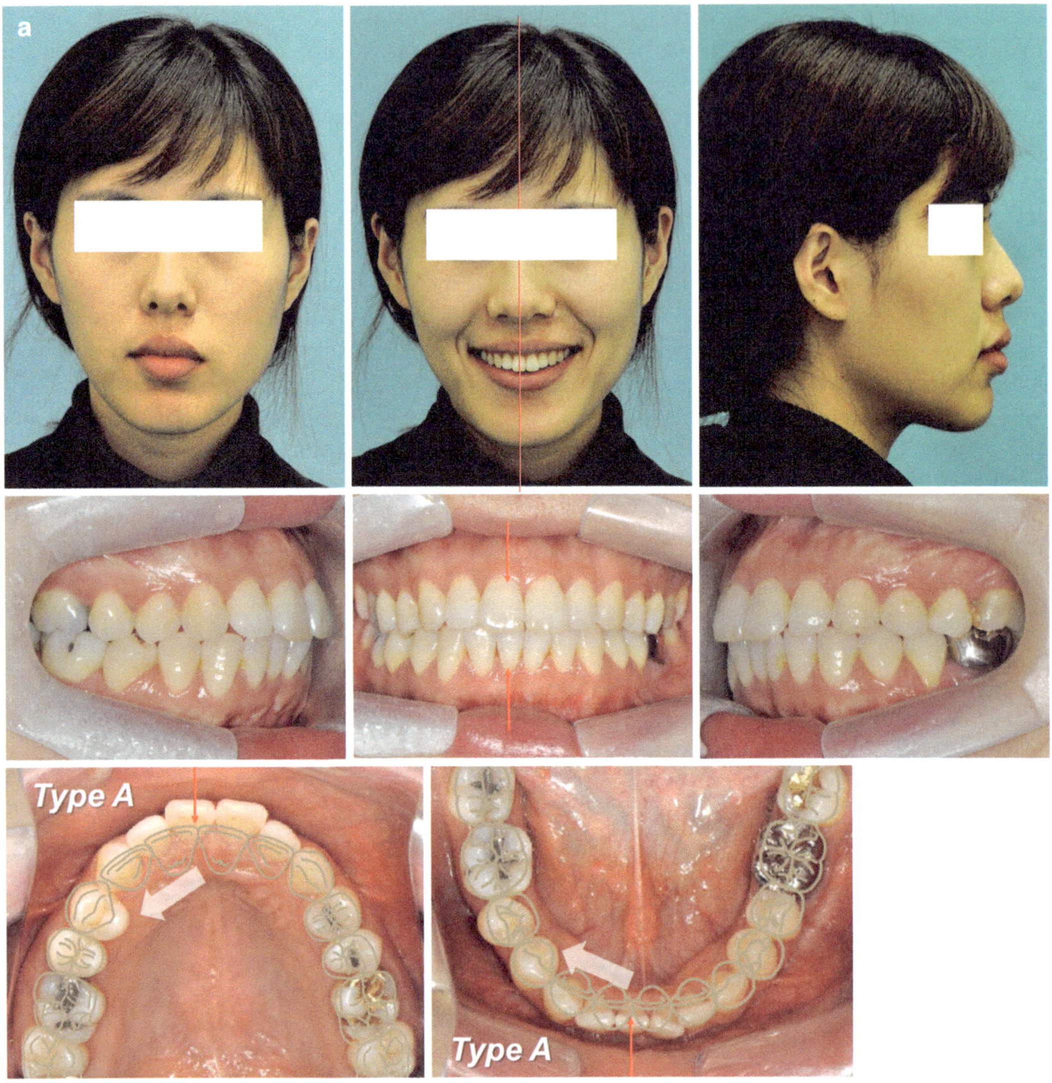

Fig. 10.6 Case 1. (**a**) Pretreatment records

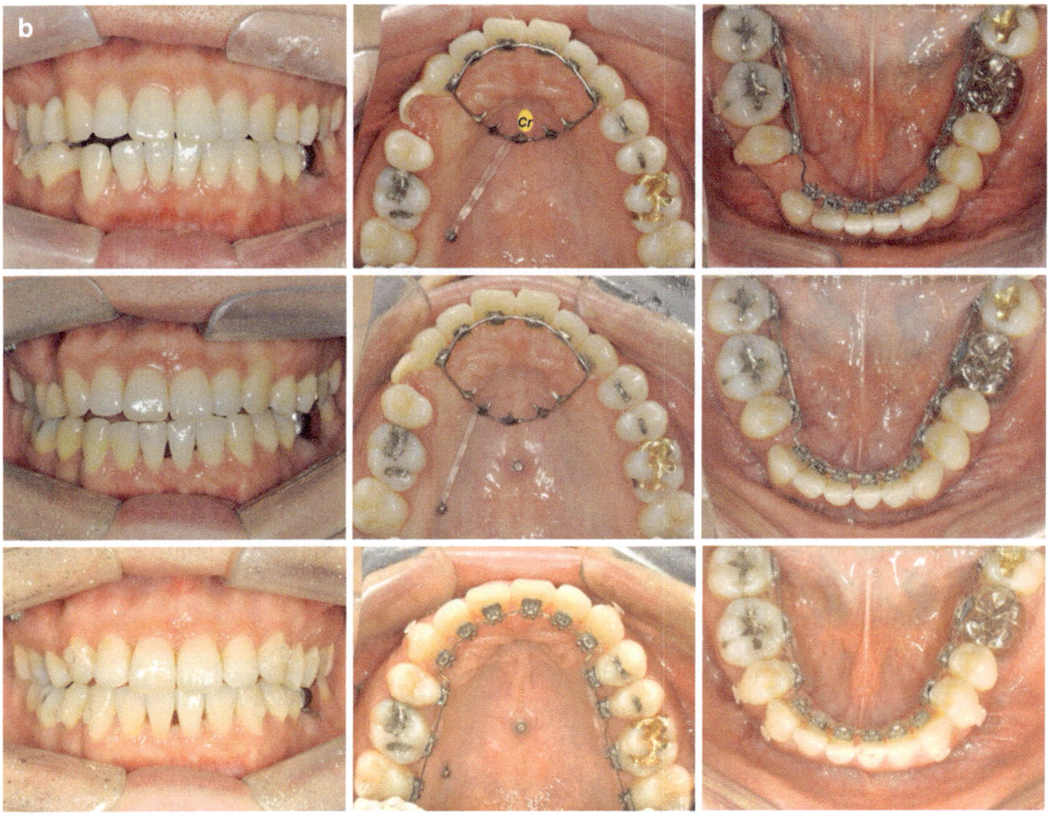

Fig. 10.6 (**b**) Progress records

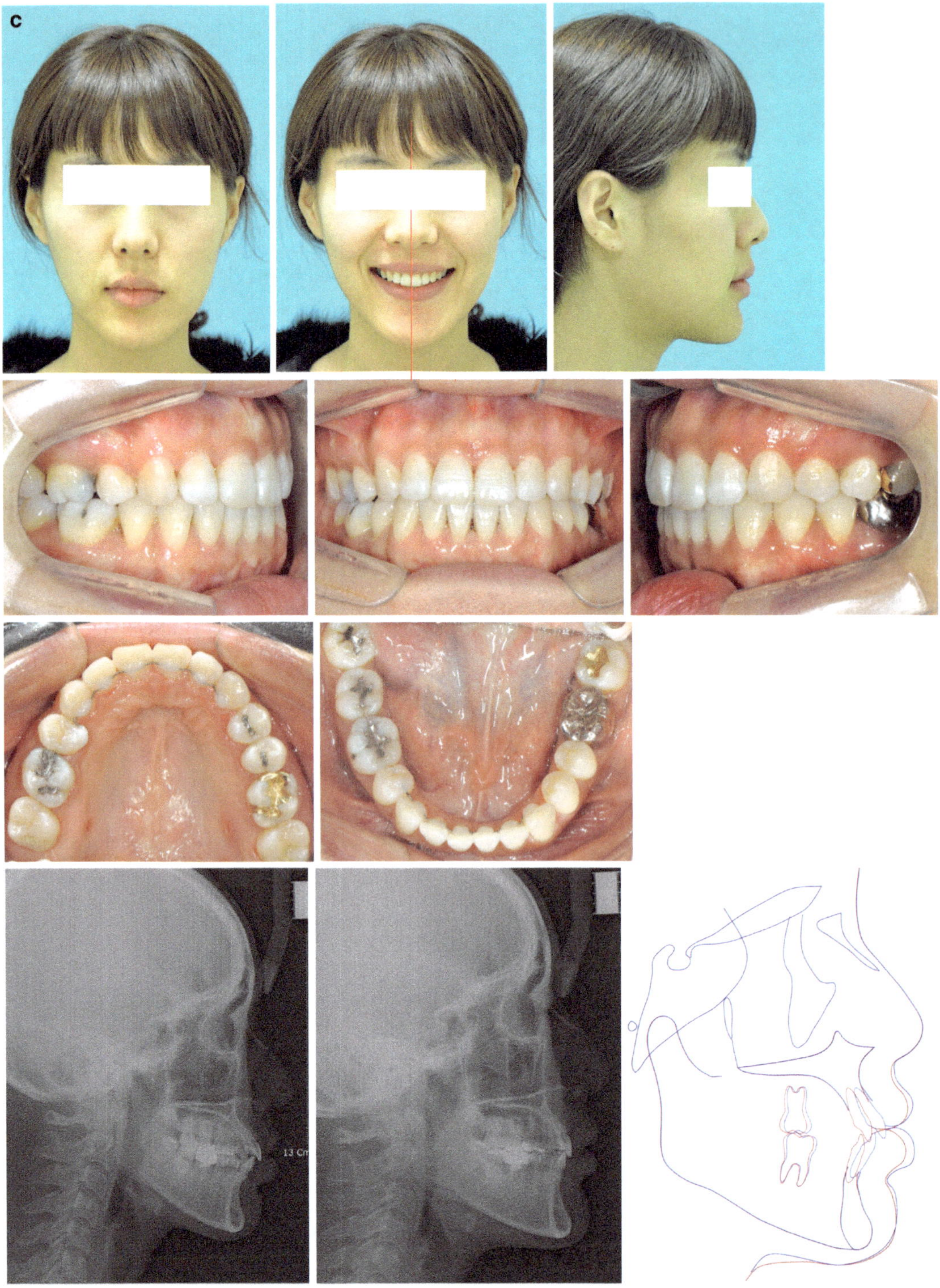

Fig. 10.6 (c) Posttreatment records

Case 2

A 39-year-old male patient was referred from prosthetic department for pre-prosthetic orthodontic treatment of anterior crossbite and poor posterior interdigitation. His initial panoramic view revealed periapical abscess on the maxillary left first molar and mandibular right first and second molars, which were subject to extraction. Mandibular left area had a cantilever crown that was to be removed. Additionally, there was a supernumerary tooth lingual to the maxillary central incisor. Particular attention was given to the generalized alveolar bone loss in the maxillary and mandibular anterior region (Fig. 10.7a).

Initial intraoral photographs were taken at the first visit to orthodontic department after extraction of hopeless teeth and the cantilever crowns. The supernumerary tooth on the lingual side of maxillary incisor was not removed due to the possible risk of alveolar bone loss. Mandibular posterior ridges remained edentulous. Anterior crossbite was not related to any functional shift, indicating a true Class III. Since the patient's main concern was to have the implant work done, he was not considering any radical procedure such as orthognathic surgery. Moreover, he did not want any appliance show on the labial side. Hence, a lingual orthodontic approach was inevitable. His initial cephalometric analysis confirmed the true Class III profile, with ANB −4° and Wits appraisal −11.0 mm.

The main issue in this case was to correct the anterior crossbite and to establish stable posterior occlusion without deteriorating the rest of the teeth displaying serious alveolar bone resorption. Insertion of a continuous archwire would definitely lead to flaring of lower incisors, which would exacerbate the negative overjet. Initial flaring and later retraction of lower incisor may leave significant recession on the labial side, as a result of unnecessary round-tripping. Therefore, preliminary segmental distalization of the mandibular posterior segment prior to lower incisor alignment was considered as safe way. The upper incisor was aligned with some flaring. Since this was minor flaring, the supernumerary tooth was not thought to hinder incisor movement. Hence, the extraction of supernumerary tooth on the lingual side was postponed indefinitely.

In order to facilitate the crossbite correction, bite resin was added on the occlusal table on the premolar segment. Upper incisors were aligned using lingual brackets (Ormco 7th generation) and 014 NiTi archwire. Additional labial-bonded elastic thread was used for rapid correction of the crossbite. In the meantime, a free gingival graft was done for tissue preparation of the implant site on the mandibular left side. A splint wire made of a 019 × 025 stainless steel was bonded to the canine and premolars segment. Miniscrews inserted in the edentulous area were used as anchorage unit for distalization of the posterior segment (Fig. 10.7b).

Following sufficient distalization, brackets were bonded in the mandibular arch as well. Alignment was not done until enough space for the specific tooth was gained. Final alignment and occlusal settling were performed. Brackets were removed after 24 months of active treatment. After treatment, there was no further alveolar bone loss except for the preexisting gingival recession (Fig. 10.7c).

The result of orthodontic treatment and the implants for maxillary left first molar and mandibular molars were maintained for the next 3 years (Fig. 10.7d).

This case demonstrated how miniscrews can be effectively incorporated to perform lingual orthodontic treatment without causing serious bone defects in a periodontally compromised patient, by enabling preliminary segmental distalization.

Case 3

A 38-year-old female patient wanted to correct her lip protrusion and crowding. Initial photographs showed convex profile and severe crowding in the upper anterior region. She also had a severe gummy smile. She had a history of temporomandibular joint disorder and related asymmetric condylar resorption, and as a result, she had significant facial asymmetry and bilateral Class II molar relation and open bite. Mandibular midline was shifted to the left by 3.0 mm. The midline deviation in the mandible was associated

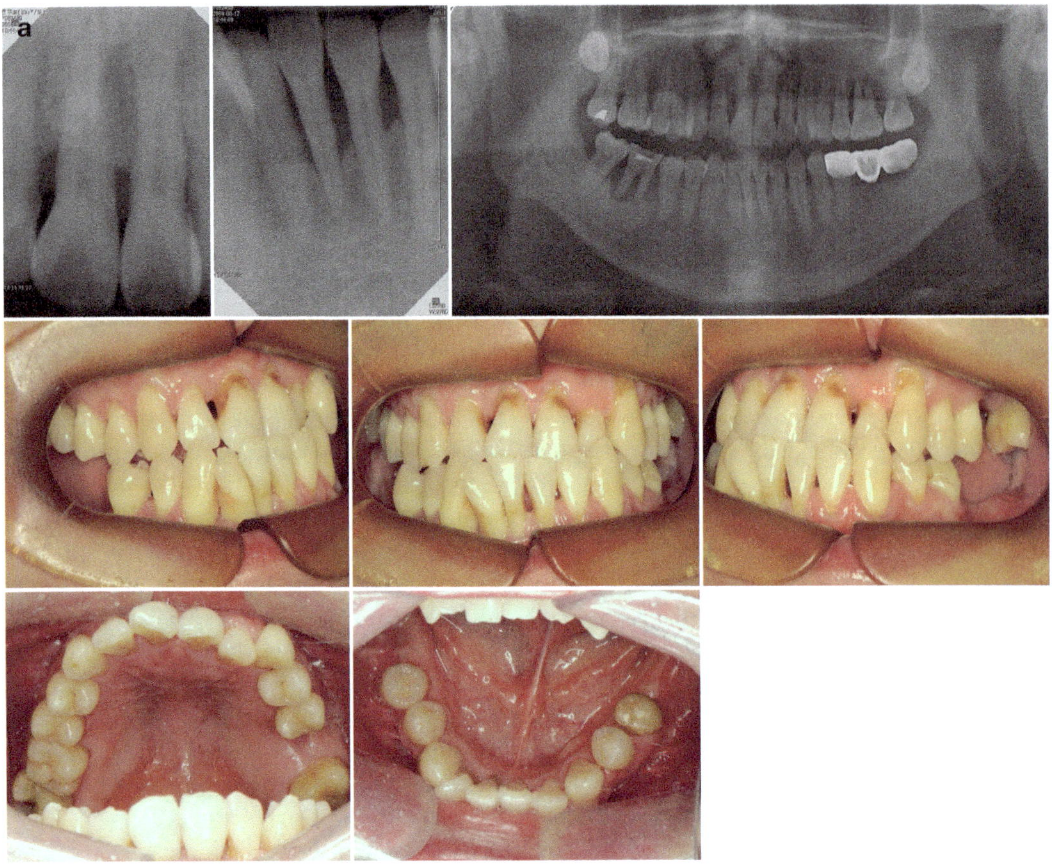

Fig. 10.7 Case 2. (**a**) Pretreatment records

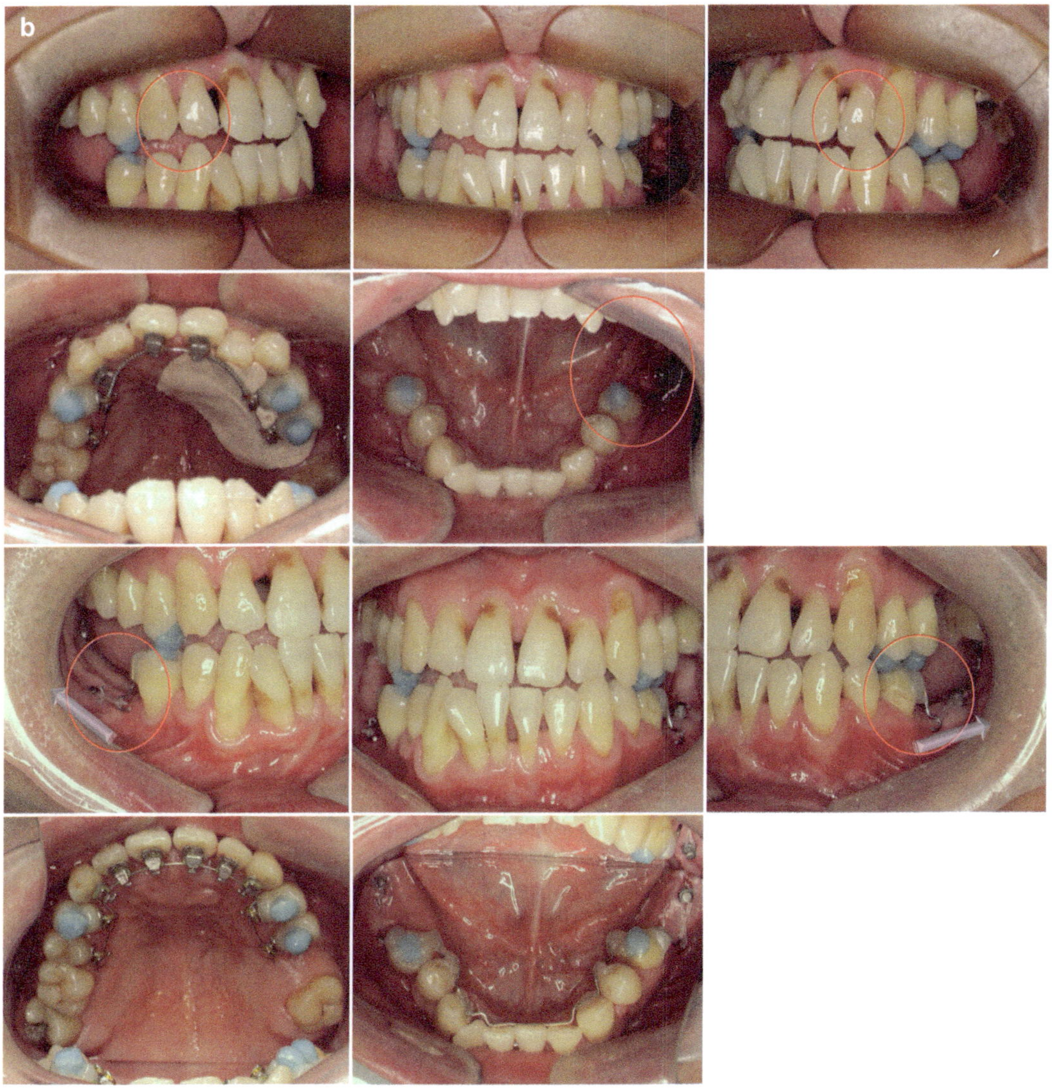

Fig. 10.7 (**b**) Progress records

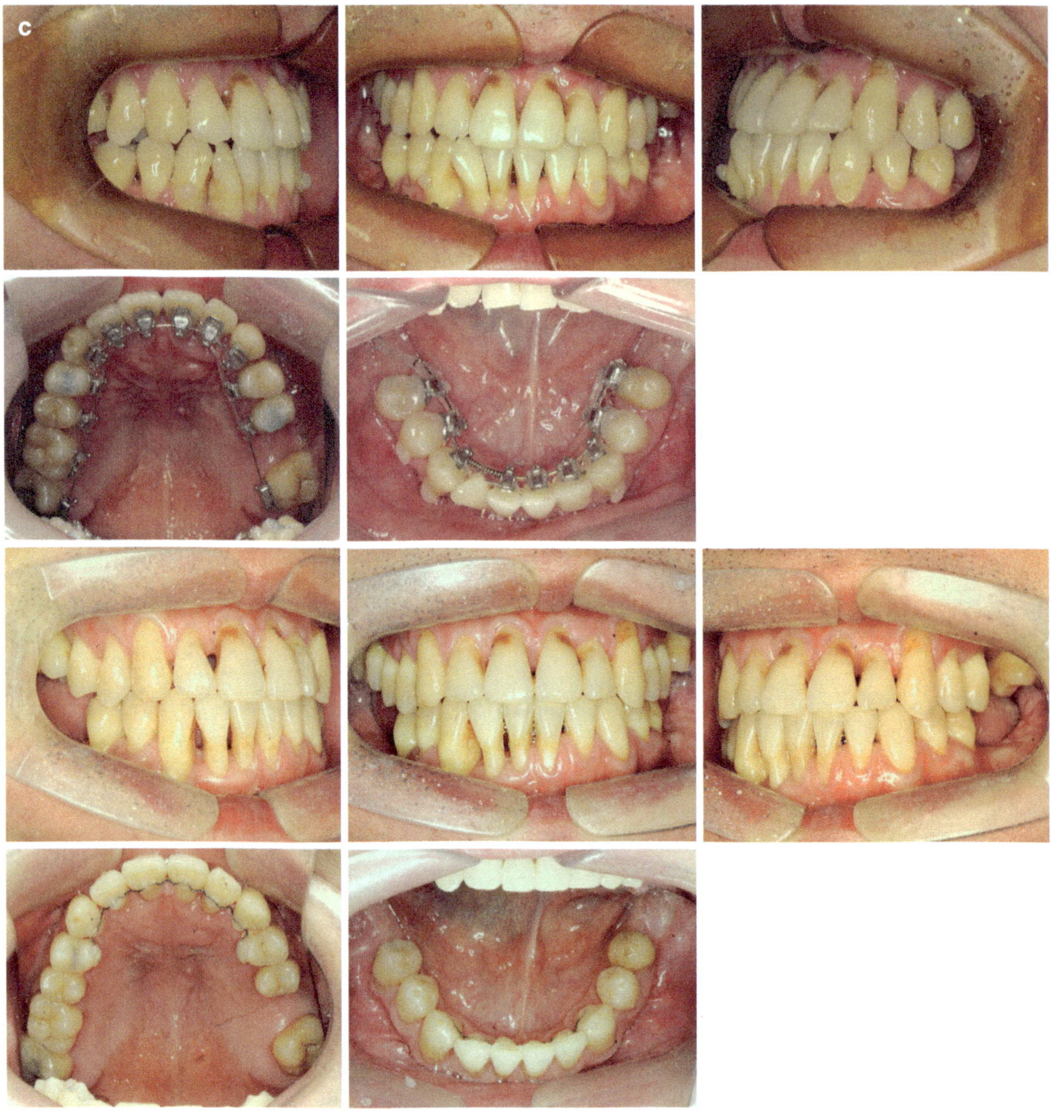

Fig. 10.7 (**c**) Progress records

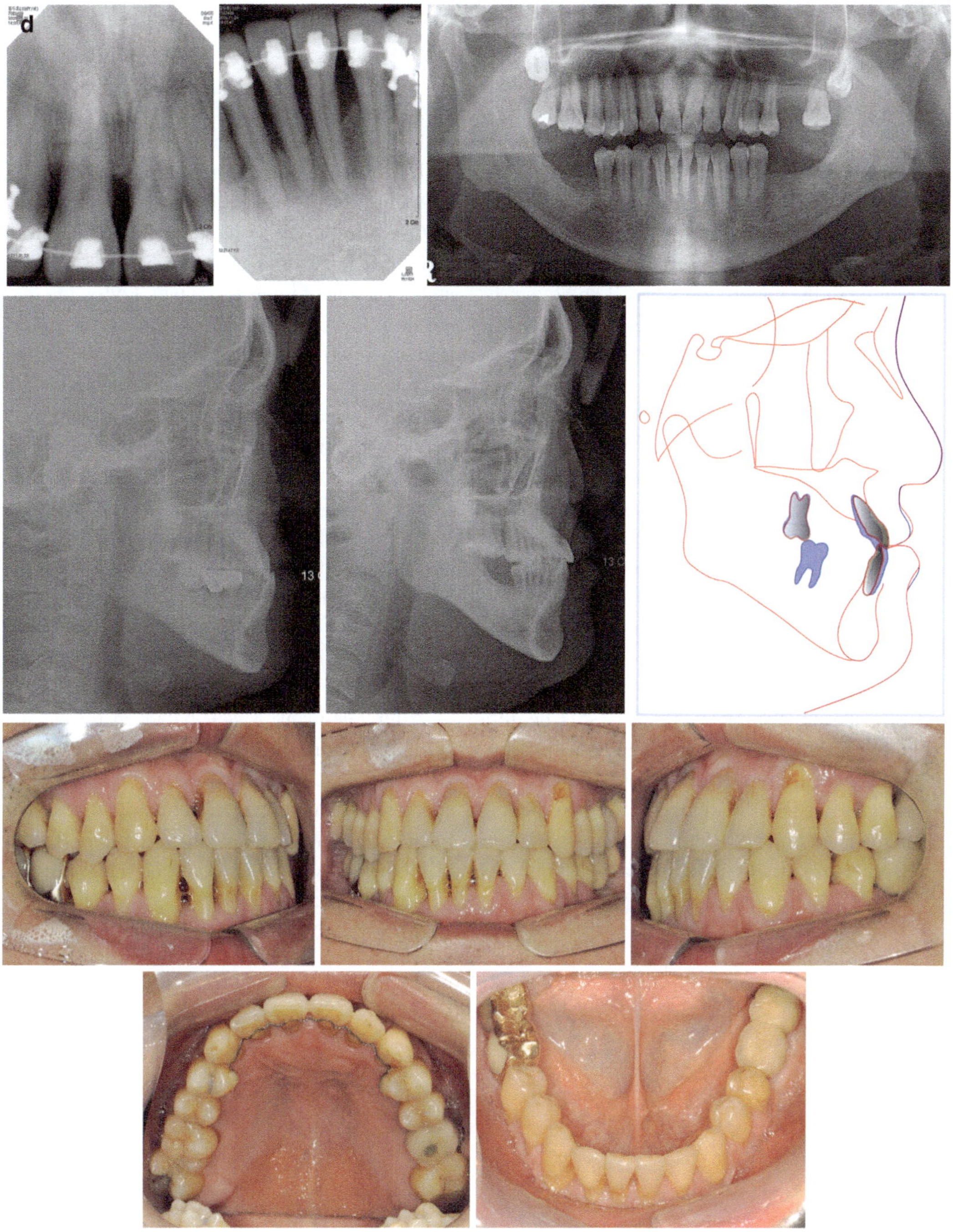

Fig. 10.7 (**d**) Posttreatment records

with previous history of enucleation of odontoma and extraction of impacted mandibular left canine, between the left mandibular lateral incisor and first premolar. However, the apical base midline deviation was not as much as that of the denture midline, indicating tipping of the mandibular incisors to the left side and the possibility of camouflage. Initial molar relation was moderate Class II both sides. Her lip protrusion was attributed to the underlying Class II and hyperdivergent face with ANB angle 8.5° and SN-MP angle 47.7°, which have been caused by the longstanding condylar resorption.

Although her skeletal discrepancy was severe, she did not want to receive surgical procedure. She did not want to show the brace in the upper anterior region, either. It has been shown that the mandibular advancement surgery in patients with previous condylar resorption possibly caused the recurrent condylar resorption [26, 27]. Therefore, the orthognathic surgery was not necessarily the treatment of choice in this present case (Fig. 10.8a).

Considering the open bite, Class II denture relation, and hyperdivergent facial type, an alternative procedure to replace the orthognathic surgery was needed. In order to compensate the retrusive mandible, maximum retraction of upper incisors via extraction of upper bicuspids was necessary. In terms of molar relation, distalization of maxillary molar and maximum anchorage in the mandible were suggested. For the overall facial profile, intrusion of posterior segment was preferred so as to induce autorotation of the mandible. Intrusive retraction of maxillary incisor segment was also essential for the gummy smile.

Overall, this case necessitated maxillary total arch intrusion, distalization of posterior segment, and retraction of incisor segment. Following incisor alignment, a splint lever arm on the palatal side of anteriors was attached. For the incisor retraction and selective intrusion of posterior segment, miniscrews were inserted, respectively, between the first and second molar, both on the buccal and palatal sides, and on the midpalate. Simultaneous intrusive distalization of posterior segment and maximum anterior retraction were performed with the miniscrews as anchor units. Mandibular midline was corrected through the extraction of right first premolar and incisor retraction, using the miniscrew on the buccal interradicular area (Fig. 10.8b).

After treatment, a well balanced profile was achieved as a result of planned total intrusion of maxillary arch, intrusive distalization of posterior segment and maximum retraction of anterior segment, was achieved. Upper and lower denture midline was coincident along the facial midline.

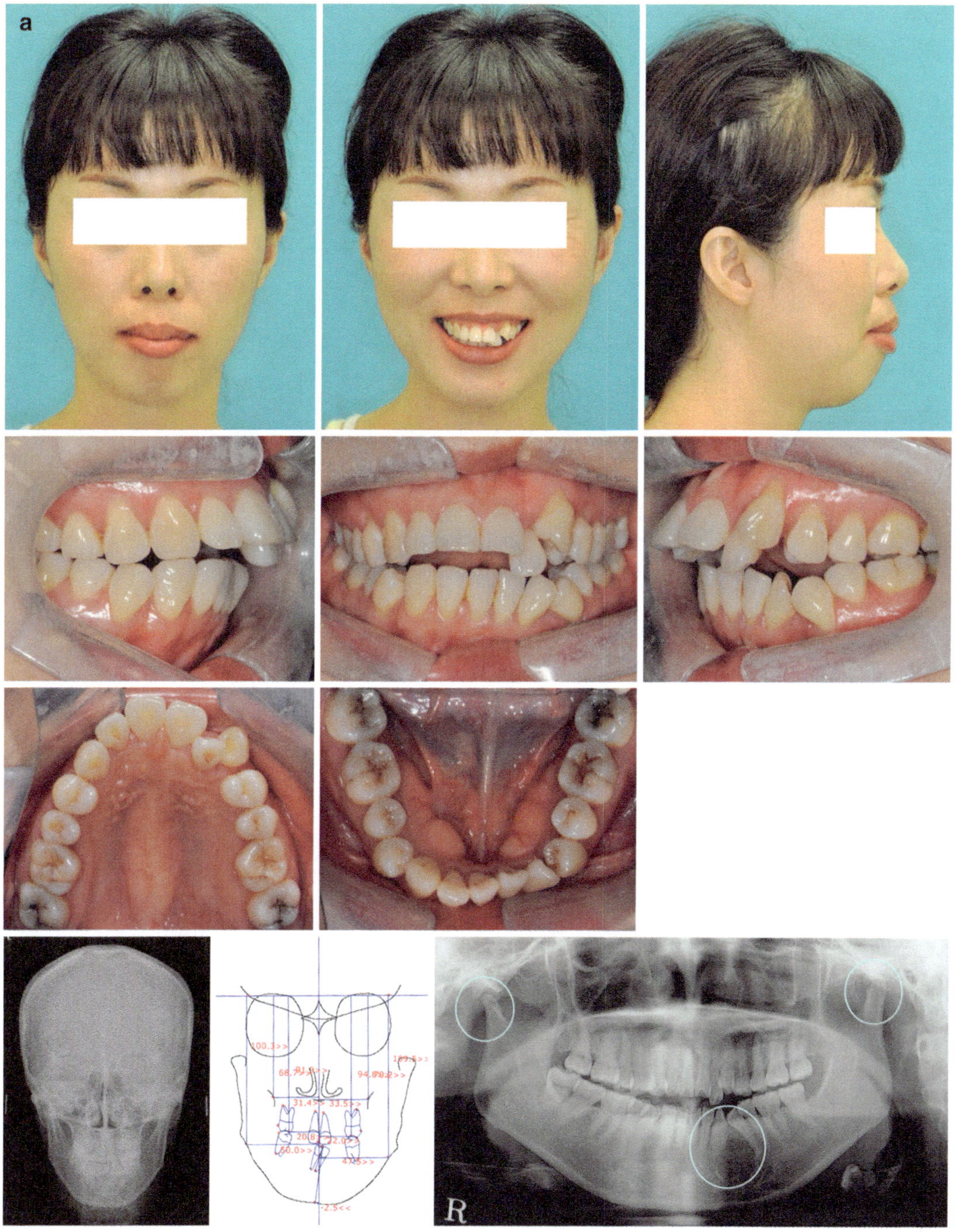

Fig. 10.8 Case 1. (**a**) Pretreatment records

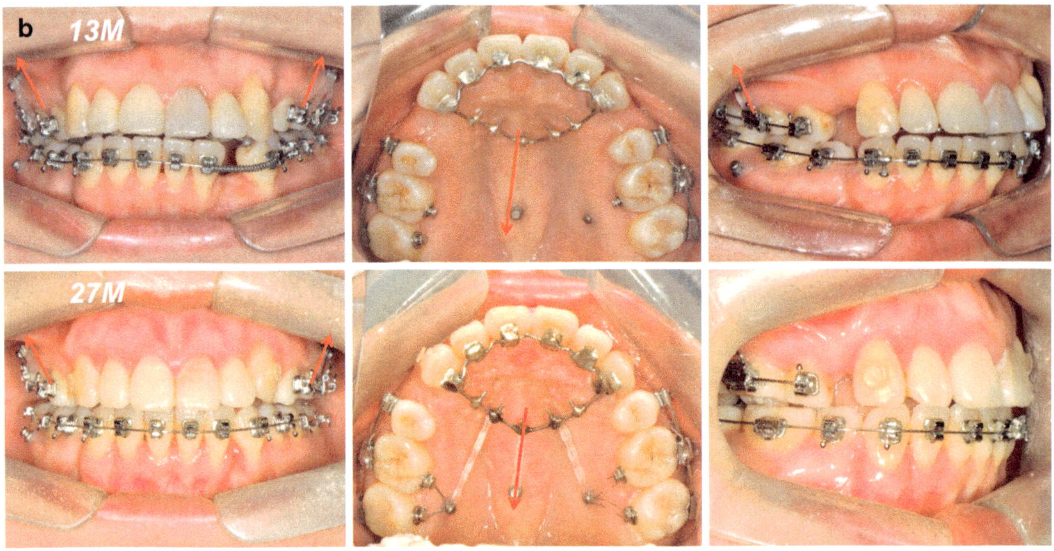

Fig. 10.8 (**b**) Progress records

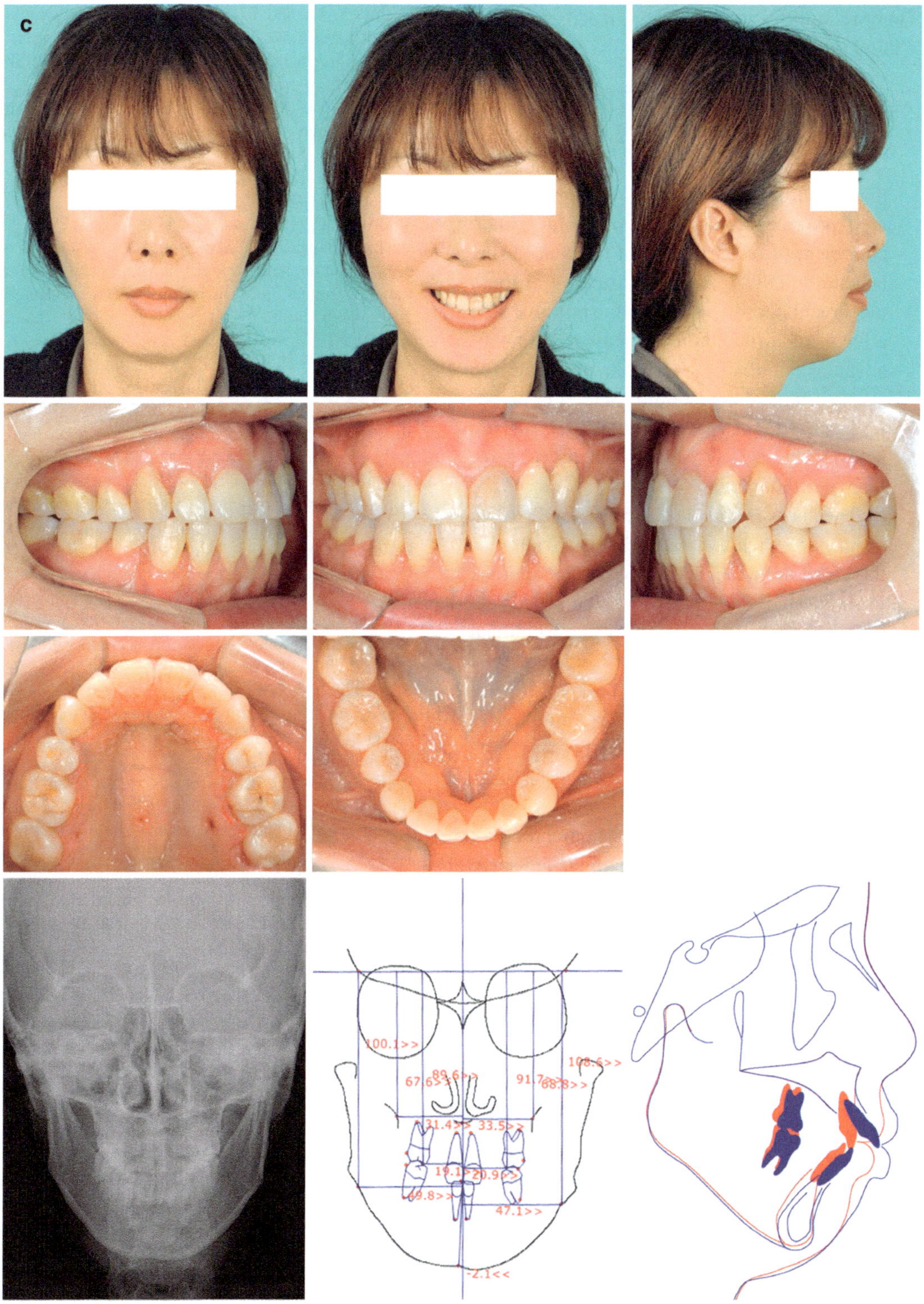

Fig. 10.8 (**c**) Posttreatment records

Gummy smile was nearly eliminated. Bilateral Class I molar relation was attained (Fig. 10.8c).

Conclusion

One of the main strengths of miniscrew implants in the lingual orthodontics may be that it allows segmental movement or total arch movement to one direction, prior to main alignment or redistribution of the space. This helps to minimize the round-tripping of tooth movement in order to reduce the possible side effects of orthodontic treatment. Another advantage is that the one can modulate the point of force application by selecting proper insertion sites. In particular, overall palatal area can be used for miniscrew insertion for lingual orthodontics.

The possibility of "inconsistent" tooth movement, such as total arch distalization or total arch intrusion, is not necessarily an issue in lingual orthodontics. In particular, correction of hyperdivergent case using conventional appliances, such as high-pull headgear, does not appear to be effective so far [28]. In contrast, total arch intrusion using miniscrews within the established alveolar housing may produce significant vertical change. Taken together, lingual orthodontic treatment is indicated mainly in adults, for whom precision movement without round-tripping is indispensible. A modified segmented arch approach combined with miniscrew implants can therefore be a useful concept in lingual orthodontics.

References

1. Salonen L, et al. Need and demand for orthodontic treatment in an adult Swedish population. Eur J Orthod. 1992;14(5):359–68.
2. Hohoff A, et al. Evaluation of the parameters underlying the decision by adult patients to opt for lingual therapy: an international comparison. J Orofac Orthop. 2003;64(2):135–44.
3. Melsen B. Current controversies in orthodontics. 1st ed. Quintessence Publishing Co. Inc, Chicago, Illinois. 1991. p. 147–56.
4. Tanne K, Koenig HA, Burstone CJ. Moment to force ratios and the center of rotation. Am J Orthod Dentofacial Orthop. 1988;94:426–31.
5. Kojima Y, Mizuno T, Fukui H. A numerical simulation of tooth movement produced by molar uprighting spring. Am J Orthod Dentofac Orthop. 2007;132:630–8.
6. Burstone CJ, Koenig HA. Force systems from the ideal arch. Am J Orthod Dentofacial Orthop. 1974;65:270–89.
7. Burstone CJ. Rationale of the segmented arch. Am J Orthod. 1962;48:805–22.
8. Shalish M, Cooper-Kazaz R, Ivgi I, Canetti L, Tsur B, Bachar E, Chaushu S. Adult patients' adjustability to orthodontic appliances. Part I: a comparison between Labial, Lingual, and Invisalign™. Eur J Orthod. 2012;34(6):724-30.
9. Kravitz ND, et al. How well does Invisalign work? A prospective clinical study evaluating the efficacy of tooth movement with invisalign. Am J Orthod Dentofacial Orthop. 2009;135:27–35.
10. Joffe L. Current products and practice, invisalign®: early experiences. J Orthod. 2003;30:348–52.
11. Egolf RJ, BeGole EA, Upshaw HS. Factors associated with orthodontic patient compliance with intraoral elastic and headgear wear. Am J Orthod Dentofacial Orthop. 1990;97(4):336–48.
12. Grauer D, Proffit WR. Accuracy in tooth positioning with a fully customized lingual orthodontic appliance. Am J Orthod Dentofac Orthop. 2011;140:433–43.
13. Mazdyasna S, Stoner JE. Factors influencing gingival recession in the lower incisor region. Proc Br Paedod Soc. 1977;7:15–7.
14. Jeong GM, et al. Finite-element investigation of the center of resistance of the maxillary dentition. Korean J Orthod. 2009;39(2):83–94.
15. Liang W, Rong Q, Xu B. Torque control of the maxillary incisors in lingual and labial orthodontics: a 3-dimensional finite element analysis. Am J Orthod Dentofac Orthop. 2009;135:316–22.
16. Sung SJ, et al. A comparative evaluation of different compensating curves in the lingual and labial techniques using 3D FEM. Am J Orthod Dentofacial Orthop. 2003;123:441–50.
17. Hong RK, Heo JM, Ha YK. Lever-arm and mini-implant system for anterior torque control during retraction in lingual orthodontic treatment. Angle Orthod. 2005;75(1):129–41.
18. Choy K, et al. Effect of root and bone morphology on the stress distribution in the periodontal ligament. Am J Orthod Dentofacial Orthop. 2000;117:98–105.
19. Wehrbein H, et al. The use of palatal implants for orthodontic anchorage. Design and clinical application of the orthosystem. Clin Oral Implants Res. 1996;7(4):410–6.
20. Park YC, et al. Lever-arm mechanics in lingual orthodontics. J Clin Orthod. 2000;34(10):601–5.
21. Kim KH, et al. Finite element analysis of effectiveness of lever arm in lingual sliding mechanics. Korean J Orthod. 2011;41(5):324–36.
22. Lee EH, et al. Three dimensional finite element analysis of continuous and segmented arches with use of orthodontic miniscrews. Korean J Orthod. 2011;41(4):237–54.

23. Lee KJ, et al. Computed tomographic analysis of tooth-bearing alveolar bone for orthodontic miniscrew placement. Am J Orthod Dentofacial Orthop. 2009;135(4):486–94.
24. Fritz U, Ehmer A, Diedrich P. Clinical suitability of titanium microscrews for orthodontic anchorage-preliminary experiences. J Orofac Orthop. 2004;65(5): 410–8.
25. Kuroda S, et al. Skeletal class III oligodontia patient treated with titanium screw anchorage and orthognathic surgery. Am J Orthod Dentofacial Orthop. 2005;127(6):730–8.
26. Arnett GW, Milam SB, Gottesman L. Progressive mandibular retrusion–idiopathic condylar resorption. Part I. Am J Orthod Dentofacial Orthop. 1996;110(1): 8–15.
27. Arnett GW, Milam SB, Gottesman L. Progressive mandibular retrusion-idiopathic condylar resorption. Part II. Am J Orthod Dentofacial Orthop. 1996;110(2): 117–27.
28. Gkantidis N, et al. Treatment strategies for patients with hyperdivergent class II division 1 malocclusion: is vertical dimension affected? Am J Orthod Dentofacial Orthop. 2011;140:346–55.

Pre-orthodontic Orthognathic Surgery (POGS) Using TADs: Evidences and Applications

11

Kee-Joon Lee

Abstract

Conventional protocol for orthodontic treatment followed by orthognathic surgery for skeletal discrepancies is not readily justified, since both procedures cause significant reduction of the overall masticatory function. In order to facilitate the procedure, a pre-orthodontic orthognathic surgery (POGS) has been suggested and practiced. One of the essential factors may be the predictability of postsurgical tooth movement. The miniscrew-type TADs enable not only individual tooth movement but also the movement of segment and total arch. Underlying biomechanical advantages of segmental movement also supports the new protocol. In case of narrow maxillary arch, a miniscrew-assisted rapid palatal expander can be effective for the preliminary transverse correction prior to surgery, which also contributes to the establishment of stable occlusion in short period of time. Therefore, the TADs are regarded indispensible for the POGS procedure.

11.1 Rationale of Presurgical Orthodontics

Conventional wisdom of surgico-orthodontic approach provides one with well-established protocol for the dentofacial deformities that cannot be camouflaged. The presurgical orthodontic treatment followed by orthognathic surgery and postsurgical orthodontic treatment has been the gold standard in conducting combined orthodontic-orthognathic surgery [1]. In order to restructure the dentition as well as the maxillomandibular basal bone, the teeth have to be decompensated prior to surgical jaw movement.

Although it is inarguable that the dental decompensation is an essential procedure for the success of orthognathic surgery, it is not clear whether the decompensation has to be carried out before surgery. The presurgical orthodontic movement has been shown to cause transient depression of the masticatory function in such as the maximum bite force and the lateral excursion, mainly due to the abrupt change in the occlusal relationship [2]. Moreover, the orthognathic surgery induces a reversible atrophy of the major

K.-J. Lee, DDS, PhD
Department of Orthodontics, Yonsei University, Yonsei-ro 50, Seodaemon-gu, Seoul 120-752, South Korea
e-mail: orthojn@yuhs.ac

K.B. Kim (ed.), *Temporary Skeletal Anchorage Devices*,
DOI 10.1007/978-3-642-55052-2_11, © Springer-Verlag Berlin Heidelberg 2014

masticatory muscles such as masseters for about a year, regardless of the surgery type [3, 4]. Therefore, in terms of rehabilitation and restoration of the orofacial muscle function, the presurgical orthodontic treatment followed by an orthognathic surgery may not be justified.

As for the tooth movement, the presurgical orthodontic treatment nearly always requires tooth movement against the existing occlusal interdigitation and/or muscular surroundings. For example, in a typical Class III patient, retraction of upper incisor against the tongue muscle and flaring of the lower incisor against lip muscles can be challenging, since artificial reduction of muscle force or tension can hardly be performed [5].

Considering the previous aspects, it is not easy to find the validity of the presurgical orthodontic treatment except that it provides stable postsurgical occlusion immediately after surgery. In order to minimize the period of reduced masticatory activity, an alternative procedure, POGS (pre-orthodontic orthognathic surgery) can be suggested as long as an adequate treatment protocol is established (Fig. 11.1).

11.2 POGS (Pre-orthodontic Orthognathic Surgery) and Prerequisites for Reliable POGS Procedure

The POGS (pre-orthodontic orthognathic surgery) refers to the orthognathic surgery conducted prior to any orthodontic tooth movement. Although the "surgery-first" approach has been introduced back in 2009 [6], this approach is not an entirely new technique, Epker and Fish stated that surgical procedures should be performed as early as possible in the overall treatment regimen [7, 8], and the strategic postsurgical leveling of the arch has already been proposed elsewhere, especially in hypodivergent cases [9].

An obvious and outstanding advantage of this procedure is that the patient gains a profile change at the initial phase of the treatment. Since the presurgical decompensation makes the profile even worse, the POGS effectively eliminates this phase. Other possible advantages such as reduction of treatment time via utilization of the so-called regional acceleration phenomenon are not proven yet [10, 11]. The regional acceleration

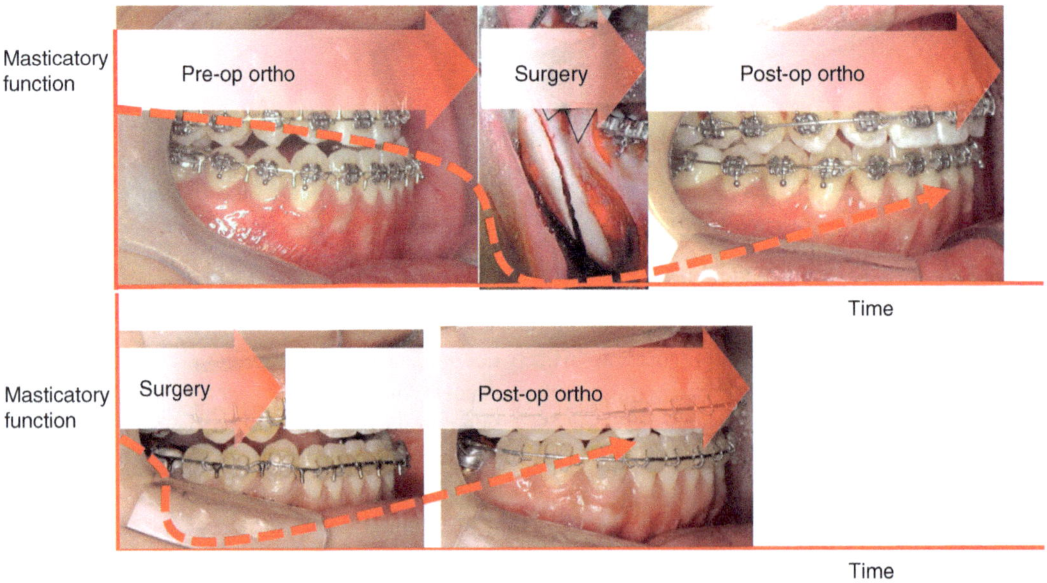

Fig. 11.1 Estimated change in the overall masticatory function according to each procedure

originally refers to local bone formation confined to the fracture area for just a few weeks and does not necessarily apply to the remote areas [12]. For example, there is no evidence yet that the osteotomy site for maxillomandibular surgery would affect the bone turnover in the alveolar area. The extent and duration of the regional acceleration related to surgical trauma needs to be explained more empirically. In contrast, unstable postsurgical occlusion and unpredictable surgical stability may hinder orthodontic occlusal structuring and extend the treatment time.

Overall, it does not mean an orthognathic surgery without the need of any orthodontic intervention. It is simply the procedure where orthodontic decompensation is conducted after surgery, for which the following are crucial (Fig. 11.2):

1. Appropriate assessment of the soft tissue with special regard to the midline
   For the POGS procedure, the presurgical treatment period becomes minimal, and the required assessment has to be made beforehand to minimize the possible errors. In particular, evaluation of the facial (soft tissue) midline is the most important. The soft tissue structure can be affected by not only the underlying hard tissue but also its counterparts. For example, the upper philtrum line can be affected by mandibular movement and the movement of the lower incisor may displace the upper lip position. Therefore, a careful presurgical assessment is a must.
2. Adequate prediction of postsurgical decompensation

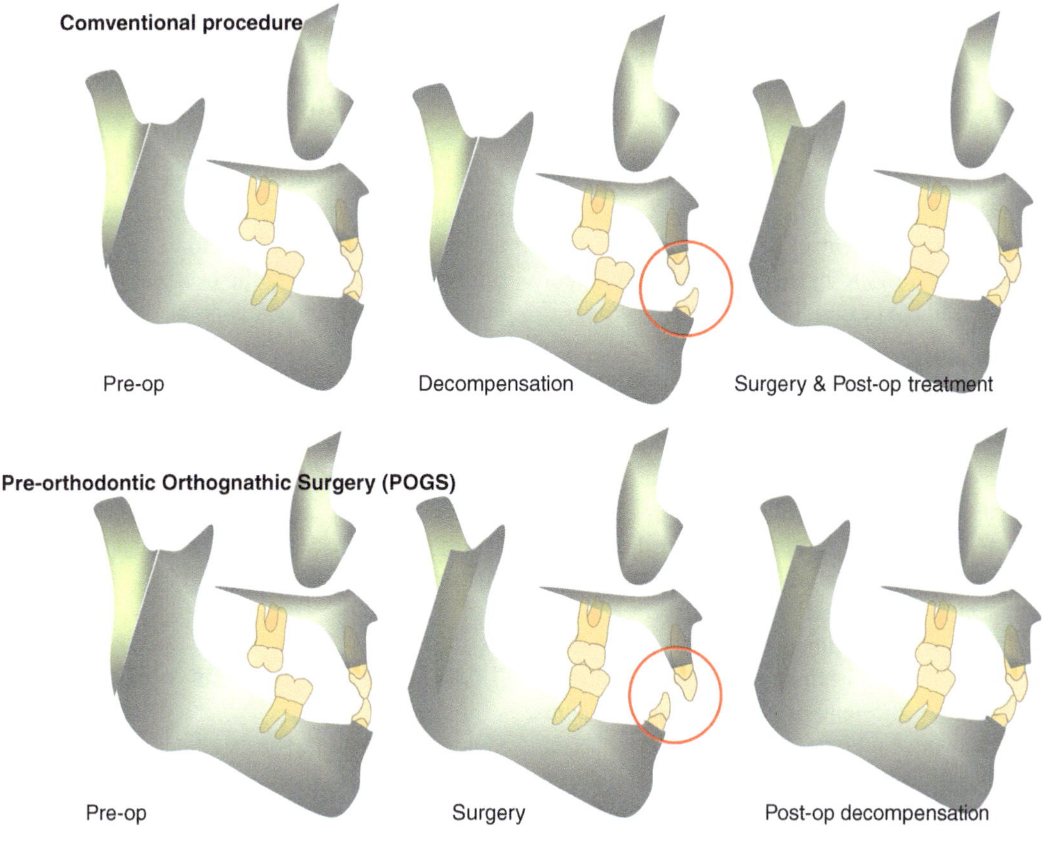

Fig. 11.2 Dental decompensation in conventional vs POGS protocol

It is not easy to precisely anticipate the pattern or amount to tooth movement. First, it is important to define the segment that has to be moved and the one that should not. Once the diagnosis is made adequately, application of miniscrews can minimize the errors by securing the anchorage segment. Previous information on the amount of possible tooth movement may help treatment planning, which will be explained further in this chapter.

3. Appropriate surgical procedure that does not cause significant postsurgical relapse or change of basal bone
A majority of the POGS cases inevitably exhibit very unstable postsurgical occlusion. Reliable and accurate surgical movement is essential. Moreover, the key factor for a reliable surgical procedure is to secure the stability of bone segment after relocation. Unfortunately, orthognathic surgery is subject to a certain degree of relapse which can hardly be anticipated before surgery [13, 14]. It is not easy to point an appropriate surgical procedure for POGS. The two known procedures for mandibular surgery, SSRO and IVRO, differ in the attachment of the pterygomasseteric sling after surgery, i.e., at the proximal segment in SSRO and at the distal segment in IVRO [15]. Therefore, the operator needs to be careful in handling the respective segment. In SSRO, the main concern of the orthodontists is the position of the proximal segment, which could affect the jaw position. Unexpected condylar dislocation or resorption following SSRO can be detrimental [16]. In contrast, elongation or extension of the pterygomasseteric sling in IVRO can lead to significant relapse of the distal segment after Class III surgery. By freeing the proximal jaw segment without rigid fixation, the IVRO has been shown to be effective in reducing the temporomandibular symptoms following surgery [17]. If one is not convinced by the condylar positioning during surgery, the IVRO may be a reliable alternative for POGS. Under any circumstances, precision relocation of the bone segments and stabilization are crucial, and the surgeon and orthodontist should closely collaborate to minimize or eliminate the possible surgical relapse (Fig. 11.3).
4. Predictable tooth movement regardless of patients' compliance
Following the surgery, the ability to move the teeth according to the plan is important. In view of the biomechanics, definition of the anchorage segment and moving segment is the key. Then the orthodontic movement is carried out according to the plan. Instead of inserting a continuous arch from the initial stage, planned movement of a specific segment or a target tooth greatly helps to minimize the unexpected tooth movement, named as round tripping. Another factor is the patients' compliance. Since the compliance for such as intermaxillary elastics is always very unpredictable, it is better advised to use intra-arch mechanics. For this, the incorporation of miniscrews will significantly increase the success of POGS.

11.3 Characteristics of Surgery Occlusion in POGS

In most non-orthodontic patients with maxillomandibular skeletal discrepancies, the dental arches are not leveled. Therefore, it is natural that the irregularities along the occlusal plane would lead to occlusal interference at certain point(s) when surgical jaw relocation was conducted. Although the initial surgical occlusion may be extremely unstable, the muscle tension is not strong enough to cause skeletal relapse immediately after surgery. Hence, timely management of the occlusion is crucial in order to establish a stable occlusion during the initial phase of the postsurgical period.

11.4 The Role of TADs in POGS

Considering that the postsurgical occlusion after POGS, in most cases, presents intermaxillary interference at some point(s) due to the lack of presurgical orthodontic treatment, early settlement of the occlusion is crucial. However, unlike in the conventional orthognathic surgery cases, use of intermaxillary elastics is strongly avoided

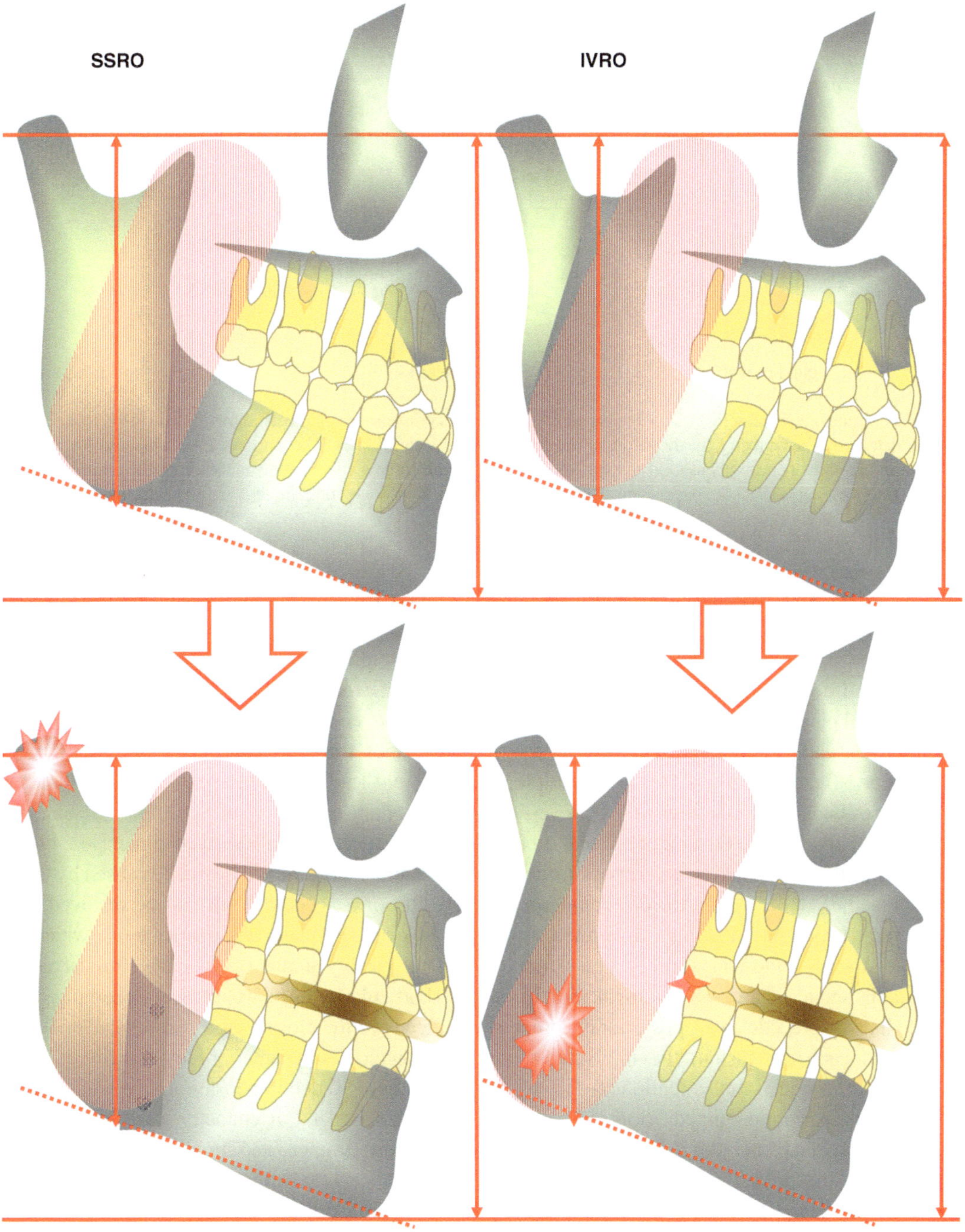

Fig. 11.3 Pattern of relocation of bone segments in SSRO and IVRO and respective attachment of pterygomasseteric sling

because the traction force may induce displacement of the proximal or distal segment of the surgically relocated maxillomandibular bones. Stable jaw position is essential for reliable POGS procedure. Therefore, instead of intermaxillary orthodontic mechanics, intra-arch mechanics is preferred for the decompensation of the denture, for which interradicular miniscrews can be very helpful since they do not require tooth anchorage (Fig. 11.4).

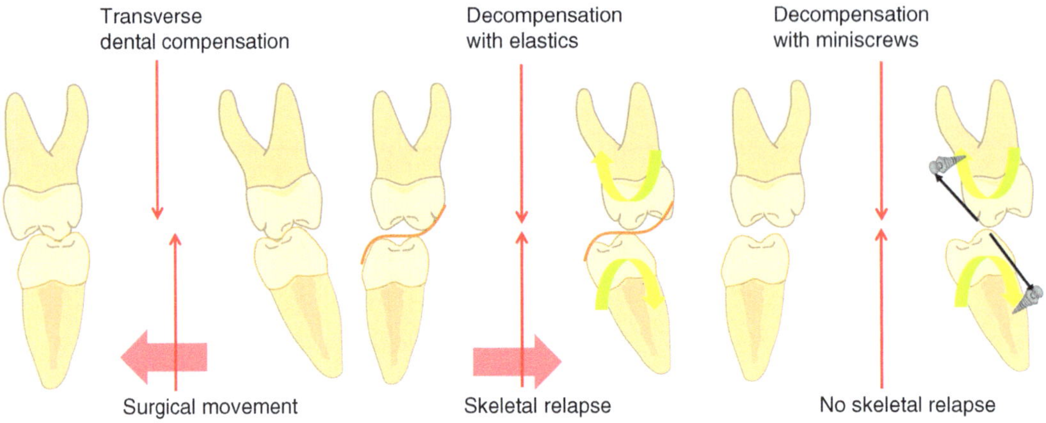

Fig. 11.4 Immediately after POGS, the occlusion is largely unstable. In case of asymmetry, the directions of the surgical relapse and the denture decompensation are opposite to each other. Intermaxillary elastics used for the transverse decompensation of the denture may lead to the relapse of the relocated bones. The transverse decompensation must be done without affecting the underlying bone using an anchorage device targeting the segment to be decompensated

11.5 Postsurgical Decompensation

Postsurgical decompensation is carried out in all three spatial planes – anteroposterior, vertical, and transverse – and it is known that a change in one dimension affects the others [1]. For example, a transverse change would influence overall vertical dimension, and a hinge closure of the mandibular body will affect the relative anteroposterior relation of the upper and lower counterparts. Therefore, it is advised to plan a stepwise orthodontic strategy following surgery. For example, an establishment of a desired vertical dimension would have to precede anteroposterior decompensation. In each dimension, the miniscrews are indicated at "inconsistent" situations (Fig. 11.5):

1. Anteroposterior decompensation
   On the sagittal plane, on a given basal bone relationship, the posterior and anterior segments may be moved to the opposite direction by reciprocal action. Alternatively, when the posterior and anterior segments have to move in the same direction, additional skeletal anchorage devices would be necessary, for which miniscrews are indicated and intermaxillary elastics are contraindicated as has been explained.
2. Vertical decompensation
   Vertical decompensation can be performed either by extrusive or intrusive measures [1]. Either Class II or Class III hypodivergent face with deep curve of Spee and deep overbite tends to leave excessive intermaxillary space between the anterior and posterior occlusal contacts, following the relocation of jawbones. According to the conventional guideline, intermaxillary elastics worn along the path of hinge closure would lead to selective extrusion of premolars and flatten the curve of Spee without deterioration of the overall vertical dimension [9]. In contrast, generalized open bite caused by extrusion of a specific tooth can be resolved by a selective intrusion of the target tooth, which can be easily attained by using miniscrew(s). Particularly, intrusive vertical decompensation leads to the closure of a mandibular body and reduction of the anterior facial height.
3. Transverse decompensation
   Many skeletal asymmetry cases have transversely compensated molars, which have to be decompensated after surgery [18]. When there is a transverse issue, one has to preliminarily define whether the problem is a relative or an absolute maxillary deficiency [1, 19]. Transverse decompensation without an absolute maxillary deficiency can be easily resolved with the use of miniscrews. In case of absolute maxillary deficiency, however, expansion of the basal bone with an appropriate device or a procedure should precede the next step, since the transverse dimension is not easy to correct and it affects both vertical and anteroposterior dimension [20, 21].

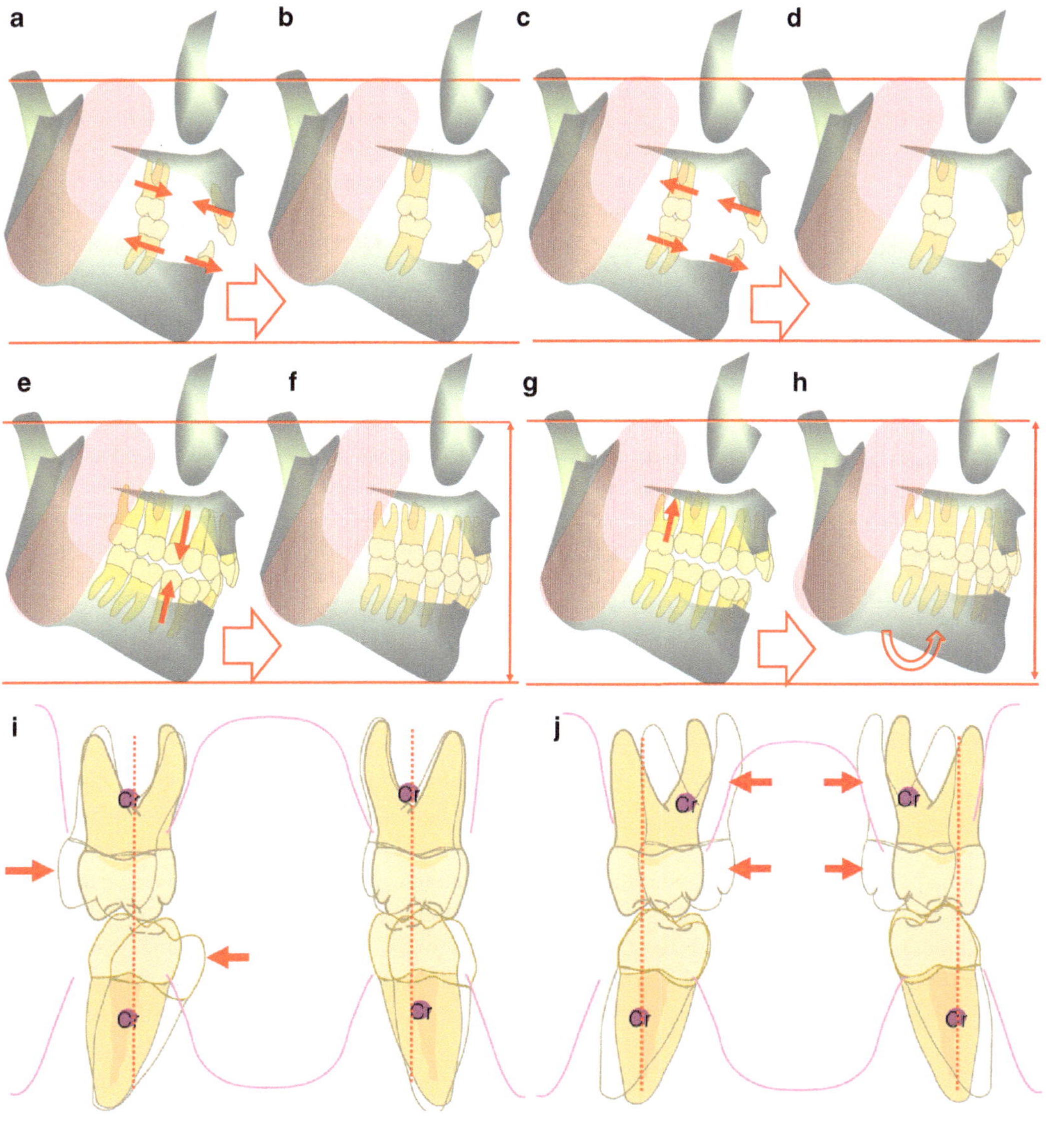

Fig. 11.5 Decompensation strategies and indication for miniscrews. (**a**, **b**) AP decompensation via reciprocal movement – miniscrews are not indicated, (**c**, **d**) AP decompensation via total arch movement – miniscrews are indicated. (**e**, **f**) Vertical decompensation via extrusion – miniscrews are not indicated. (**g**, **h**) Vertical decompensation via selective intrusion – miniscrews are indicated. (**i**) Transverse decompensation without absolute transverse deficiency – miniscrews are indicated, (**j**) Transverse decompensation with absolute transverse deficiency – transverse issue has to be resolved via surgical or nonsurgical measures, including miniscrew-assisted RPE

11.6 Useful Mechanics for Predictable Tooth Movement

Since the interradicular miniscrews and elastic chains introduce relatively constant intrusive force vector(s) [22], intrusive mechanics for effective intrusion of extruded tooth or teeth is necessary. The monocortical miniscrew-type TADs are used for the following purposes:

1. Single tooth intrusion

   In many of the skeletal Class III patients, the maxillary second molars tend to be extruded due to the lack of occlusal contact with their mandibular counterpart. In particular, a

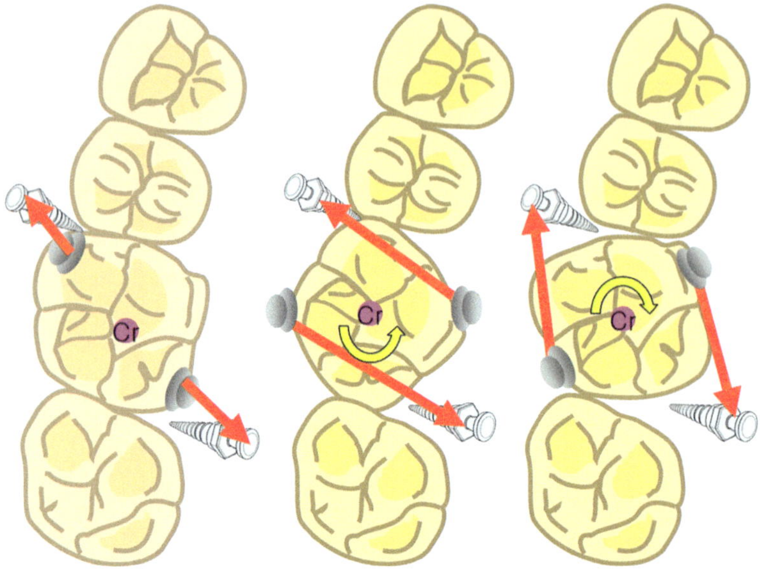

Fig. 11.6 Depending on the position of the miniscrew and the attachment on the tooth, various combination of tooth movement may be resulted. Intrusion, mesial, or distal tipping and/or rotation can be possible

prominent palatal cusp may hinder adequate interdigitation between the surgically relocated jaw segments. In terms of occlusal settling, selective intrusion of the extruded tooth or cusp can be more efficient than the overall extrusion of the rest teeth in the arch. Either a palatal or buccal interradicular miniscrew would induce rotational intrusion of the target tooth. In order to induce pure intrusion along the vertical axis of the tooth, bilateral miniscrews are helpful (Fig. 11.6).

2. Buccolingual tipping of a single tooth
   Transverse compensation of the dental arch is commonplace especially in the skeletal asymmetry, with typical buccal inclination of the maxillary posterior segment and lingual inclination of the mandibular segment and vice versa, in the respective deviated side of the chin point and the opposite side. This uneven inclination of the buccal segment results in unilateral contact occlusion after POGS procedure, for which early transverse decompensation without causing shifting the basal bone is crucial. The surgery occlusion is established with unequal buccal overjet between the deviated and opposite side, and the immediate decompensation is conducted using either palatal interradicular miniscrew(s) in the maxilla and/or buccal interradicular miniscrews in the mandible at the initially deviated side.

Case 1

A 20-year-old male presented with facial asymmetry. Initial extraoral view revealed severe facial asymmetry caused by mandibular deviation. In the intraoral view, the mandibular denture midline was deviated to the left by 7.5 mm (Fig. 11.7a).

Following the diagnosis, a two-jaw orthognathic surgery, including posterior rotation of the maxilla, was planned. Due to the underlying transverse deviation and related dental compensation, the surgery occlusion was finally established with greater buccal overjet on the left side. The extruded maxillary right second molar was thought to be a major interference; hence, the replacement of the second molar using the impacted third molar was chosen. Interradicular miniscrews were inserted before surgery on the palatal slope of the maxillary left side, between the first and second premolars and between the first and second molars, respectively (Fig. 11.7b).

Four weeks after surgery, immediate transverse decompensation was performed to secure a stable bilateral occlusal contact. The treatment was finished in 12 months, with proper eruption of the maxillary right third molar in place. The patient obtained balanced and a symmetric face after the treatment (Fig. 11.7c).

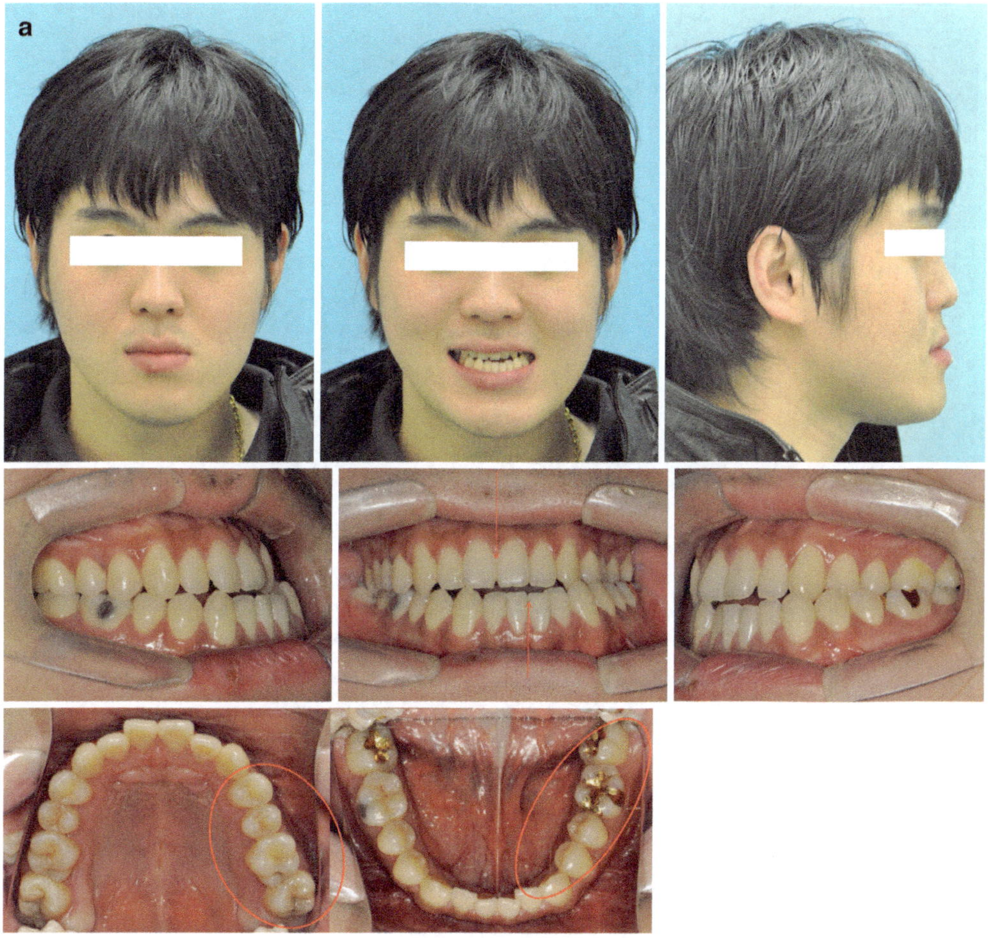

Fig. 11.7 Case 1. (**a**) Pretreatment records. (**b**) Progress records. (**c**) Posttreatment records

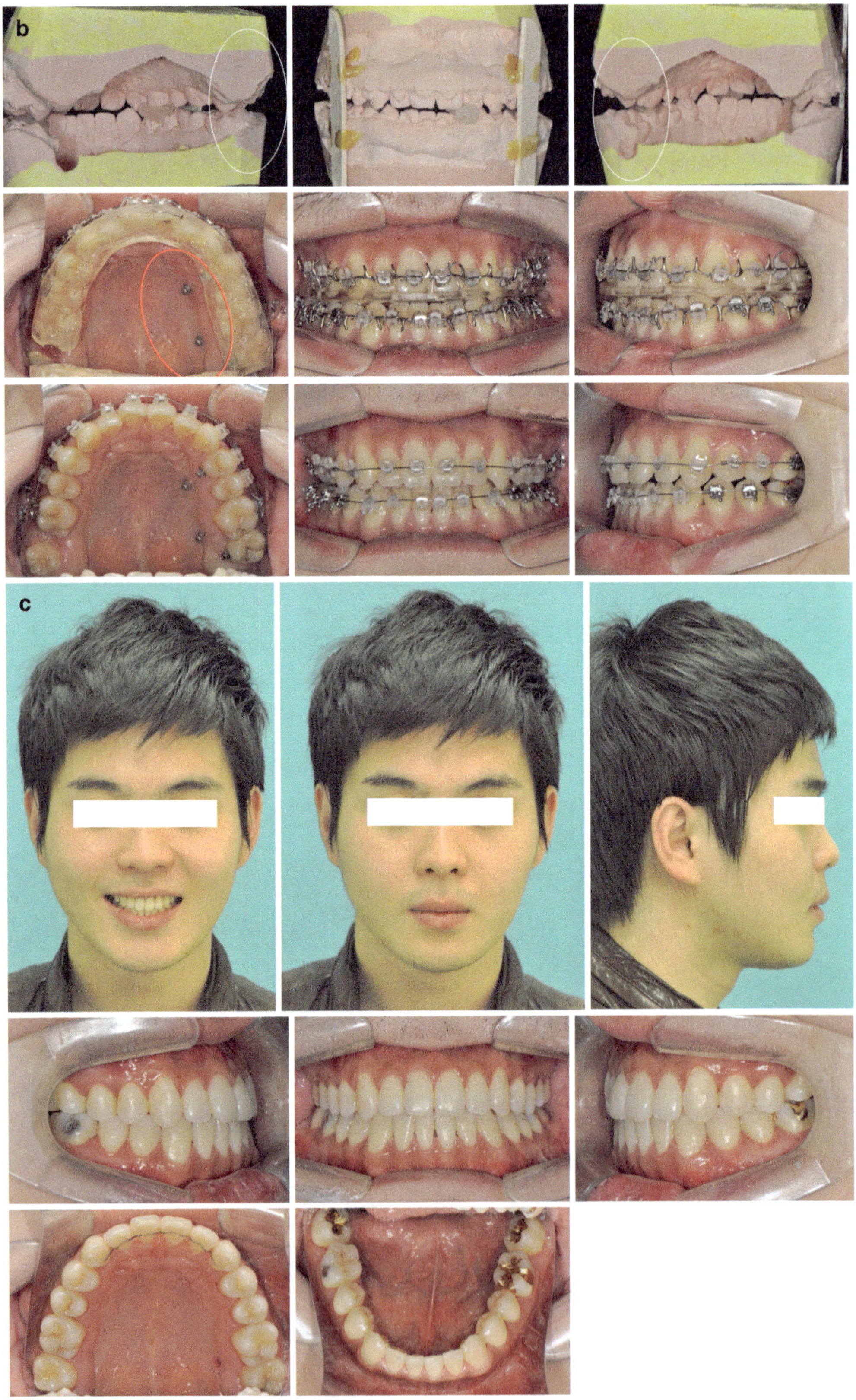

Fig. 11.7 (continued)

3. Segmental distalization
   In the majority of the surgery cases, the amount of crowding is not necessarily symmetric between the right and left sides, which calls for differential movement at each side. If the amount of crowding was not severe, selective distalization of the posterior segment would enable the alignment of the anterior teeth without jeopardizing the denture midline. Interradicular miniscrews on the buccal side effectively distalize the posterior segment by 2–3 mm without significant rotation or tipping of the segment [23]. A segmented arch extending from the second molar to the first premolar can be used for this type of movement, and the incisors are not aligned until sufficient molar relation is attained. This way, one can still use the denture midline as the reference for the basal bone position and the early detection of surgical relapse. Once the jaw relationship is established, the alignment can be complete using a regular leveling wire. The reason why miniscrews are essential is because they do not cause burning anchorage for the distalization of molars. Interradicular miniscrews either on the buccal or palatal side are more useful than the midpalatal miniscrew(s) because they do not require an additional connecting structure. The elastic chains are strained between the miniscrew head and the archwire hooks.
   In order to facilitate the molar distalization in the maxilla, one may choose to extract the upper second molar allowing substitution with the third molar (Fig. 11.8).
4. Anterior retraction
   The "decompensation" of the incisors indicates retraction of the upper incisors and flaring of the lower incisors in Class III surgical patients and vice versa in Class II patients. Premolar extraction is often chosen to effectively retract upper incisors in the conventional surgico-orthodontic procedures. In POGS cases, the anteroposterior decompensation has to be performed without causing significant displacement of relocated bones. Hence, the use of intermaxillary elastics is largely contraindicated, and adequate movement should take place using some anchorage devices within each arch. Based on our previous clinical trials, the anteroposterior movement of the incisors using miniscrews following extraction of premolars is a function of the position of the interradicular miniscrews in terms of anteroposterior and vertical displacement. Interradicular miniscrews placed between the second premolar and the first molar induced maximum retraction of the upper incisors without a significant vertical change in the incisal edge, while miniscrews between the first and second premolars introduced a more significant intrusion of incisors as well as retraction. The axis change before and after retraction was related to the bracket-wire play, leading to an average of 10 ° of reduction of incisor angles during retraction [22]. Those can be used to establish a reliable surgery occlusion and to estimate the amount and pattern of orthodontic tooth movement in cases involving premolar extraction.
5. Total arch movement
   It has been shown that not only the posterior segment but also the anterior segment can be distalized simultaneously, which can be referred to as the "total arch movement" [25, 26]. This notion is clinically meaningful because the total arch movement can be effectively applied to some borderline cases between extraction and nonextraction. It appears that the amount and pattern of displacement may differ depending on the number and position of the miniscrews and dual miniscrews induced significantly greater distalization of the arch, i.e., 2.91 mm at the first molar and 2.41 mm at the incisor, than those of a single miniscrew [22]. This intra-arch movement can be used for the correction of generalized Class II or Class III relationship after surgery. It can also be useful to resolve some unexpected movement or shift of the basal bone as a result of surgical relapse (Fig. 11.9).

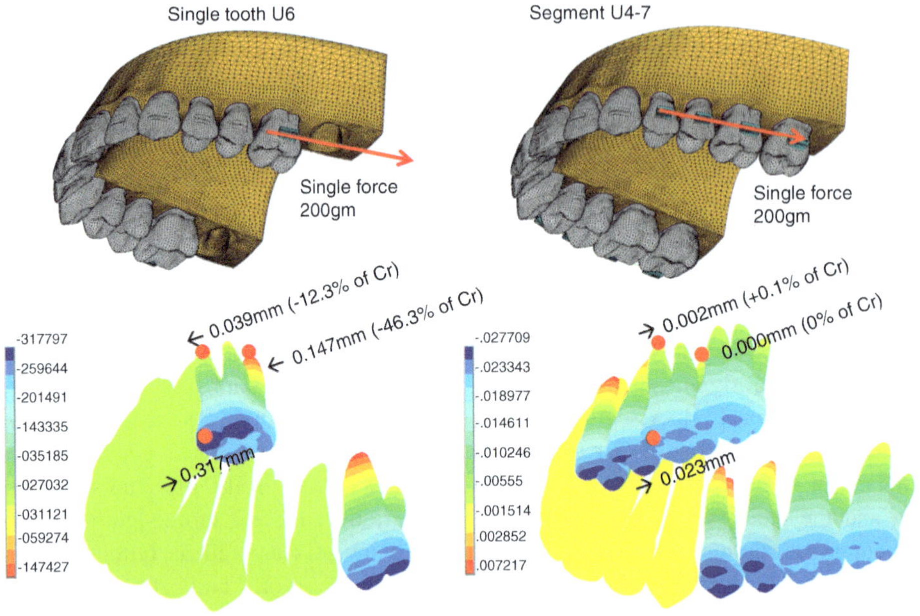

Fig. 11.8 A three-dimensional simulation using finite elements shows that a single tooth distalization using a single line of force causes significant rotation of the molar. Instead, segmentation of the posterior segment reduces the rotational effect due to the configuration of the target segment. An anteroposteriorly long segment would exhibit greater resistance to tipping in response to a single distalizing force due to the greater s2 value [24]

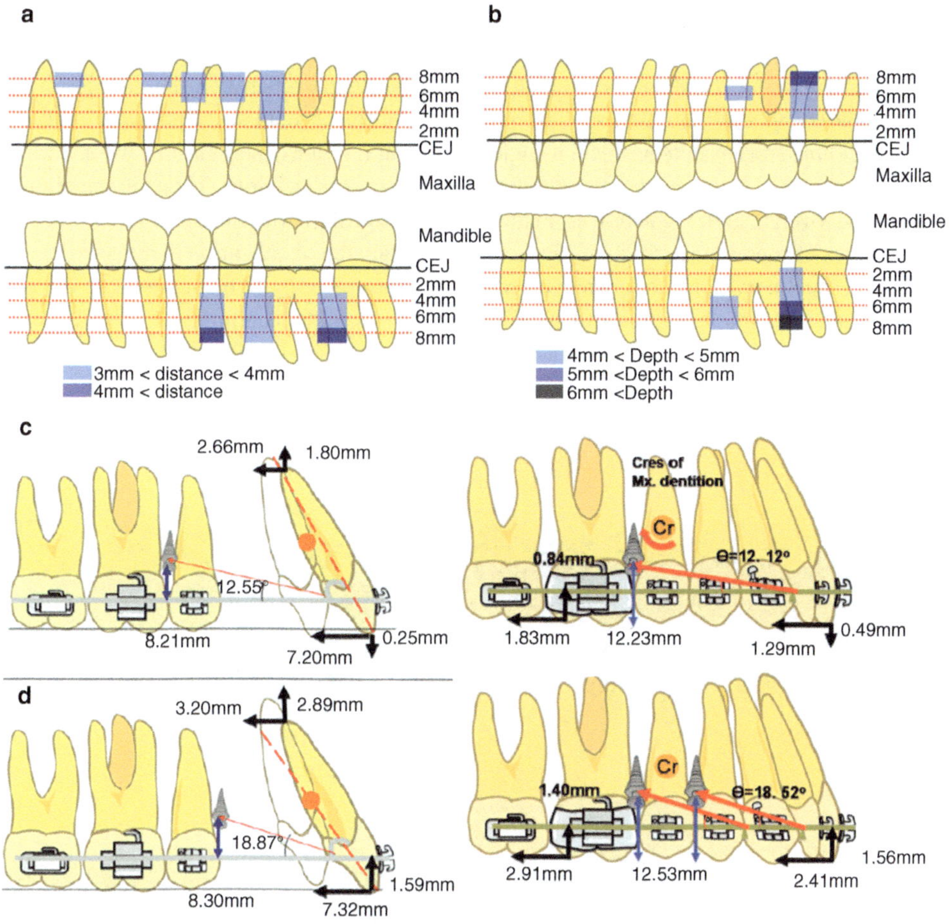

Fig. 11.9 Insertion sites in the maxillary and mandibular buccal interradicular region display sufficient space [27]. Possible amount of displacement of anterior segment and total arch depending on the position and number of interradicular miniscrews [22, 26]. (**a**) Areas with interradicular space greater than 3 mm. (**b**) Areas with safety depth greater than 4 mm. (**c**) Single miniscrew: distalization and rotation. (**d**) Dual miniscrews: distalization and intrusion

Case 2

A 28-year-old female patient visited the orthodontic department with a chief complaint of mandibular prognathism. Initially she had a severely protrusive mandible and an acute nasolabial angle. An intraoral view showed the overall crossbite along with the overall arch, which was mainly caused by a severe anteroposterior jaw discrepancy. Absolute maxillary deficiency was not evident from the initial intermolar widths. Considering the hypodivergent face and the short anterior facial height, a two-jaw surgery was planned to induce a clockwise rotation of the mandible (Fig. 11.10a).

Surgery occlusion was constructed to allow extrusion of the premolars, leaving some intermaxillary space between the anterior and posterior occlusal contact. Following the surgery, vertical intermaxillary elastics were worn only to level the curve of Spee. Then the remaining Class II relationship was finally resolved by inducing the total arch distalization in the maxilla and total arch protraction in the mandible, respectively, using interradicular miniscrews in the posterior segments (Fig. 11.10b). A final occlusion and a straight profile were gained after the whole procedure (Fig. 11.10c).

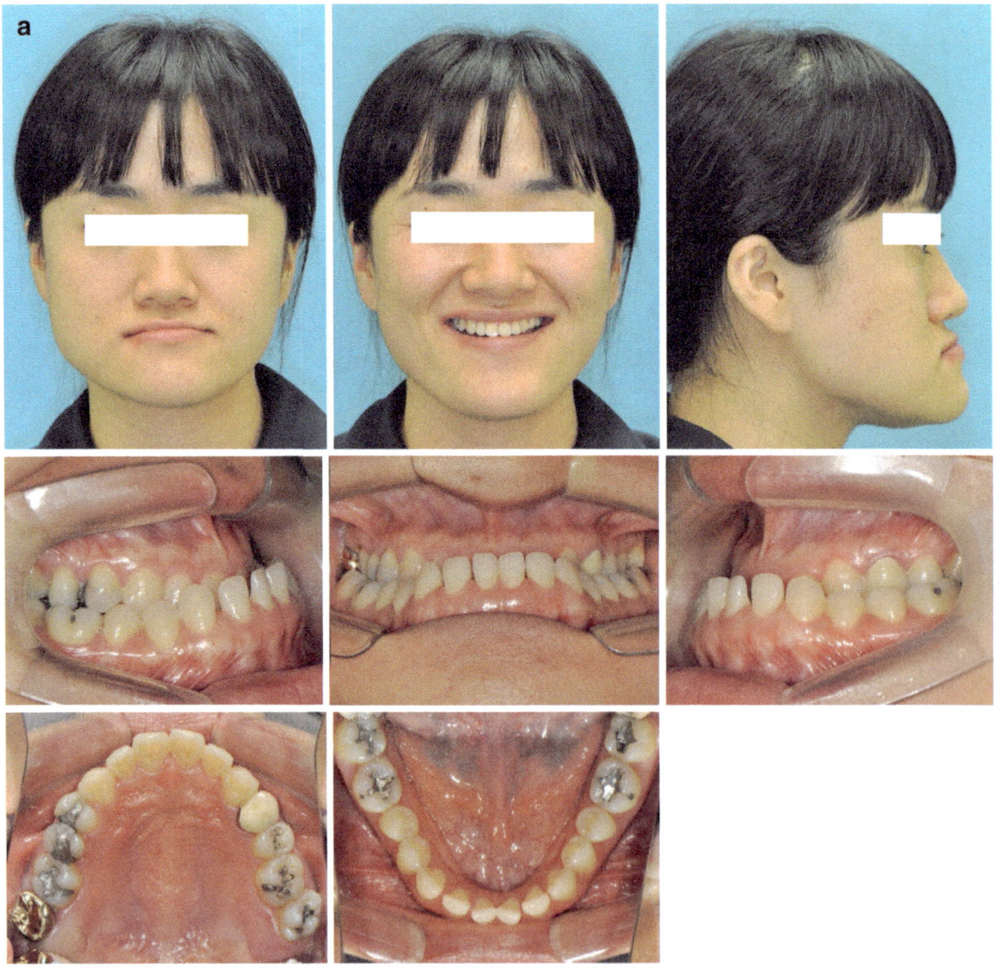

Fig. 11.10 Case 2. (**a**) Pretreatment records. (**b**) Progress records. (**c**) Posttreatment records

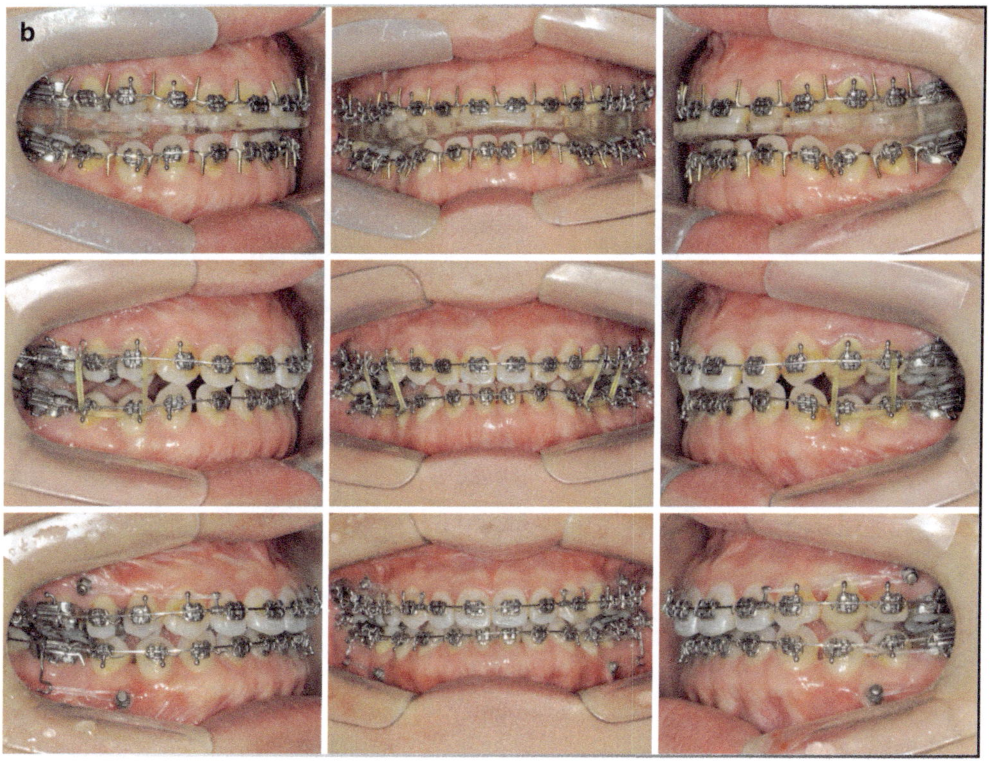

Fig. 11.10 (continued)

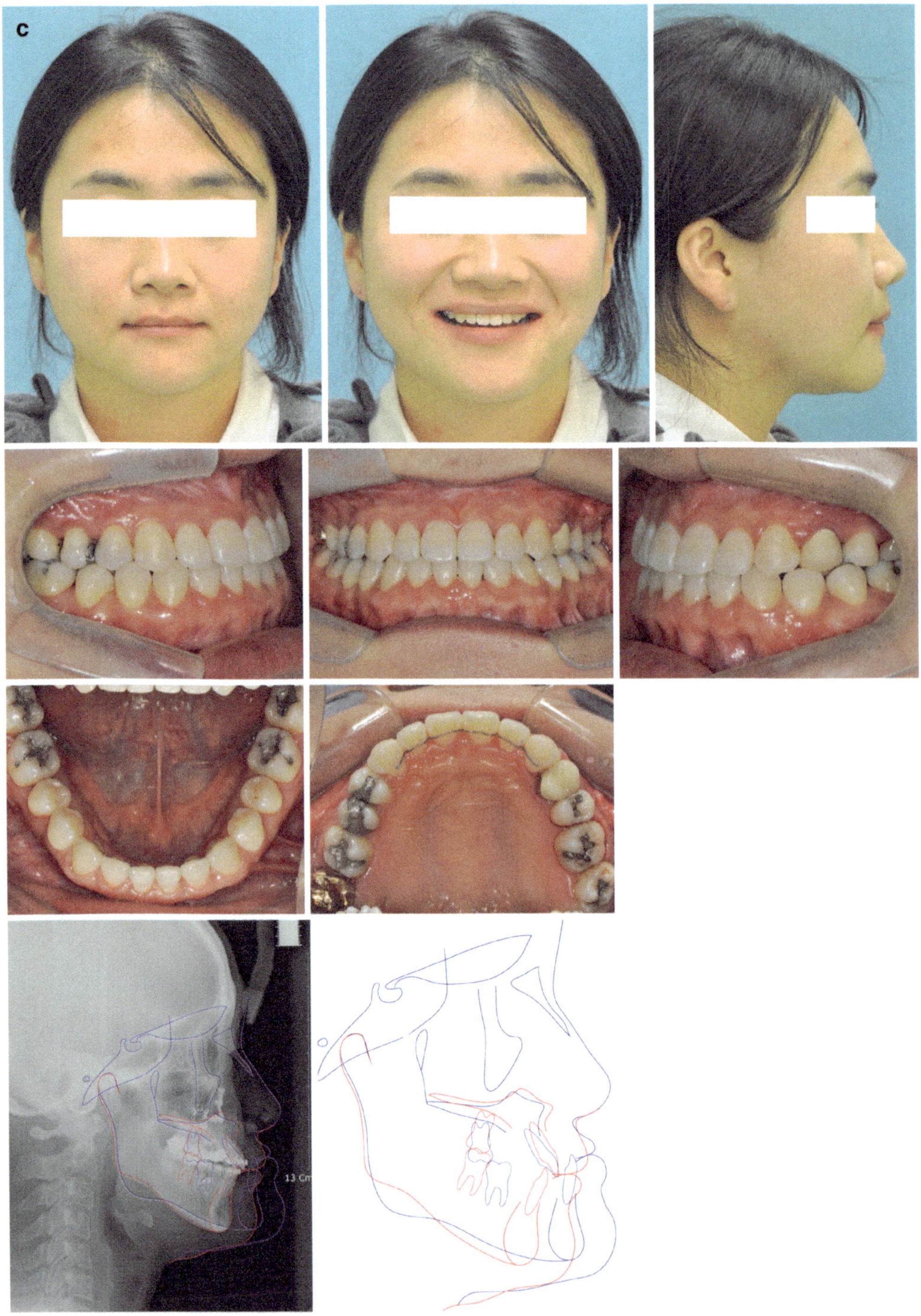

Fig. 11.10 (continued)

6. Maxillary expansion using MARPE
Transverse correction is a major issue not only in the conventional procedure but also in the POGS procedure. Many skeletal Class III patients have a posterior crossbite partly caused by the relative anteroposterior jaw position, as well as anterior crossbite. The so-called relative transverse deficiency needs to be distinguished beforehand [1]. In terms of the denture relation, the difference between maxillary and mandibular intermolar widths is estimated to be at least 5 mm [28]. Even in the case of sufficient difference, excessive buccal tipping of the maxillary posterior teeth is a sign of transverse compensation. Once the "absolute" transverse deficiency is diagnosed, adequate action has to follow to resolve the issue. Rapid palatal expansion is a reliable and common solution for narrow maxilla in prepubertal children, while transverse correction in the mandibular arch is very limited [29]. However, in adults, nonsurgical maxillary expansion is presumed to be difficult, and surgical intervention such as surgically assisted rapid palatal expansion (SARPE) or segmental surgery are suggested as substitutes [30]. The SARPE in the orthognathic surgery cases, however, tends to lead to a two-stage SARPE followed by double-jaw surgery, which may increase the morbidity [31]. Single-stage maxillary expansion via a multipiece segmental osteotomy is subject to a serious relapse of the relocated bony segment [32].
Therefore, using an alternative appliance, miniscrew-assisted RPE (MARPE) can be an option [33]. The combined use of hyrax RPE and the attached miniscrews can be effective in terms of delivering the force to the basal bone during expansion and allowing sufficient bone formation along the separated suture. Effective nonsurgical maxillary expansion is a radical solution for the orthognathic surgery cases showing maxillary transverse deficiency, for which miniscrews are easily incorporated.

Case 3

A 21-year-old male wanted to correct his prognathic profile. He had a Class III skeletal pattern with mandibular prognathism. There was moderate crowding in the upper arch, with an arch length discrepancy of 5.5 mm. His incisor axis relative to the SN plane was 100 °. In addition, obvious maxillary transverse deficiency was diagnosed with respective intermolar widths of 47.0 and 45.0 mm and a significant buccal tipping of maxillary molars (Fig. 11.11a).

Putting those factors together, both the extraction and the nonextraction of premolars were considered. Since extraction of premolars and retraction of upper incisors and additional clockwise maxillary jaw rotation were expected to overly upright the incisors, extraction was not readily chosen. However, a nonextraction option would definitely require transverse correction, for which additional surgical procedures such as SARPE or segmental maxillary surgery were considered. Again, the SARPE, once performed, would need to be followed by additional LeFort I osteotomy. On the other hand, the single stage segmental maxillary expansion would not secure postsurgical stability. Hence, a preliminary MARPE was inserted, and following the maxillary suture separation in 4 weeks, a surgical archwire was inserted. A regular two-jaw orthognathic surgery was performed, and an immediate molar intrusion of selective maxillary second molars, using palatal miniscrews, and arch alignment were followed (Fig. 11.11b). The incisor axis did not change significantly, and a proper transverse occlusal relationship was achieved after treatment (Fig. 11.11c1, c2).

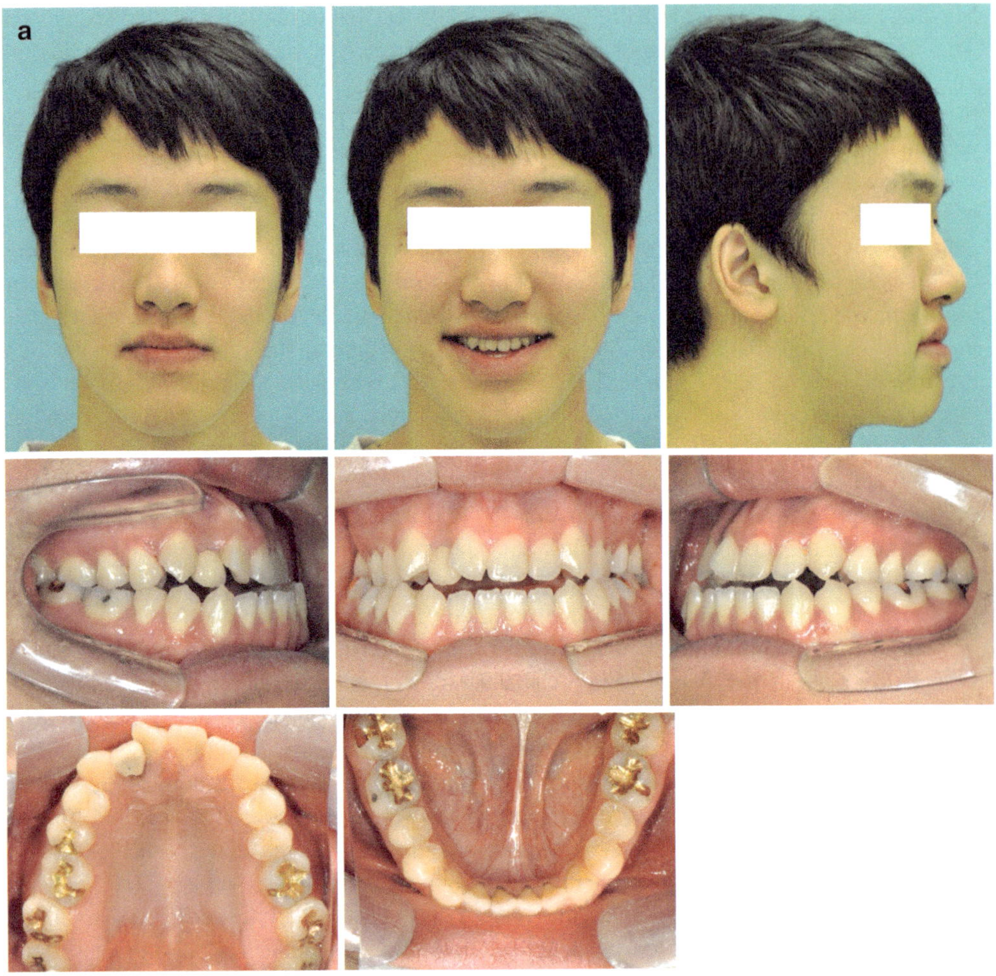

Fig. 11.11 Case 3. (**a**) Pretreatment records. (**b**) Progress records. (**c1**, **c2**) Posttreatment records

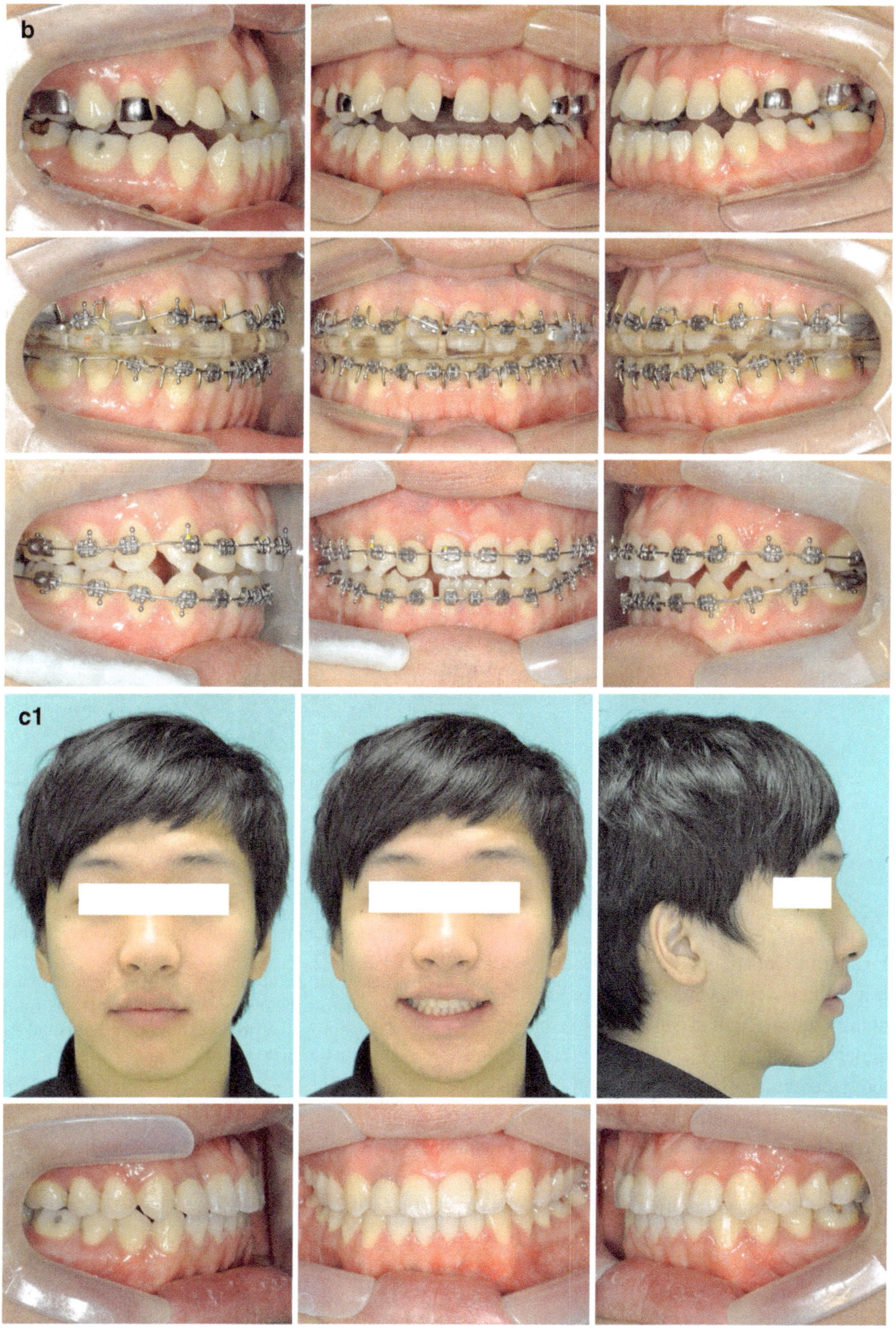

Fig. 11.11 (continued)

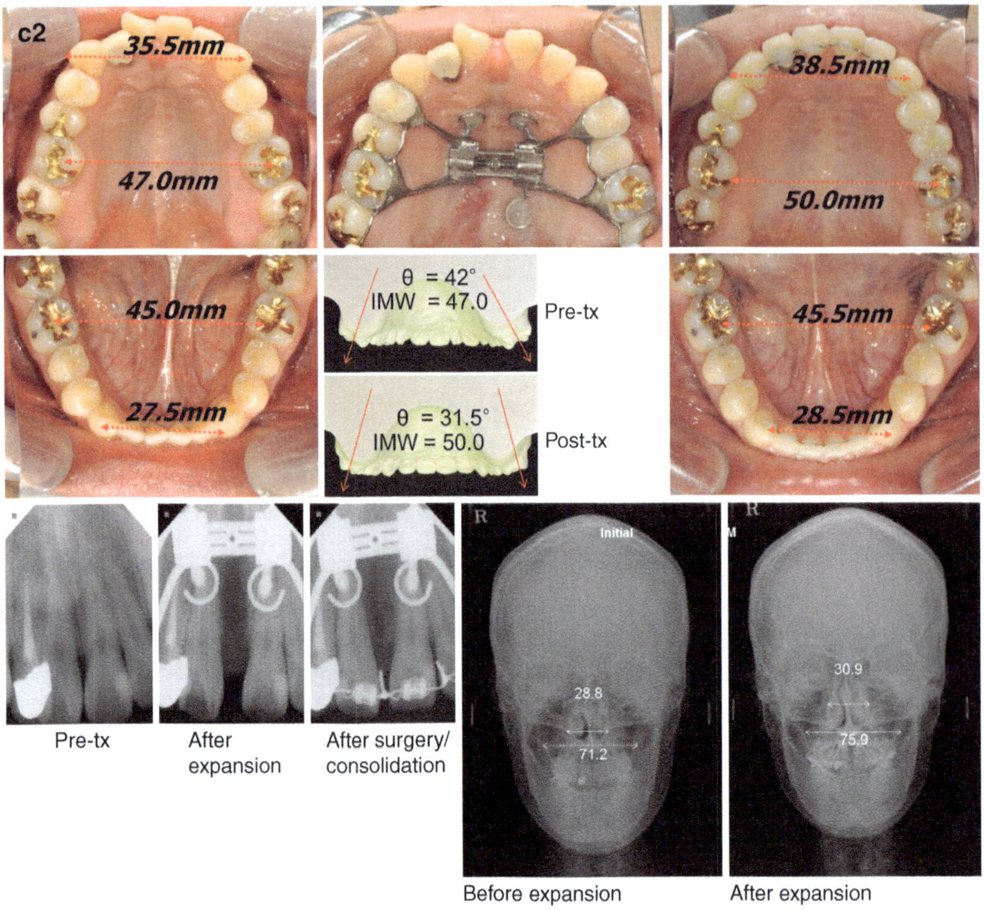

Fig. 11.11 (continued)

Conclusion

It is hard to imagine a POGS procedure without using miniscrews. Considering the complexity of the pattern of dental compensation in the three dimensions, and the diversity of the required tooth movement, the versatility of the miniscrew may add great strength in conducting the POGS procedure, compared to other types of skeletal anchorage devices, such as miniplates, for which insertion sites are rather limited [34]. Particularly, accurate insertion of the miniscrews in the inter-radicular area is essential.

References

1. Jacobs JD, Sinclair PM. Principles of orthodontic mechanics in orthognathic surgery cases. Am J Orthod. 1983;84(5):399–407.
2. Thomas GP, et al. The effects of orthodontic treatment on isometric bite forces and mandibular motion in patients before orthognathic surgery. J Oral Maxillofac Surg. 1995;53:673–8.
3. Katsumata A, et al. 3D CT evaluation of masseter muscle morphology after setback osteotomy for mandibular prognathism. Oral Surg Oral Med Oral Pathol Oral Radiol Endod. 2004;98(4):461–70.
4. Trawitzki LVV, et al. Masseter muscle thickness three years after surgical correction of Class III dentofacial deformity. Arch Oral Biol. 2011;56:799–803.
5. Nicolet C, et al. Lip competence in Class III patients undergoing orthognathic surgery: an electromyographic study. J Oral Maxillofac Surg. 2012;70: e331–6.
6. Nagasaka H, et al. "Surgery first" skeletal Class III correction using the skeletal anchorage system. J Clin Orthod. 2009;43(2):97–105.
7. Epker BN, Fish L. Surgical-orthodontic correction of open-bite deformity. Am J Orthod. 1977;71(3):278–99.
8. Lee RT. The benefits of post-surgical orthodontic treatment. Br J Orthod. 1994;21:265–74.
9. Watted N, Witt E, Bill JS. A therapeutic concept for the combined orthodontic surgical correction of angle Class II deformities with short-face syndrome: surgical lengthening of the lower face. Clin Orthod Res. 2000;3:78–93.

10. Liou EJ, et al. Surgery-first accelerated orthognathic surgery: orthodontic guidelines and setup for model surgery. J Oral Maxillofac Surg. 2011;69(3):771–80.
11. Liou EJ, et al. Surgery-first accelerated orthognathic surgery: postoperative rapid orthodontic tooth movement. J Oral Maxillofac Surg. 2011;69(3):781–5.
12. Mueller M, et al. A systematic acceleratory phenomenon (SAP) accompanies the regional acceleratory phenomenon (RAP) during healing of a bone defect in the rat. J Bone Miner Res. 1991;6(4):401–10.
13. Kitahara T, et al. Hard and soft tissue stability of orthognathic surgery. Angle Ortho. 2009;79:158–65.
14. Joss CU, Vassalli IM. Stability after bilateral sagittal split osteotomy setback surgery with rigid internal fixation: a systematic review. J Oral Maxillofac Surg. 2008;66:1634–43.
15. Ueki K, et al. The effects of changing position and angle of the proximal segment after intraoral vertical ramus osteotomy. Int J Oral Maxillofac Surg. 2009;38:1041–7.
16. Navarro R d L, et al. Histologic and tomographic analyses of the temporomandibular joint after mandibular advancement surgery: study in minipigs. Oral Surg Oral Med Oral Pathol Oral Radiol Endod. 2009;107:477–84.
17. Jung HD, Jung YS, Park HS. The chronologic prevalence of temporomandibular joint disorders associated with bilateral vertical ramus osteotomy. J Oral Maxillofac Surg. 2009;67:709–803.
18. Brunelle JA, Bhat M, Lipton JA. Prevalence and distribution of selected occlusal characteristics in the US population, 1988–1991. J Dent Res. 1996;75(Spec No):706–13.
19. Betts NJ, et al. Diagnosis and treatment of transverse maxillary deficiency. Int J Adult Orthodon Orthognath Surg. 1995;10(2):75–96.
20. Altug Atac AT, Karasu HA, Aytac D. Surgically assisted rapid maxillary expansion compared with orthopedic rapid maxillary expansion. Angle Orthod. 2006;76(3):353–9.
21. Alpern MC, Yurosko JJ. Rapid palatal expansion in adults with and without surgery. Angle Orthod. 1987;57(3):245–63.
22. Lee KJ, et al. Displacement pattern of the maxillary arch depending on miniscrew position in sliding mechanics. Am J Orthod Dentofacial Orthop. 2011; 140(2):224–32.
23. Park HS, Lee SK, Kwon OW. Group distal movement of teeth using microscrew implant anchorage. Angle Orthod. 2005;75(4):602–9.
24. Choy K, et al. Effect of root and bone morphology on the stress distribution in the periodontal ligament. Am J Orthod Dentofacial Orthop. 2000;117:98–105.
25. Yamada K, et al. Distal movement of maxillary molars using miniscrew anchorage in the buccal interradicular region. Angle Orthod. 2009;79:78–84.
26. Bechtold TE, et al. Distalization pattern of the maxillary arch depending on the number of orthodontic miniscrews. Angle Orthod. 2013;83:266–73.
27. Lee KJ, et al. Computed tomographic analysis of tooth-bearing alveolar bone for orthodontic miniscrew placement. Am J Orthod Dentofacial Orthop. 2009;135(4):486–94.
28. Uysal T, et al. Dental and alveolar arch widths in normal occlusion, Class II division 1 and Class II division 2. Angle Orthod. 2005;75:941–7.
29. Melsen B. Palatal growth studied on human autopsy material. A histologic microradiographic study. Am J Orthod. 1975;68(1):42–54.
30. Koudstaal MJ, et al. Surgically assisted rapid maxillary expansion (SARME): a review of the literature. Int J Oral Maxillofac Surg. 2005;34(7):709–14.
31. Bailey LJ, et al. Segmental LeFort I osteotomy for management of transverse maxillary deficiency. J Oral Maxillofac Surg. 1997;55(7):728–31.
32. Phillips C, et al. Stability of surgical maxillary expansion. Int J Adult Orthodon Orthognath Surg. 1992; 7(3):139–46.
33. Lee KJ, et al. Miniscrew-assisted nonsurgical palatal expansion before orthognathic surgery for a patient with severe mandibular prognathism. Am J Orthod Dentofacial Orthop. 2010;137(6):830–9.
34. Sugawara J, et al. Distal movement of mandibular molars in adult patients with the skeletal anchorage system. Am J Orthod Dentofacial Orthop. 2004;125(2):130–8.

Index

K.B. Kim (ed.), *Temporary Skeletal Anchorage Devices*,
DOI 10.1007/978-3-642-55052-2, © Springer-Verlag Berlin Heidelberg 2014

GPSR Compliance

The European Union's (EU) General Product Safety Regulation (GPSR) is a set of rules that requires consumer products to be safe and our obligations to ensure this.

If you have any concerns about our products, you can contact us on ProductSafety@springernature.com

In case Publisher is established outside the EU, the EU authorized representative is:

Springer Nature Customer Service Center GmbH
Europaplatz 3
69115 Heidelberg, Germany

Batch number: 10732675

Printed by Printforce, the Netherlands